Systems Thinking Analyses for Health Policy and Systems Development

Health systems are fluid and their components are interdependent in complex ways. Policymakers, academics and students continually endeavour to understand how to manage health systems to improve the health of populations. However, previous scholarship has often failed to engage with the intersections and interactions of health with a multitude of other systems and determinants. This book ambitiously takes on the challenge of presenting health systems as a coherent whole, by applying a systems-thinking lens. It focuses on Malaysia as a case study to demonstrate the evolution of a health system from a low-income developing status to one of the most resilient health systems today. A rich collaboration of multidisciplinary academics working with policymakers who were at the coalface of decision-making and practitioners with decades of experience, provides a candid analysis of what worked and what did not. The result is an engaging, informative and thought-provoking intervention in the debate. This title is Open Access.

JO. M. MARTINS is Adjunct Professor at the International Medical University, Kuala Lumpur, Malaysia.

INDRA PATHMANATHAN is Principal Visiting Fellow in the International Institute of Global Health, United Nations University, Kuala Lumpur, Malaysia.

DAVID T. TAN is Head of Experimentation in the United Nations Development Programme.

SHIANG CHENG LIM is Country Technical Lead for Better Health Programme Malaysia at RTI International (Malaysia Office).

PASCALE ALLOTEY is Director of the International Institute for Global Health at United Nations University.

Systems Thinking Analyses for Health Policy and Systems Development

A Malaysian Case Study

Edited by

JO. M. MARTINS
International Medical University
INDRA PATHMANATHAN
United Nations University International Institute for Global Health
DAVID T. TAN
United Nations University International Institute for Global Health
SHIANG CHENG LIM
United Nations University International Institute for Global Health
PASCALE ALLOTEY
United Nations University International Institute for Global Health

CAMBRIDGE
UNIVERSITY PRESS

CAMBRIDGE
UNIVERSITY PRESS

University Printing House, Cambridge CB2 8BS, United Kingdom

One Liberty Plaza, 20th Floor, New York, NY 10006, USA

477 Williamstown Road, Port Melbourne, VIC 3207, Australia

314–321, 3rd Floor, Plot 3, Splendor Forum, Jasola District Centre, New Delhi – 110025, India

103 Penang Road, #05–06/07, Visioncrest Commercial, Singapore 238467

Cambridge University Press is part of the University of Cambridge.

It furthers the University's mission by disseminating knowledge in the pursuit of education, learning, and research at the highest international levels of excellence.

www.cambridge.org
Information on this title: www.cambridge.org/9781108845205
DOI: 10.1017/9781108954846

When citing this work, please include a reference to the DOI 10.1017/9781108954846

First published 2021

A catalogue record for this publication is available from the British Library.

Library of Congress Cataloging-in-Publication Data
Names: Martins, Jo. M., 1936– editor.
Title: Systems thinking analyses for health policy and systems development : a Malaysian case study / edited by Jo. M. Martins, Indra Pathmanathan, David T. Tan, Shiang Cheng Lim, Pascale Allotey.
Description: Cambridge, United Kingdom ; New York, N.Y. : Cambridge University Press, 2021. | Includes bibliographical references and index.
Identifiers: LCCN 2020053664 | ISBN 9781108845205 (hardback) | ISBN 9781108949675 (paperback) | ISBN 9781108954846 (ebook)
Subjects: LCSH: Medical policy – Malaysia. | Integrated delivery of health care – Malaysia. | Medical care – Malaysia.
Classification: LCC RA395.M35 S97 2021 | DDC 362.109595–dc23
LC record available at https://lccn.loc.gov/2020053664

ISBN 978-1-108-84520-5 Hardback

UNITED NATIONS UNIVERSITY
UNU-IIGH
International Institute for Global Health

Contents

Figures

Tables

Boxes

Biographies of Editors and Contributors

The twenty-member editorial-cum-authors team that designed and produced this innovative and insightful view of health systems have an interesting mix of talents. They have professional backgrounds in public health, economics, social science, engineering, mathematics, systems thinking, medical sciences, and pharmaceuticals. Together, they combine insights gained during decades of personal experience of working in and managing national programmes in the Malaysian health system with a breadth of vision acquired through international public health work and the scientific rigour of academic publications. In delightful contrast to most publications in this field, the editors of this book guided active and iterative interaction between the authors, and between the authors and a wide range of Malaysian stakeholders. This process enriched and deepened the understanding of the workings of health systems.

The team consists of four categories, namely:

- Editorial team. The editorial team designed the parameters of the book, guided the chapter authors, reviewed the chapters, and derived key messages for all chapters. Most members of the team also authored one or more chapters.
- Lead authors for chapters.
- Lead authors for case studies.
- Co-authors for chapters or case studies.

Editorial Team cum Lead Authors for One or More Chapters

Jo. M. Martins

Professor (adjunct), International Medical University, Malaysia

Jo. M. Martins was a senior finance officer in a large corporation before entering public service in Australia. His work has included the design and implementation of community health services and the rationalisation of hospital services in Australia. He has been an advisor and consultant to the World Health Organization. He was a task manager for health projects for the World Bank, including the first World Bank–funded health project in Malaysia. He has held professorial positions and continues his association with university teaching and research in Australia and at the International Medical University in Malaysia. He is an assistant editor of the *Asia Pacific Journal of Health Management* and the author/editor of books, book chapters, peer reviewed articles, and official reports.

Indra Pathmanathan

Principal Visiting Fellow, International Institute of Global Health, United Nations University, Kuala Lumpur, Malaysia

ORCID ID: 0000–0003-4781–2199

Indra Pathmanathan has fifty years' experience as a public health specialist. Working initially in Malaysia in academia, research, education of health personnel, and managing health programmes, she witnessed at first hand many of the key milestones cited in this book and took a lead role in establishing national programmes for health systems research and quality assurance. Her international experience includes consulting in health systems research for the World Health Organization, Geneva, to support programmes in several countries; serving in the World Bank, Washington, as team leader for reproductive health in the South Asia region; and evaluating health policies and programmes in Bangladesh, Ethiopia, and Sri Lanka. She has authored several books and peer-reviewed papers.

David Tat Ui Tan

United Nations Development Programme, Head of Experimentation

ORCID ID: 0000–0003-4820–2878

David Tan uses systems thinking for transdisciplinary research, organisational learning and development, and co-creation of narratives. He is currently with United Nations Development Programme Accelerator Labs, bringing innovation, learning, and safe-to-fail experiments to the development process. Prior to this, he was a health policy researcher at the United Nations University International Institute for Global Health studying health systems and the health-urban development interface.

Shiang Cheng Lim

Strategic Programme Manager and Monitoring, Research and Evaluation Lead, RTI International (Malaysia Office)

Shiang Cheng Lim is an applied researcher with more than fifteen years of research and programme experience in solving practical interdisciplinary problems in the field of global health, especially in areas related to sexual and reproductive health (SRH), abortion, HIV, gender-based violence (GBV), ageing, cognitive function and impairment, non-communicable diseases (NCDs), and health systems. Her research largely focuses on how complex contextual factors influence people's health-related behaviour and decisions and how it can be improved through a multidimensional approach through health system strengthening, strategic partnership management, and participatory engagement.

Pascale Adukwei Allotey

Director, United Nations University, International Institute for Global Health (UNU-IIGH)

ORCID ID: 0000–0002-6942–5774

Pascale Allotey, as Director of UNU-IIGH, is interested in furthering the knowledge base in topics such as the application of systems thinking to improve understanding of health systems and increase the effectiveness of health policies globally. Her research over the last twenty-five years has focused on health equity, health and human rights, gender and social determinants of health, forced migration and marginalisation, sexual and reproductive health, infectious diseases, and non-communicable diseases. The engagement of communities in research and policy has been central to defining her areas of research. She has authored and edited several books and authored over 150 peer-reviewed articles.

Lead Authors for Other Chapters

David Christopher Ariam McCoy

Professor of Global Public Health and Director of the Centre for Global Public Health, Institute of Population Health Sciences, Queen Mary University of London

David McCoy is Professor of Global Public Health. He is Director of the Centre for Global Public Health in the Institute of Population Health Sciences at Queen Mary University of London. He qualified as a medical doctor from the University of Southampton and spent six years as a clinician in the UK and South Africa before entering a career in public health. Since returning to the UK, he has worked as a public health specialist in the NGO sector, academia, and the NHS.

Edward Barry Newell

Honorary Associate Professor, Fenner School of Environment and Society, the Australian National University, Canberra, Australia

Barry Newell is a physicist who focuses on the practical and theoretical aspects of policymaking in complex adaptive systems. He has a particular interest in the use of systems thinking to support effective cross-sector communication and adaptive policymaking in situations dominated by uncertainty. This work has led to the practical systems thinking and modelling approach called *Collaborative Conceptual Modelling* (CCM) that he has developed in collaboration with Katrina Proust. CCM is focused on putting systems thinking to work. He is co-author, with Robert Dyball, of the textbook *Understanding Human Ecology: A Systems Approach to Sustainability*.

Mukundan Sugunan Pillay

Managing Director, TSI Healthcare Sdn Bhd, Malaysia

Datuk Dr Mukundan Pillay is a civil engineer with additional qualifications (masters and doctorate) in public health. He was a pioneer public health engineer in the Ministry of Health, Malaysia, and had a key role in providing technical leadership for upgrading both rural and urban sanitation and water supply in the country. He became director of engineering services of the Ministry of Health Malaysia and then deputy director general of the ministry in charge of research and technical support. He was also a pioneer in contracting private sector entities to undertake functions previously confined to the public sector. He shared his experience internationally, serving as Senior Health Adviser with the WHO in Beijing and as Senior Health Specialist with the World Bank in Bahrain.

Chiu-Wan Ng

Professor of Public Health, University of Malaya, Malaysia

ORCID: 0000–0002-7687–2310

Chiu-Wan Ng graduated in Medicine from the National University of Singapore and obtained her MPH in Health Systems Management and her PhD in Health Economics from the University of Malaya. Her main research interests include health systems, financing, and economics, in particular efforts to achieve universal health coverage in low- and middle-income countries in the Asia Pacific region. She is the Malaysian country investigator for the EQUITAP (Equity in Asia Pacific Health Systems) and GNHE (Global Network on Health Equity) research collaborations.

Thomas Paraidathathu

Executive Dean and Professor, Faculty of Health and Medical Sciences, Taylor's University, Malaysia

ORCID: 0000–0002-8834–9623

Thomas Paraidathathu is a pharmacist with an MS and a PhD in Pharmacology/Toxicology. Serving in the Ministry of Health, Malaysia, Thomas worked initially as a hospital pharmacist and later in drug regulatory affairs, where he gained first-hand experience in building national capacity to improve the safety of medical and traditional products marketed in the country. Subsequently as an academic, he built human resource capacity and is currently an emeritus professor. He has been a member of the Pharmacy Board of Malaysia, council member and vice president of the Malaysian Pharmaceutical Society, and a founding member of the Malaysian Academy of Pharmacy.

Nuraidah binti Mohd Marzuki

Public Health Physician, Health Informatics Section, Planning Division, Ministry of Health Malaysia, Putrajaya, Malaysia

Nuraidah Marzuki is a public health physician with the Health Informatics Centre, Ministry of Health, Malaysia. She has more than fifteen years of experience in government-led e-health initiatives. She previously served at the e-Health Section, Planning Division as Project Manager for the Malaysia Health Information Exchange (MyHIX). She received her MBBS and graduated with a Doctorate in Public Health from the University of Malaya.

Lead Authors for Case Studies

Kuan Joo Lim

Retired public health officer

Kuan Joo Lim is a medical officer with a post-graduate qualification in public health, MPH (health planning). He served in the Ministry of Health for twenty-nine years and has experience in hospital management (public and private sectors), health planning, hospital planning, healthcare financing, health information including IT, quality assurance, training, research and disease control, and medical ethics. He served as a short-time consultant to the World Health Organization and the Islamic Development Bank.

Debbie Siru

Consultant

Debbie Siru has extensive experience in the field of environmental health, primarily in the areas of drinking water quality and medical waste management. She has personal experience in building national capacity in medical waste management in the public and private sectors in Malaysia. She has an MSc in Water and Environmental Management from the University of Warwick, UK, and was the first person outside the US to obtain a Certificate in Healthcare Environmental Management from ECRI, USA. She has also been engaged by the World Health Organization on four separate occasions to provide consultancy on various aspects of environmental health.

Chee Han Lim

Senior Researcher, Third World Network

Chee Han Lim is a founding member of the Agora Society Malaysia, a senior researcher at the Third World Network, and formerly a senior analyst at the Penang Institute. He holds a PhD in Infection Biology from Hannover Medical School, Germany, an MSc in Immunology, and a BSc in Biotechnology from Imperial College London. Health and socio-economic policies are his current concerns. He believes that a nation can advance significantly if policymaking and research are taken seriously.

Other Contributors

Katrina Margaret Proust

Honorary Senior Lecturer, Fenner School of Environment and Society, the Australian National University

Katrina Proust has a background in environmental and applied history and complex social-ecological systems. Her work focuses on the historical factors and the feedback dynamics that shape relationships between humans and their environment. She is particularly interested in the interconnected systems that comprise urban communities. With Barry Newell she has developed *Collaborative Conceptual Modelling*, an approach to complex social-ecological issues that provides a conceptual framework to help a group undertake a systems project.

Safurah Jaafar

Professor of Community Medicine, International Medical University, Malaysia

ORCID ID: 0000–0001-6834–7885

Safurah Jaafar currently holds the position of Head of Division Family and Population Health and also Programme Director of the MBA in Healthcare Management at the International Medical University. She was instrumental in reforming PHC delivery in Malaysia, with an interest in safeguarding the equitable distribution of care in achieving universal health coverage, while serving the Ministry as Director, Family Health Development Division, Ministry of Health, Malaysia from 2007 to 2017.

Milton Siew Wah Lum

Consultant Obstetrician and Gynaecologist, Alpha Specialist Centre and Damansara Specialist Hospital, Petaling Jaya, Malaysia

Milton S. W. Lum, who studied at the Royal Military College and University of Malaya, is a Fellow of the Royal College of Obstetricians and Gynaecologists, Royal Society of Medicine, and Academy of Medicine of Malaysia. He has held leadership positions at national and international medical and speciality organisations, membership of the boards of various hospitals, membership of the Council of University Tunku Abdul Rahman, and was previously FIGO Visiting Professor. He has served as an elected member of the Malaysian Medical Council since 1994 and is currently Chairman of the Board of Governors of Perdana University and Trustee of Nanyang Press Foundation.

Anuar Zaini bin Md. Zain

Professor of Internal Medicine, Jeffrey Cheah School of Medicine and Health Sciences, Monash University Malaysia

ORCID ID: 0000–0001-7007–5743

Dr Anuar Zaini is currently Professor of Internal Medicine and founding Head of Jeffrey Cheah School of Medicine and Health Sciences, Monash University Malaysia (2005–2017). He is also resident Consultant Endocrinologist at Beacon Hospital in Petaling Jaya. After graduating from the University of Malaya (UM) in 1973, he pursued training in clinical endocrinology at the Royal Victoria Infirmary, Newcastle-upon-Tyne, UK (1976–1978) and at Prince Henry Hospital and Monash Medical Research Centre, Melbourne (1983–1985). He was Dean of UM's Medical Faculty for more than a decade (1986–2000) and also concurrent Director of the University Malaya Medical Centre during 1998–2000. He was appointed UM Vice-Chancellor, a post which he held from 2000 to 2003. He is a member of the Royal College of Physicians (UK) and a fellow of the Royal College of Physicians, Edinburgh, and of the Royal Australasian College of Physicians (Australia).

Fazilah binti Shaik Allaudin

Senior Deputy Director, Medical Care Quality Section, Medical Development Division, Ministry of Health, Malaysia

Dr Fazilah has had various roles in strategic leadership positions at the Ministry of Health in Malaysia. A significant portion of her career has been in digital health. Since 2010, she has been leading digital strategy for the national health system transformation agenda and involved in digital health and innovation strategies and implementation in both the public and the private sector. She has been actively pursuing e-health collaborations domestically, regionally, and internationally.

Tharani Loganathan

Medical Lecturer, Department of Social and Preventive Medicine, Faculty of Medicine, University of Malaya, Malaysia

ORCID ID: 0000–0001-6690-000X

Tharani Loganathan is a public health medical specialist and medical lecturer at the University of Malaya. She teaches undergraduate medical students and postgraduate MPH and DrPH students in Global Health, Law and Health, and Management and Health subjects in the Health Policy and Management Unit at the Department of Social and Preventive Medicine, Faculty of Medicine, University of Malaya. She has a particular research interest in migrant health and health systems and policy research on advancing the health system goal of achieving universal health coverage. Tharani Loganathan is an Atlantic Fellow for Health Equity in South East Asia.

Supathiratheavy Rasiah

Senior Lecturer, Community Medicine Department, School of Medicine, International Medical University, Malaysia

ORCID ID: 0000–0002-3451–5024

Supathira has worked with the Ministry of Health Malaysia, gaining expertise in the implementation and commissioning of EMR systems at various levels of hospitals, health facility planning and development, country health planning and evaluation, and telehealth project implementation. Her achievements also include improvements in health service delivery while serving as a hospital director at a 1,000-bed tertiary care hospital and a regional 400-bed secondary-level care hospital in Sabah, Malaysia. She is currently a senior lecturer at the International Medical University, involved in undergraduate and post-graduate programmes. Her research interests are in the fields of health informatics, improving care for type 2 diabetes mellitus, and trust in healthcare.

Faizul Nizam bin Abu Salim

Special Officer to the Director General of Health, Ministry of Health Malaysia; PhD student, Department of Community Health, National University of Malaysia

ORCID ID: 0000–0003-2827–8867

Dr Faizul Nizam Abu Salim has served as the Special Officer to the Director General of Health Malaysia since May 2016. Being directly involved in assisting the Director General in his governance role over the technical arm of Ministry of Health Malaysia, which cut across six different technical programmes and fifteen State Health Departments, Dr Faizul has amassed knowledge and experience of public health, health management, and leadership. Within this role he has developed a niche area of interest and expertise in strategic communication for health, especially in relation to crisis and risk communication. He is currently pursuing his PhD (Community Health) on this subject at the National University of Malaysia.

Foreword

Health and development are inextricably linked. Countries require robust health systems to enable the delivery of quality health services and to ensure access to health as a public good while both balancing national budgets and providing protection against individual catastrophic spending on healthcare. Getting this balance right remains a problem for most countries, particularly in resource-constrained settings. Training resources available to address the development of health systems often take a narrow, singular, linear approach which fails to engage with the intersections and interactions of health with a multitude of systems and determinants. Although there is general guidance and technical support for countries from multilateral agencies like the World Health Organization and the World Bank, the importance of local contexts in building and strengthening health systems adds a layer of complexity to the task. The publications by de Savigny and colleagues on systems thinking for health systems strengthening and applied systems thinking for health systems research (de Savigny and Taghreed, 2009; de Savigny, Blanchet and Taghreed, 2017) provide the analytical approach and the tools to use systems thinking to understand the multiplicity of factors involved. However, texts seldom demonstrate how the systems thinking approach has been applied across an entire health system.

This book is timely for several reasons. Health systems, particularly in resource-constrained settings, are progressing from approaches driven largely by disease-related vertical programmes to a greater focus on strengthening the foundations of the system with people at the centre. Simultaneously, lower-income countries are reclaiming control of priority-setting for health, all with the imperative to achieve Universal Health Coverage – to ensure that access to quality care is available to and accessible by all. The scholarship for health systems strengthening is increasingly robust, with a growing body of evidence to help inform decisions. However, the decisions also need to be grounded in the historical, political, economic, and social context of the country. Even with new ideas and great will, implementation needs to draw on an understanding of the past to forge the path for the future. And this is the approach taken by this book, skilfully edited by Martins et al.

This book presents a case study of a country – Malaysia – that is transitioning from low income (1957) to the cusp of high income as one of the more successful countries in South East Asia. The case is presented from the perspective of health system development. Systems thinking feedback loops are applied throughout the narrative of the different health systems building blocks as a model for understanding feedback pathways. The approach is engaging and works as a mechanism for critical analysis, as well as drawing out the relevant learning points and contexts that allow for the lessons to be generalised.

The authors highlight the social functions of health systems and the political economy underlying decision making; these are often ignored in more theoretical texts. The engagement of authors and other stakeholders who were historically involved in decisions provides a biographical perspective – again, a refreshing and reflective approach that does not detract from the rigour of the analysis.

The book is comprehensive, covering from traditional medicines to digital technology; from contact tracing of tuberculosis and field epidemiology in remote hamlets to the establishment of the national institutes of health; from training of the human resources for health to health technology assessment; and management of communicable and non-communicable diseases. A reading of this text provides a good background to understanding the ability of the health system to manage the 2020 COVID-19 outbreak – and the final two chapters present an excellent analysis of both the value of the systems thinking approach to the analysis and the transferrable lessons for other countries and the settings of both successes and pitfalls.

Personally, and as Executive Director of the Alliance for Health Policy and Systems Research, this text gives me immense pleasure and pride, because this is the first application of systems thinking at the national level since the Alliance launched the Systems Thinking Report in 2009. I hope this book will be useful and used by the policy, research, and teaching communities in other parts of the world as a real-life example of systems thinking.

DR ABDUL GHAFFAR
Executive Director, *Alliance for Health Policy and Systems Research*

Foreword

Systems thinking has been applied to many specific health issues, but this book represents the first attempt to apply it to an entire heath system. Furthermore, this book recognises that health systems are open systems that mutually interact with other systems. The Ministry of Health, Malaysia is proud to have participated actively with UNU-IIGH in the analytic process. It has been a highly beneficial mutual learning process. We have gained insights into critical elements in our past development, acquired better appreciation of our own strengths and limitations, and recognised opportunities to address the challenges we face.

The book highlights Malaysia's historical success in dealing with numerous health issues, mainly communicable disease and family/ child health. Fortuitously, this book was completed in January 2020, coinciding with the onset of the COVID-19 pandemic. Fortunately, the lessons from our past successes were within living memory and provided the foundation on which the health system in Malaysia was able to build rapidly, engage with government, and respond effectively. The outbreak certainly tested the links between the various components of our health system – public health; laboratories; primary, secondary, and tertiary services; pharmaceutical and engineering (environmental health) services; human resources; and information, as well as governance and leadership. It has been a real-life verification of the importance of the analysis outlined in this manuscript – the links were strong and mutually supportive.

Malaysia continues to learn and to strengthen its health system to ensure the health of the population. I hope the key messages outlined in this book will be useful to policy makers and academics around the world. Further, I would recommend that engaging in an analytic process such as this would be a good learning process for staff in all health systems.

This was an ambitious venture, and I commend UNU-IIGH for the partnership and the rigour with which the process was undertaken. I am immensely proud of the past and present staff of the Ministry of Health who contributed to the effort.

DR NOOR HISHAM ABDULLAH
Director General, Ministry of Health Malaysia

Preface

This book demonstrates a novel approach to analysing the development of health systems. Using a country case study, it applies systems thinking across an entire health system, engaging with the intersections and interactions of health with a multitude of systems and determinants.

How did we do this? This preface provides a brief summary in the hope that it will be helpful to others who might wish to replicate the process in other-country settings.

The process of producing this analysis was complex, with three phases. First, we required an authenticated account of the historical development of the health system, with evidence of health outcomes. Next, we applied systems thinking analysis to the evolution. Finally, we derived generic 'lessons' that would have applications in other-country contexts. We found that the process provided an opportunity for practice-based and reflective learning across policy makers, academics, practitioners, and researchers, encompassing the government (public) sector, the private sector, and non-government organisations.

Challenges abounded. As with most developing countries, Malaysia is not rich in data and documentation, particularly for the earlier decades of its development. Furthermore, the public sector dominates the healthcare system and holds most of the more recent documentation in archives that are not readily accessible to those outside the public sector. To address this challenge, stakeholder engagement and partnership building between the United Nations University International Institute for Global Health (UNU-IIGH) and the Ministry of Health was critical for negotiating access to documents and data. Additionally, one of the criteria for the selection of chapter authors and stakeholders was their personal historic participation in various phases of the development of the health system. Thus they were able to locate key documents and use personal linkages to interact with key individuals to authenticate and elaborate the available documentary evidence.

Another challenge was the in-built reluctance for open discussion between various stakeholders, such as the public with the private sector or between academicians and practitioners. Additionally, the vocabulary and concepts of systems thinkers are strange to healthcare professionals. The interaction process required a 'safe space'. UNU-IIGH provided such a safe space. Being a neutral organisation with the mandate to support analyses, evidence generation, and capacity strengthening in global health within the UN and member states, UNU-IIGH was ideally placed to co-ordinate the process of production and contribute to the analysis. As one of fourteen institutes in the UNU system, UNU-IIGH retains intellectual independence from the UN and is able to host rigorous academic debate and analysis. Malaysia hosts UNU-IIGH because of the strength and the ethos of the Malaysian health system, which facilitated access to both content and engagement and made for a rich mutual learning experience.

Various health system experts needed to interact repeatedly with analytic systems thinkers. Chapter 2 describes how this process enriched the analysis. This safe space also encouraged key stakeholders (listed in our acknowledgements) to review and comment on the initial analysis and tentative conclusions in each chapter. Subsequent analysis integrated their inputs.

Finally, the editorial team participated actively with chapter authors and stakeholders throughout this process. Thus, as a team, the editors were able to derive the generic key messages shown in each chapter, and these reflect the various components of the system as well as the system as a whole.

We hope the outcomes of the analysis will be useful not only to further the science of applying systems thinking to health systems but also to support policy makers as they seek to better understand their own health systems and address current problems.

Indra Pathmanathan
Co-editor
Pascale A. Allotey
Director
United National University International Institute for Global Health

Acknowledgements

This book would not have been possible without the support of and genuine partnership with the Ministry of Health Malaysia. The Director General of the Ministry of Health, Datuk Dr Noor Hisham Abdullah, enabled access to documents and data and encouraged active participation by key staff in the stakeholder consultations that reviewed earlier drafts of the book. Additionally, the Director General and key officials shared their unique perspectives and experience, which were invaluable in supplementing and contexualising documented information. Our analysis was greatly enriched by the information and by the subsequent review provided by key stakeholders. The stakeholders are listed below, and the names of representatives from each stakeholder are given in Appendix IV. The Special Officer in the Director General's office, Dr Faizul Nizam Abu Salim, was the key co-ordinator between the authors, the editorial team, and the MoH officers, and his efforts contributed significantly to the timely completion of the book.

Stakeholder	Organisations/agencies/individuals
Ministry of Health (MoH)	Director General (DG) and Deputy DGs
MoH Divisions and Departments	• Planning, including Health Policy and Plan, National Health Financing, National Health Accounts, Health Informatics Centre, eHealth Planning • Family Health Development • Medical Development • Disease Control • Engineering Services

(*cont.*)

Stakeholder	Organisations/agencies/individuals
	• Pharmaceutical Services • Food quality and safety • Finance • Traditional and Complementary Medicine
MoH National Institutes of Health	• Institute of Health Systems Research • Institute of Health Management • Institute of Clinical Research • Institute for Public Health
Political leaders	Two former Ministers of Health
Professional leaders	Former Secretary General, Ministry of Finance Two former Director Generals of Health
Previous key officers in the MoH	• Five Deputy Director Generals • Six Directors of Divisions and Departments • Two Directors of Research Institutes
World Health Organization	• Representatives of the Office for Malaysia, Brunei Darussalam, and Singapore
Academia (universities)	• University Malaya • National University of Malaysia • Monash University Malaysia • International Medical University
Professional medical associations	• Malaysian Medical Association • Federation of Private Medical Practitioners' Association
Pharmaceutical private sector agencies	• Malaysian Organization of Pharmaceutical Industries (MOPI) • Pharmaceutical Association of Malaysia (PhAMA)
Managed care organisation	• PMCare Sdn Bhd

Abbreviations

A&E	Accident and emergency
ADR	Adverse drug reactions
AIDS	Acquired immune deficiency syndrome
AMCHAM	American Malaysian Chamber of Commerce
APEC	Asia-Pacific Economic Cooperation
APPL	Approved products purchase list
ARAC	ASEAN Risk Assessment Centre for Food Safety
ARV	Antiretroviral
ASEAN	Association of Southeast Asian Nations
ASIS	Asset and services information system
ASMA	Alam Sekitar Malaysian Sdn Bhd
BAKAS	Bekalan Air dan Kebersihan Alam Sekeliling
BCG	Bacille Calmette-Guerin
BSE	Breast self-examination
CAT	Cultural adaptation template
CDC	Centers for Diseases Control and Prevention
CDCR	Control of Drugs and Cosmetics Regulations
CDs	Communicable diseases
CFS	Certificate of free sale
CGPs	Clinical practice guidelines
CHE	Catastrophic health expenditure
CLD	Causal loop diagram
CMIS	Computerised central management information system
CORFIS	Community-based cardiovascular risk factor intervention strategies
CPGs	Clinical practice guidelines
CPP	Certificate of pharmaceutical product
CRC	Clinical Research Centre
CT	Computed tomography
CWMS	Clinical Waste Management System

DAA	Direct-acting antivirals
DALY	Disability-adjusted life year
DCA	Drug Control Authority
DDT	Dichlorodiphenyltrichloroethane
DEC	Diethylcarbamazine
DG	Director General
DNDi	Drugs for Neglected Diseases Initiative
DOC	Department of Chemistry
DOE	Department of Environment
DoS	Department of Statistics
DOSH	Department of Occupational Safety and Health
DPT	Diphtheria, pertussis, and tetanus
DRG	Diagnosis-related group
DRGD	Drug registration guidance document
DUNas	Dasar Ubat Nasional
EHS	Environmental health services
EIA	Environmental impact assessment
EPF	Employees' Provident Fund
EPU	Economic Planning Unit
EQA	Environmental Quality Act 1974
ESRD	End-stage renal disease
EU	European Union
FCTC	Framework Convention on Tobacco Control
FDA	Food and Drug Administration
FFPAM	Federation of Private Medical Practitioners Associations
FHDD	Family Health Development Division
FMS	Family medicine/Family medicine specialist(s)
FOMEMA	Foreign Workers' Medical Examination
FPAs	Family planning associations
FRHAM	Federation of Reproductive Health Associations, Malaysia
FSWs	Female sex workers
G6PD	Glucose-6-phosphate dehydrogenase
GDP	Gross domestic product
GLCs	Government-linked companies
GMP	Good manufacturing practice
GMS	Government Medical Store
GNP	Gross national product

GP	General practitioner(s)
GU	Government Use Licence
HCV	Hepatitis C virus
HEs	Health experts
HFMD	Hand, foot, and mouth disease
HIA	Health impact assessment(s)
HIC	Health Informatics Centre
HIV	Human immunodeficiency virus
HIV/AIDS	Human immunodeficiency virus infection and acquired immune deficiency syndrome
HMIS	Health and management information system
HMO	Health Maintenance Organisation
HO	House officers
HPRA	Health Policy Research Associates
HPV	Human papillomavirus
HR	Human resources
HRH	Human resources for health
HRWG	Harm Reduction Working Group
HSC	Health sub-centre
HSFS	Health services financing study
HSIP	Hospital-specific implementation plan
HSR	Health systems research
HTA	Health technology assessment
IAQ	Indoor air quality
ICD	International Classification of Diseases
ICT	Information and communication technology
IDs	Influence diagrams
IDUs	Injecting drug users
IHP	Institute for Health Policy
IHSR	Institute for Health Systems Research
ILO	International Labour Organization
IMR	Institute for Medical Research
IPH	Institute for Public Health
IPR	Intellectual property rights
ISO	International Organisation of Standardisation
IT	Information technology
IWK	Indah Water Konsortium
JICA	Japan International Cooperation Agency
JSC	Japan Sanitation Consortium

LB	Live births
LEHAPs	Local Environmental Health Action Plans
LMICs	Low- and middle-income countries
MAB	Medicine Advertisements Board
MAC	Malaysian AIDS Council
MAD	Mutual acceptance of data
MADRAC	Malaysian Adverse Drug Reactions Advisory Committee
MaLRA	Malaysian Leprosy Relief Association
MAP	Master Agreed Procedures
MAPTB	Malaysian Association for the Prevention of Tuberculosis
MBS	Modified budgeting system
MCDA	Multi-criteria decision analysis
MCH	Main health centre/maternal and child health/maternal and child healthcare
MCOs	Managed care organisations
MCQ	Midwife clinic quarters
MDG	Millennium Development Goals
MDT	Multiple drug therapy
MHC	Main health centre
MHLG	Ministry of Housing and Local Government
MHSR	Malaysia Health Systems Research
MHTC	Malaysia Healthcare Travel Council
MIMS	Monthly Index of Medical Specialities
MLT	Medical laboratory technologist
MMC	Malaysian Medical Council
MMR	Measles, mumps, rubella (Chapter 6)/Mass miniature radiography (Chapter 6)/Maternal mortality ratio (Chapter 8)
MMT	Methadone maintenance treatment
MNHA	Malaysia National Health Accounts
MO	Medical officer
MoE	Ministry of Education
MoF	Ministry of Finance
MOH/MoH	Ministry of Health
MOHA	Ministry of Home Affairs
MOHMF	Ministry of Health Medicines Formulary
MPF	Malayan Pharmaceutical Factory

MPP	Medicines patent pool
MPR	Median price compared to international reference price
MPS	Master agreed procedures
MQA	Malaysian Qualifications Authority
MSF	Médecins Sans Frontières
MSM	Men who have sex with men
MSQH	Malaysian Society for Quality in Health
MTAAG+	Positive Malaysia Treatment Access and Advocacy Group
MVP	Medicines, vaccines, and pharmaceuticals
MyCC	Malaysia Competition Commission
MyHDW	Malaysian health data warehouse
MyIPO	Intellectual Property Corporation of Malaysia
MYR	Malaysian ringgit
MYSA	Malaysian Space Agency
NCD	Non-communicable disease
NDWQSP	National Drinking Water Quality Monitoring and Surveillance Programme
NEHAP	National Environmental Health Action Plan
NGO	Non-governmental organisation
NHA	National health accounts
NHMS	National Health and Morbidity Survey(s)
NHMS III	Third National Health and Morbidity Survey 2006
NIH	National Institutes of Health
NKF	National Kidney Foundation
NMCS	National Medical Care Surveys
NMP	National Medicine Policy
NPC	National Pharmaceutical Control Bureau
NPCL	National Pharmaceutical Control Laboratory
NPRA	National Pharmaceutical Regulatory Agency
NSEP	Needle and syringe exchange programme
NSP	National Strategic Plan
OECD	Organisation for Economic Co-operation and Development
OOP	Out of pocket
OOPPs	Out-of-pocket payments
OPDs	Outpatient departments
OTC	Over-the-counter

PAM	Penicillin with 2 per cent aluminium monostearate
PAP	Papanicolaou
PEPAS	Promotion of Environmental Planning and Applied Studies
PET	Positron emission tomography
PHC	Primary healthcare
PhRMA	Pharmaceutical Research and Manufacturers of America
PIC/S	Pharmaceutical Inspection Co-operation Scheme
PIN	Personal identification number
PMD	Prime Minister's Department
PMTCT	Prevention of mother-to-child transmission
PROSTAR	Program Sihat Tanpa AIDS untuk Remaja
PSD	Public Services Division
PSOs	Private sector operators
PVHI	Private voluntary health insurance
PWD	Public Works Department
QAP	Quality assurance programme
QMP	Quality management system
QUALICOPC	Quality and Costs of Primary Care
REAP	Reviewed approach
REAP-WISE Reviewed approach:	wellness, illness, support services, emergency information
RESP	Rural environmental sanitation programme
RHS	Rural health service
RM	Malaysian ringgit
RRT	Renal replacement therapy
SARS	Severe acute respiratory syndrome
SDG	Sustainable Development Goal
SEHAPs	State environmental health action plans
SIR	Susceptible infected recovered
SITC	Standard International Trade Classification
SOCSO	Social Security Organisation
SPAN	National Water Services Commission
SPUB	Sistem Pendispensan Ubat Bersepadu
SSD	Sewerage Services Department
STC	Secondary and tertiary care

STs	Systems thinkers
SWD	Solid Waste Department
T&CM	Traditional and complementary medicine
TAPS	Treatment and adherence support programme
TB	Tuberculosis
TBA	Traditional birth attendants
TBIS	Tuberculosis information system
TCM	Traditional and complementary medicine/traditional Chinese medicine
TEH	Total expenditures on health
TG	Transgender people
TGA	Therapeutic Goods Administration
THE	Total health expenditure
TMs	traditional medicines
TPAs	Third-party administrators
TPC	Teleprimary Care
TRIPS	Trade-related aspects of intellectual property rights
TRPI	Technical requirements and performance indicators
TWGs	Thematic working groups
UHC	Universal health coverage
UK	United Kingdom
UN	United Nations
UNCT	UN Country Team
UNDP	United Nations Development Programme
UNFPA	United Nations Population Fund
UNICEF	UN Children's Fund
US	United States
USA	United States of America
WHO	World Health Organization
WIPO	World Intellectual Property Organization
WISE	Wellness, illness, support, emergency and information
WTO	World Trade Organization
YLD	Years of life lost due to disability
YLL	Years of life lost

SECTION I

1 An Introduction to Health Systems

DAVID MCCOY AND PASCALE ALLOTEY

1.1 Introduction

Health systems are complex. For one, they are made up of multiple inter-acting components. Indeed, according to the World Health Organization (WHO), a health system consists of all 'organizations, people and actions whose primary intent is to promote, restore or maintain health'. They are also usually defined as country-level entities, rendering them large, encompassing both rural and urban areas, public and private systems as well as formal/allopathic and informal/traditional systems of health provision.

Health systems perform multiple functions in society – they do not merely deliver healthcare services and other interventions aimed at maintaining or improving health. They play a role in protecting households from the financial impacts of both illness and the costs of healthcare. It is important to note that health systems also perform an economic function in society (Sachs, 2001). For example, there is some evidence that the health of a population can influence economic productivity, while for many health workers and businesses, the health system is an economic sector that provides employment, wages and business opportunities. Health systems are also social and cultural institutions that play a function in helping establish 'a wider set of societal norms and values' (Gilson, 2003).

Health systems are open systems that exist in a dynamic relationship with their wider context. Indeed, they are diffuse systems with poorly defined and often porous boundaries and are thus adaptive and continuously evolving in response to multiple factors. For this reason, the social, political and economic context of any health system has to be considered when assessing its structure and performance.

Finally, health systems are sites of competition and contestation between actors with different needs and wants. There is contestation over how health priorities are set, how health systems are financed and how resources are allocated within the system. There are often ideologically and politically contrasting visions of what role a health system should play in society and what role the state and the market should play within health systems.

These different aspects of the complexity of health systems are rarely addressed simultaneously and in an inter-disciplinary manner. The truth is that health systems can only be comprehensively studied and understood through multiple disciplinary lenses, including those of history, economics, medicine, epidemiology, politics, law, ethics, anthropology and sociology.

This book presents a comprehensive and critical analysis of health systems within the context of local politics, history and socio-economic development. In the following sub-sections, we unpack some of the different dimensions of health systems complexity. First, we look at the different societal functions performed by the health system. We then investigate how health systems are also sites of contestation between different ideas and values as well as different interest groups. We then examine a variety of approaches to constructing health systems frameworks and typologies and how these can be used to describe and understand the functioning and performance of health systems. The next section discusses the open and contextual nature of health systems and the relationship between the health system and a variety of external factors, including shifts in international health policy-making. The chapter concludes with a brief discussion of systems thinking, which is discussed in greater detail in Chapter 2.

1.2 The Different Societal Functions of a Health System

For most, the obvious function of a health system is to deliver a variety of services and interventions. These services may be 'personal' services (delivered to individuals or families) or 'non-personal' services (typically public health interventions targeted at entire populations or the environment in which people live). Clearly, this is a primary function of health systems, and most evaluations of health systems performance are based on how well these personal and non-personal services are delivered in terms of their effectiveness, accessibility, fairness, efficiency and affordability.

However, health systems are more than just a vehicle for delivering health services. For example, health systems can help define and shape the identity of countries. For many post-colonial countries, health systems development is an important ingredient in nation-building, with the construction of health facilities and the extension of healthcare to rural populations viewed as indicators of progress and modernisation that are sources of national pride. Similarly, the health systems of the United Kingdom, Germany and Canada are often viewed emblematically as a national characteristic.

Perhaps more importantly, health systems play an essential social function in both shaping and reflecting relations amongst groups of people in a society. For example, national health systems reflect the depth and breadth of the social contract between governments and citizens by determining the scope of health-related rights and entitlements afforded to the citizens or residents. They also shape and reflect the relationship between the different socio-economic segments of society by either reinforcing or mitigating the relationship between social inequalities and health inequalities. The degree to which healthcare is affordable, accessible and responsive is also a critical determinant of social mobility.

Furthermore, much research and evidence have demonstrated how health systems play a significant role in defining the lived experience of being poor, socially disadvantaged or infirm. For example, studies from multiple countries have described how sub-standard and abusive treatment from healthcare providers are viewed as core defining features of what it is to be poor (WHO & World Bank, 2002). Similarly, the chronic anxiety and fear produced by the lack of protection from the costs of illness, injury and disability are a feature of relative poverty in the USA, even for working families (Himmelstein et al., 2005; Whitehead et al., 2001). The International Labour Organization (ILO) defines social health protection as the provision of organised measures to mitigate the distress caused by the reduction of productivity, stoppage or reduction of earnings, or the cost of necessary treatment that can result from ill health (ILO, 2008).

By shaping how medical services are organised, regulated and delivered, health systems also play a key cultural role in society. Indeed, by helping to define the experience and significance of core human experiences such as birth, death and illness, health systems can legitimately be viewed as cultural institutions in their own right, interacting with other cultural institutions such as religion and the arts.

Finally, health systems are also economic institutions. Many health systems incorporate markets of various kinds and sizes, as well as market actors who view health systems through a commercial lens. And, as already noted, investments in health systems are also investments in economic development. Not only are they central to the production of healthy and productive workers, they are also a source of employment and can stimulate growth in other industrial sectors.

There is a tendency to gloss over the fact that health systems have multiple identities and roles and instead view them narrowly in mechanistic terms as a structure or instrument designed to deliver health services. However, a fuller understanding of health systems would place greater emphasis on their social, cultural and economic significance and on the fact that they represent a terrain for the contestation of different ideas and interests.

1.3 Contestation within Health Systems

Certain competing ideas and interests are particularly important for determining the design, structure, performance and evolution of health systems. These include different ideological positions about the role and responsibility of the state in guaranteeing access and providing healthcare to all, the role and degree of freedom afforded to markets within health systems, and the degree to which individuals are responsible for their own state of health and wellbeing.

Health policy is also affected by competition and contestation between different groups in society over how the costs and benefits of health systems are shared. Indeed, many authors have noted the fundamentally political nature of healthcare reform and policy-making processes that determine the allocation and distribution of resources and the setting of priorities within the health sector (Barker, 1996; Grindle & Thomas, 1991; Walt & Gilson, 1994).

Of particular importance are competing views on how health systems should be financed and to what degree financing is regressive or progressive. Determining the extent to which health systems facilitate the sharing of risk and the costs of healthcare across the whole of society is fundamentally a normative process based on views regarding the obligations of higher-income populations to cross-subsidise the needs of lower-income groups, and of the young, fit and healthy to help insure against the costs of being old, disabled and unwell.

Evans (1997) identifies conflicts of interest in health systems financing as being grouped around three main axes. He describes the first as being between 'those who pay for services, and those who are paid for them' and centred around the fact that healthcare *expenditure* is always translated into healthcare *incomes* (to those who are paid to provide healthcare). As a consequence, there is always a tension between actors who want to contain costs (taxpayers and governments) and those who want to maximise expenditure (health professionals, pharmaceutical companies, etc). In practice, overall expenditure can be grown by increasing public health budgets and/or expanding the inflow of private health finance through direct out-of-pocket payments or private insurance systems.

It is also the case that different provider groups within the health system will compete with each other to capture healthcare expenditure as income for themselves. Thus doctors may promote ideas and policies to safeguard the pre-eminence of medicine within health systems and stave off competition from other types of healthcare provider. Pharmaceutical companies will promote policies and practices that increase the consumption of proprietary medicines; private insurance companies will lobby against social or national health insurance models and against any regulation of insurance markets that would impinge on their ability to generate profits. While these tensions may be the result of legitimate technical disagreements about the most effective and equitable use of resources in a health system, they may also be the result of competing interests.

The second axis of conflict, according to Evans, is between different groups of payers, and it is mainly centred around the choice of method of health financing and how this determines what share of any given level of health spending will be borne by different groups in society. As financing from general taxation generally places a larger burden on people with higher incomes in contrast to private financing, which places a greater burden on those who become (or are at most risk of becoming) ill, Evans argues that it is no surprise that 'higher-income people tend to support private finance, whereas lower-income people do not'.

Evans' third and final axis of conflict is over access to services and the choice between a universal and equitable public sector health system and a mixed public–private system. This conflict is between a single system that limits the advantage to people with higher incomes in accessing better care and a mixed system that gives some people the opportunity to 'buy their way to the front of the queue and to ensure that any "rationing" is imposed on someone else'.

The three axes of conflict can also reinforce each other. For example, pressure from higher-income groups to ensure that they can access higher-quality care in the private sector can be reinforced by provider groups lobbying against cost containment and restrictions within a universal system as a way of increasing overall health expenditure.

Finally, it is important to note that while the choices between different health financing models and policies can be framed in political and ideological terms, they can also be framed in non-political and technocratic ways. For example, universal systems of healthcare financing and provision can also be promoted as enabling health systems efficiencies through economies of scale and monopsony power. Equally, mixed systems of financing and provision can be advocated as efficiency measures by creating market competition and encouraging greater levels of individual responsibility for health. This point is pertinent because there is a tendency to cast many debates about health policy and healthcare reforms in technocratic terms to obscure or downplay political and ideological differences.

1.4 Health Systems Frameworks and Typologies

Given the complexity of health systems, it is not surprising to find that several frameworks have been developed to help study and evaluate them. Many are designed to help describe and understand the various components that contribute to the primary function of delivering health services.

For example, the WHO 'building blocks' framework comprises six building blocks consisting of 'leadership and governance'; four intermediate blocks consisting of 'financing', 'the health workforce', 'medical products, vaccines and technologies', and 'health information systems'; and a final block consisting of 'service delivery'. A framework used by Roemer (1993) similarly conceptualises four functional components that combine to enable service delivery: (1) financing; (2) production of inputs (e.g. personnel, facilities and pharmaceuticals); (3) organisation and structure of the health system; and (4) management.

These and other frameworks tend to share a pattern of having a component related to an organising function of some sort (variously labelled as 'governance', 'stewardship', 'management', 'leadership' and 'regulation'), which is then combined with various categories of inputs required to deliver services (e.g. finance and personnel).

However, while such frameworks describe the various components involved in producing health services, they do not provide a useful basis for understanding the social, political and economic dimensions of health systems. For example, the WHO building blocks framework does not allow for the description or assessment of a health system according to the core issues of how health financing, resource allocation and benefits distribution are structured and organised.

Thus it is necessary also to consider frameworks that speak more to these issues, especially political economy frameworks that are focused on describing the determinants of how the costs and benefits of health systems are distributed across society. Such political economy frameworks typically integrate an analysis of how different stakeholders relate to each other *and* to certain key functions. Many focus on the roles and powers of government and other public institutions in defining the relationship between financing and healthcare delivery, and determining the mandates, opportunities and powers of other actors, and use this as a basis for creating a typology of health systems (Böhm et al., 2013; Field, 1973; Wendt et al., 2009).

One such approach by Rothgang et al. (2005) highlights the core regulatory function of structuring the relationships between financing agencies, healthcare providers and potential beneficiaries and classifies health systems according to who is involved in carrying out this function. They also break down regulation into six objects: (1) determining which parts of the population are included in the public and/or private system (coverage); (2) determining the system of financing; (3) determining how providers are remunerated; (4) determining which providers have access to markets and financing agencies; (5) determining how patients access providers; and (5) determining the content and range of services available to patients (Rothgang et al., 2005).

Another political economy framework is one used by Roemer to classify health system policies into four broad types: (1) entrepreneurial and permissive; (2) welfare-oriented; (3) universal and comprehensive;

and (4) socialist and centrally planned (Roemer, 1991). The Organization for Economic Cooperation and Development has also categorised health systems according to three features: (1) whether the prime funding source consists of payments that are made voluntarily or that are compulsory; (2) whether services are provided by direct ownership (e.g. the ministry of health or social insurance agency provides the services itself), by contractual arrangements (e.g. the ministry of health or social insurance agency contracts providers to deliver services), or simply by private providers (paid by direct out-of-pocket payments); and (3) whether services are paid for prospectively or retrospectively (Böhm et al., 2013).

As a final example of the many ways in which health systems can be described and understood, we draw attention to the selection of a set of five key descriptors suggested by Mills and Ranson (2012):

- The dominant method of financing (e.g. tax, social insurance, private insurance, out-of-pocket payments).
- The underlying political philosophy (e.g. capitalist, socialist).
- The nature of state intervention (e.g. to cover the whole population or only the poor).
- The level of gross national product (e.g. low, middle, high).
- Historical or cultural attributes (e.g. industrialised, non-industrialised, transitional).

1.5 The Open and Contextual Nature of Health Systems

As noted earlier, health systems are social institutions that can help inform wider social and political norms and attitudes such as those that relate to the relationship between the state and inhabitants or between different segments of society. However, health systems are also clearly affected and influenced by social, economic and political forces that are highly contextual.

For example, the end of the Second World War in western Europe and the end of direct colonialism in Africa and Asia were political events that helped produce an environment that sustained strong government commitment to the idea of universal public sector health systems. Conversely, the collapse of the Soviet Union and the shift from a socialist to a capitalist political system precipitated the collapse of the universal health system in many parts of the former Soviet Union.

Other examples of political systems influencing the design of health systems include the racist and fragmented structures of the apartheid health system in South Africa and the communitarian health system of Cuba.

We can also see how ideologies and value systems such as democracy and human rights can shape the design of health systems. For example, many countries now have constitutions in which governments have duties to ensure the progressive realisation of human rights, including access to essential healthcare. At the same time, health systems are also affected by political and economic changes. For example, economic recession and a debt crisis in Africa, Asia and Latin America in the 1980s and 1990s led to structural adjustment programmes that produced a set of health sector reforms that included public sector budget cuts and a shifting of the burden of healthcare costs onto households through the use of user fees and private healthcare.

Similarly, neoliberal policies and globalisation have combined to produce a set of political dynamics that have had profound influence on the design and evolution of health systems. These include an increase in cross-border flows of finance, goods and services affecting the health sector and the general adoption of policies aimed at deregulating the health sector, outsourcing healthcare services liberalisation and promoting privatisation. Some of these changes have also been enhanced by technological developments that have facilitated the faster and freer flow of finance and information across national borders.

Any understanding of the evolution, design and performance of a health system must therefore include an analysis of its social, economic and political context. It is also important to examine the wider context when considering policies to develop, strengthen or reform health systems for the future. While health systems are subjected to a variety of external forces and changing circumstances, ideally they should be capable of anticipating new external forces and changes to the context in which they operate. For example, developments in medicine that are driven by technological advances in artificial intelligence, gene therapy, robotics, nanotechnology, cybernetics and telecommunications are likely to create a variety of demands on health systems and healthcare services that can be accommodated either in a planned or an unplanned manner. Similarly, we can anticipate that global warming and climate change, coupled with the likely accompaniment of mass population displacements, will exert pressure on healthcare systems in different parts of the world. Other transitions that are currently underway include demographic and nutrition transitions that will probably increase the number of people living in old age and with chronic diseases.

1.6 Malaysia as a Case Study

This book tells the story of the evolution of Malaysia's health system. The story is worth telling because it is a health system that has been successful, to a large extent, in having achieved universal health coverage and significant progress in health outcomes of the population. At the same time, Malaysia, like other countries, continues to face a number of complex challenges, including emerging infectious and non-communicable diseases. In telling the story of Malaysia's health system, this book also critically examines the robustness of the foundations of the health system to meet these challenges.

To do so, we have applied a systems-thinking analytical approach. Systems thinking has emerged as an area of health systems research and analysis designed specifically to help decipher the complexity of health systems and inform the design and evaluation of health systems–strengthening interventions (De Savigny & Adam, 2009). The practice of systems thinking has developed as we recognise the complexity and interconnectedness of our problems. As a solution to a complex problem and a tool that cuts across disciplines, systems thinking is itself complex. Thus it evades a simple, concise definition and has been subject to multiple definitions and redefinitions (Arnold & Wade, 2015). For our purposes, we describe systems thinking as an approach to recognising that events take place in the context of a system and that systems are composed of elements that are interconnected through feedback loops – such that solely following a linear analysis of cause and effect will fail to capture important understandings of the system. By studying the system as a whole, and not just the sum of its parts, the practice of systems thinking leads to better understanding and better decision-making. We detail our approach and methodology in Chapter 2.

The application of systems thinking and theory to the health sector has received growing attention in recent years. This has resulted in part from frustrations over the limited success of interventions for strengthening and improving the performance of health systems. It also comes from a growing appreciation of the fact that health systems are complex adaptive systems in which interactions between system components are typically non-linear, not easily controlled, unpredictable and characterised by unintended effects, paradoxical behaviour and multiple feedback loops (De Savigny & Adam, 2009; Dorner, 1997; Tan et al., 2005; Rickles et al., 2007; Paina & Peters, 2011). As such, the WHO has encouraged systems thinking as a way of enabling researchers, funders and policy-makers to improve their understanding of what works in health systems strengthening and 'catalyse conceptual thinking regarding health systems, system-level interventions, and evaluations of health system strengthening' (De Savigny & Adam, 2009).

We aim to demonstrate several ways that systems methodologies can contribute to health system strengthening. Systems thinking is a useful means of exploring problem spaces and boundaries, including linkages within and beyond the health system. Health system problems and interventions do not respect categorical or highly structured categories, such as health system building blocks, nor disciplinary and organisational boundaries, such as the various departments in a health ministry. In tracing the feedback loops to describe a system surrounding a problem, systems thinking helps us re-evaluate our assumptions about what is and isn't relevant. It helps us think about contexts as dynamic and interactive rather than as a static background that remains unchanged in an intervention. It also draws our attention to the deep connections between societies and health systems and the ways they shape one another.

The systems' interactions in health systems are inherently complex. The visual representation of causal pathways in systems thinking can help us understand and communicate such complexity. Likewise, the emphasis on feedback loops as system drivers focuses our attention on the self-corrective and adaptive capacities of systems and away from deceptively simple narratives of linear cause and effect. By providing a framework and language for thinking and speaking about complexity, systems thinking increases our capacity to engage meaningfully with it.

Finally, by redefining problem spaces and facilitating conversation about complex systems, systems thinking fosters interdisciplinarity and co-production for health systems strengthening. The systems analysis and visualisation in this book came out of extensive research, consultation and dialogue with a wide range of stakeholders that fed into an iterative process of sense-making between subject matter experts and systems thinkers. The process of co-production not only makes the knowledge generated more holistic and robust but also increases the likelihood of use and acceptance due to buy-in and the creation of an output that is understandable to all partners involved.

The book is divided into three sections. Section I consists of two introductory chapters. The first unpacks the multiple dimensions of a 'health system' and discusses the different ways in which a health system is complex. It describes health systems from a number of dimensions, including the technocratic, social, cultural, political, economic and normative. In doing so, it describes a variety of health systems frameworks and typologies. It also discusses the importance of contextualising any description and analysis of any health system and understanding how health systems thinking and policy have evolved over time internationally. The second introductory chapter presents the aspects of systems thinking and systems theory that are the focus of this book. It describes the growing interest in applying systems thinking to the study of health systems, the challenges faced, and the dual approach of case studies and whole-systems analysis taken herein.

In Section II, we present the story of the development of the Malaysian health system, its changes over time and the challenges it faces today and looking forward. It begins with a historical overview of the health system in Chapter 3, followed by separate chapters on each of the WHO health systems building blocks. The service delivery building block is divided into four sections: primary care, secondary and tertiary care, disease control, and environmental health. In each chapter, systems thinking is applied to examine the development of each building block and their linkages with each other as well as the drivers, enablers and obstacles outside the health system. The division of thematic areas into building blocks is purely instrumental.

Finally, Section III presents some generic lessons that can be used to guide future action and future change in both Malaysia and elsewhere. Chapter 13 summarises and discusses a number of issues and observations that cut across the various chapters in Section II and considers the challenges facing the Malaysian health system today and in the future. The chapter also highlights lessons that may be applicable to other countries in Asia and Africa. Chapter 14 presents lessons on the functioning and behaviour of health systems through reflections on the development of the case studies and an analysis of the key feedback processes that shape health systems.

References

Arnold, R. D. and Wade, J. P. (2015). A definition of systems thinking: a systems approach – ScienceDirect. *Procedia Computer Science*, 44, 669–78.

Barker, C. (1996). *The Health Care Policy Process*. Thousand Oaks, CA: Sage.

Böhm, K., Schmid, A., Götze, R., Landwehr, C. and Rothgang, H. (2013). Five types of OECD healthcare systems: empirical results of a deductive classification. *Health Policy*, 113, 258–69.

De Savigny, D. and Adam, T. (2009). *Systems Thinking for Health Systems Strengthening*. Geneva: World Health Organization.

Dorner, D. (1997). *The Logic of Failure: Recognizing and Avoiding Error in Complex Situations*. New York: Basic Books.

Evans, R. G. (1997). Health care reform: who's selling the market, and why? *Journal of Public Health*, 19, 45–9.

Field, M. G. (1973). The concept of the 'health system' at the macrosociological level. *Social Science & Medicine*, 7, 763–85.

Gilson, L. (2003). Trust and the development of health care as a social institution. *Social Science & Medicine*, 56, 1453–68.

Grindle, M. S. and Thomas, J. W. (1991). *Public Choices and Policy Change: The Political Economy of Reform in Developing Countries*. Baltimore, MD: Johns Hopkins University Press.

Himmelstein, D. U., Warren, E., Thorne, D. and Woolhandler, S. (2005). Illness and injury as contributors to bankruptcy. *Health Affairs*, 24, W5-63.

International Labour Organization. (2008). *Social Health Protection: An ILO Strategy towards Universal Access to Health Care*. Geneva: International Labour Organization.

Mills, A. J. and Ranson, M. K. (2012). The design of health systems. In M. H. Merson, ed., *Global Health: Diseases, Programs, Systems, and Policies*. Burlington, MA: Jones & Bartlett Learning, pp. 615–48.

Paina, L. and Peters, D. H. (2011). Understanding pathways for scaling up health services through the lens of complex adaptive systems. *Health Policy and Planning*, 27, 365–73.

Rickles, D., Hawe, P. and Shiell, A. (2007). A simple guide to chaos and complexity. *Journal of Epidemiology & Community Health*, 61, 933–7.

Roemer, M. I. (1991). *National Health Systems of the World*. Vol. I. Oxford: Oxford University Press.

Roemer, M. I. (1993). *National Health Systems of the World*. Vol. II. Oxford: Oxford University Press.

Rothgang, H., Cacace, M., Grimmeisen, S. and Wendt, C. (2005). The changing role of the state in healthcare systems. *European Review*, 13, 187–212.

Sachs, J. D. (2001). *Macroeconomics and Health: Investing in Health for Economic Development*. Geneva: World Health Organization.

Tan, J., Wen, H. J. and Awad, N. (2005). Health care and services delivery systems as complex adaptive systems. *Communications of the ACM*, 48, 36–44.

Walt, G. and Gilson, L. (1994). Reforming the health sector in developing countries: the central role of policy analysis. *Health Policy and Planning*, 9, 353–70.

Wendt, C., Frisina, L. and Rothgang, H. (2009). Healthcare system types: a conceptual framework for comparison. *Social Policy & Administration*, 43, 70–90.

Whitehead, M., Dahlgren, G. and Evans, T. (2001). Equity and health sector reforms: can low-income countries escape the medical poverty trap? *The Lancet*, 358, 833–6.

World Health Organization and World Bank. (2002). *Dying for Change: Poor People's Experience of Health and Ill-Health*. Washington, DC: World Bank.

2 *Systems Thinking for Health System Improvement*

BARRY NEWELL, DAVID T. TAN AND KATRINA PROUST

2.1 Current Challenges in Health Systems Analysis

There has been a rapid growth of interest in the application of systems thinking and system science to health systems improvement (Adam, 2014; Chughtai & Blanchet, 2017). The Alliance for Health Policy and Systems Research produced *Systems Thinking for Health Systems Strengthening* (de Savigny & Adam, 2009) in 2009. This landmark document (1) called for greater use of system principles, including dynamic thinking, systems as causes, and feedback effects in understanding health systems; (2) illustrated how a single health intervention is mediated by and impacts on the wider health system; and (3) provided guidance on how systems thinking might be used to facilitate multisectoral planning and the evaluation of health system interventions. Since then, there have been several major publications, including 'Systems Thinking for Health Systems Strengthening in LMICs: Seizing the Opportunity', a special issue of *Health Policy and Planning*; 'Advancing the Application of Systems Thinking in Health Systems' in *Health Research Policy and Systems*, *Applied Systems Thinking for Health Systems Research: A Methodological Handbook* (de Savigny et al., 2017); and *Health Systems Thinking: A Primer* (Johnson et al., 2019). These papers describe system methodologies intended to improve understanding, planning and evaluation in health systems.

Despite this interest, there are relatively few examples of the application of systems thinking to health systems strengthening (Wilkinson et al., 2018). This is reflected in the large proportion of papers on the subject advocating the use of systems approaches for health systems improvement without actually applying them (Carey et al., 2015), reflecting gaps that need to be bridged to support practice. Lack of capacity and resources for such novel and complex methods is certainly a barrier, especially in low- and middle-income countries (LMICs) (El-Jardali et al., 2014). However, well-funded efforts at operationalisation in developed countries have also faced major difficulties (Sautkina et al., 2014).

The escalating calls for a systems thinking approach to health systems improvement demand a practical response. We have identified two key challenges that need to be addressed. First, while system methodologies are necessary for addressing complex problems, in practice such methods require collaboration between many stakeholders, most of whom will have no familiarity with systems thinking. It follows that implementing system methodologies requires not only technical systems know-how but also a well-developed capacity to facilitate cross-sector communication and engagement. One way of minimising the engagement barriers, and therefore advancing the use of systems thinking at health system level, is to adopt system methods that are concrete and as easily accessed as possible.

A second challenge is the lack of a usable systemic model of the overall health system. The relationships between the World Health Organization (WHO) building blocks, emphasised by de Savigny and Adam (2009), provide a natural point of entry to systems thinking. However, there is limited evidence of the use of feedback between health system building blocks in the analysis of interventions (Baugh Littlejohns et al., 2018; Mutale et al., 2017). This highlights the need to further develop the concepts first put forward in *Systems Thinking for Health Systems Strengthening* to make them usable by a wider range of health researchers and practitioners. A methodological approach capable of supporting efforts to integrate the wide range of situations, observations and policies that typify health systems is essential in efforts to address these two challenges.

Stephen Boyden (1986) outlined six essential characteristics of a methodology that can facilitate the development of a systemic model (Box 2.1). As Boyden's focus was broadly 'culture-nature systems', of which health systems are a part, his criteria can be used essentially unchanged to guide efforts in health systems improvement.

Consideration of the Boyden criteria led us to select *system dynamics* as the methodological basis for the case studies presented in this book. System dynamics is a method for learning in and about complex systems (Sterman, 2000). It is a mature discipline that, as pointed out by Newell (2015), meets all of Boyden's methodological requirements. As described more fully in Section 2.2, system dynamics is built on fundamental principles concerning the way system structure (i.e. the

Box 2.1 The Boyden criteria

A methodology capable of supporting the development of an integrated health system model needs to perform the following functions:

1. It should provide a rational basis for *organising information* relating to different aspects of the [health] system under consideration.
2. It should provide a structure for *analysing, visualising and communicating* about the interactions between the different aspects (natural and cultural) of human situations.
3. It should facilitate recognition and consideration of fundamental principles relating to the interactions between variables of different kinds.
4. It should encourage consideration of the *full spectrum of variables* which may be relevant in any particular situation under investigation. [In particular, it should ensure that full consideration be given to intangible aspects of reality as well as aspects that are tangible and easily quantified.]
5. It must encourage consideration of *changes over time* in the system under investigation as well as a sense of perspective with respect to rates of change and the scale of societal activities and impacts.
6. It must be *flexible*. That is to say, while it must be useful in the organisation of information and in communication, it should also encourage speculation and the formulation of new ideas; it must *never dictate* our way of thinking about human situations.

Adapted from Boyden (1986, 198) – italics in the original. The criteria have been numbered for ease of reference.

network of interactions between key state variables) drives system behaviour over time (thus meeting criteria B3 and B5). It is flexible in that it deals in elementary building blocks (stocks, flows, feedback loops) that can be combined, Lego™-like, to represent system structure in essentially any context (B6). Because of this versatility, it provides a means of organising information from different disciplines and thereby supports the development of practical integrative approaches

(B1, B4). The generic nature of its concepts encourages consideration of a wide range of variables when teams formulate their 'dynamic hypotheses' (tentative identification of system structures that can generate observed behaviour). It provides practical tools (such as causal loop diagrams (CLDs) and stock-and-flow maps and models) that can be used to facilitate the visualisation, testing and communication of these hypotheses (B2). Finally, while system dynamics rests on powerful mathematical foundations, in practice its basic concepts are usually expressed in terms of simple metaphors that can be easily understood by people with a wide range of backgrounds.

System dynamics methods are not confined to quantitative modelling – in fact the discipline supports a seamless progression from systems thinking to dynamical modelling (Forrester, 1961; 1968; 1969; 1990). The book *Thinking in Systems: A Primer* (Meadows, 2009) is a readable introduction. Elsewhere, Sterman (2000) provides a thorough discussion in *Business Dynamics: Systems Thinking and Modelling for a Complex World.*

2.2 System Dynamics Concepts and Tools

The accessibility of system dynamics concepts depends on the discipline's use of easily understood conceptual metaphors (Lakoff & Johnson, 2003; Newell, 2012). For example, the notion of 'stocks and flows' is usually introduced in terms of the bathtub metaphor (Table 2.1). In this metaphor, the bathtub stands for a specific component of a complex system. At any particular time, the 'state' of the component is represented by the amount ('stock') of water that has accumulated in the tub. Changes in this variable (seen as changes in the water level) represent changes in the state of the system component. The processes that change the state of the component are represented by the 'flows' of water into and out of the tub. Stocks can be tangible quantities like water, money or the number of people infected with a virus, and they can be intangible quantities like social capital, political will or happiness.

System dynamics provides a disciplined visual language that can be used to communicate assumptions about the interactions between the parts of a system. This language includes stock-and-flow maps. A simple example is shown in Figure 2.1. In this diagram, the boxes represent the levels of variable quantities ('stocks') that indicate the

Table 2.1 ***The bathtub metaphor***

A bathtub	→	[1]A system component
The water in the tub	→	An accumulation, a 'stock', a variable that represents the current state of the system component
The amount of water in the tub	→	The amount accumulated, the 'level' of the stock, the state of the system component
Water entering the tub from the tap	→	An 'inflow', a state-change process that increases the amount accumulated
Water leaving the tub through the drain	→	An 'outflow', a process that decreases the amount accumulated
Water leaving the tub by splashing	→	Another outflow that decreases the amount accumulated

Source: Newell (2012).
[1] The arrows represent the expression 'corresponds to'.

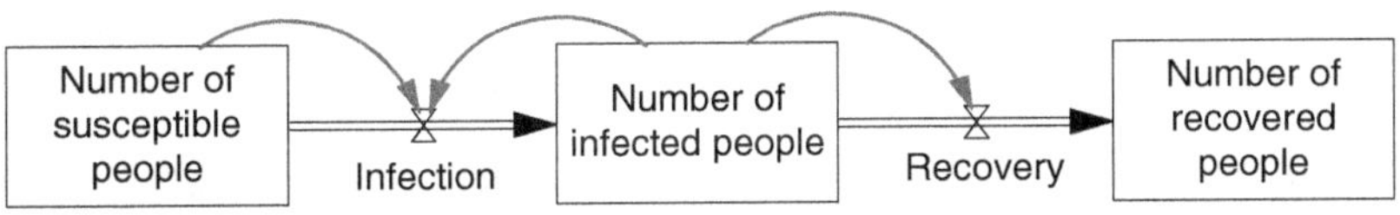

Figure 2.1 The susceptible–infected–recovered (SIR) system. This stock-and-flow map represents the causal structure of the system that governs the spread of infectious diseases. In epidemiological practice, this structure is known as the SIR model. The three stocks shown in the map are connected by two flows that represent the processes of infection and recovery, respectively. The rates of these state-change processes are controlled by the levels of the stocks.

current state of the system of interest. The double-line arrows represent state-change processes ('flows') that can alter the stock levels (i.e. change the state of the system). The tap symbols in the arrows represent process 'flow rates'. The single-line arrows represent 'influence links' whereby stock levels control process flow rates.

CLDs can play a useful role in situations where a stock-and-flow model is not required or cannot be easily constructed. An example is shown in Figure 2.2. In this type of diagram, blocks of text represent the levels of state variables (stocks). The arrows are 'influence links' that represent the state-change processes (flows). A change in the level of the driver variable (at the tail of the arrow) causes a change in the

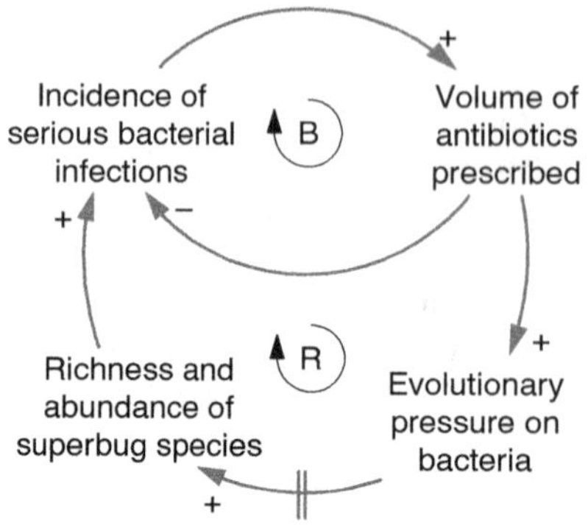

Figure 2.2 A causal loop diagram (CLD). This diagram depicts the story of the fight against increasingly prevalent antibiotic-resistant bacteria. An increase in the incidence of serious bacterial infections leads to an increase in the volume of antibiotics prescribed. The prescription of antibiotics leads to a reduction in the incidence of serious infections. At the same time, however, the increased use of antibiotics increases the evolutionary pressure on bacterial populations, leading to an eventual increase in the richness and abundance of drug-resistant species and a consequent increase in the incidence of serious infections. While the latter effect takes time to appear, it eventually dominates.

level of the affected variable (at the arrowhead). The plus and minus signs are link 'polarities'. A positive polarity (+) indicates that an increase in the level of the driver variable will cause the level of the affected variable to eventually rise above the level it otherwise would have had, and that a decrease in the level of the driver variable will cause the level of the affected variable to eventually decrease below the level it otherwise would have had. A negative polarity (–) indicates that the relationships are inverse. The small parallel lines crossing one arrow are a 'delay mark' – they indicate that the effect of a change in the level of the driver variable will take a relatively long time to appear. The encircled 'B' indicates a balancing feedback loop, and the encircled 'R' indicates a reinforcing feedback loop. Provided that these rules of 'visual grammar' are followed, CLDs can help articulate dynamic hypotheses that account for the response of a health system to imposed policy and management initiatives.

From a system dynamics point of view, '[the] feedback loop is the . . . basic unit of analysis and communication of system behaviour' (Richardson, 1991). There are just two types of feedback: reinforcing loops that amplify change and balancing loops that resist change. The

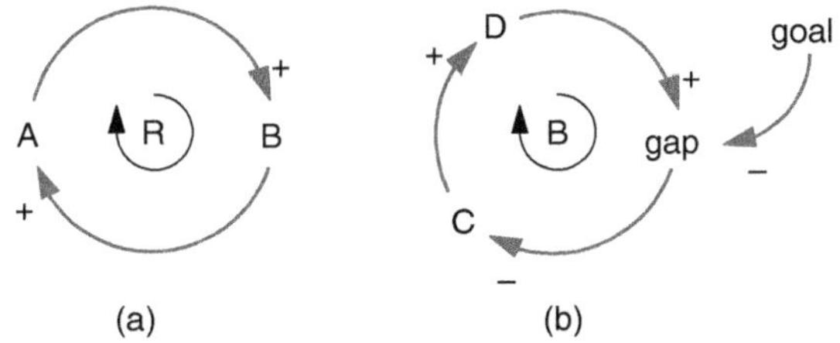

Figure 2.3 Two types of feedback structure: (a) reinforcing feedback; (b) balancing feedback. In general, a dynamic hypothesis that aims to explain the behaviour of a real-world system will comprise a network of competing reinforcing and balancing loops.

generic structures shown in Figure 2.3 illustrate these cases. In panel (a), reinforcing feedback exists when an increase/decrease in the level of variable A causes an increase/decrease in the level of variable B, which causes a further increase/decrease in A, and so on, around the loop. This causal structure drives accelerating growth (or accelerating collapse) of both A and B. In panel (b), balancing feedback occurs when management efforts (or natural processes) work to hold the level of variable D close to a particular goal. The case shown represents the situation where D lies *above* the goal. An increase in C causes an increase in D. This change in D increases the gap between D and the goal, which triggers mechanisms that work to reverse the change in C and so bring D back towards the goal. The goal may be deliberately set (e.g. the chosen setpoint on a thermostat), an outcome of the collective interactions among many actors (e.g. how much money one is expected to spend on a birthday present) or a systemic level that may be natural or anthropogenic (e.g. the body temperature maintained by homeostasis).

Influence diagrams (IDs) (Figure 2.4) are the simplest systems thinking tool offered by system dynamics. They are similar to CLDs but do not have polarities assigned to their causal links. This makes them suitable for initial discussions where some polarities may be uncertain and difficult to determine.

IDs provide a flexible means of articulating assumptions about cause–effect structure. Thus they can function as a visual cause–effect language supporting a team's early efforts to co-develop knowledge. Individual team members can use IDs to describe their assumptions about the boundaries and causal structure of their system of interest.

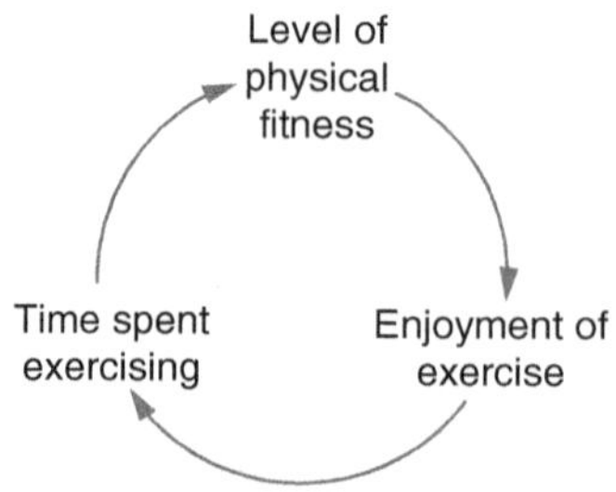

Figure 2.4 An influence diagram (ID). This example represents a feedback loop where *Time spent exercising* affects *Level of physical fitness*. This change affects *Enjoyment of exercise*, which leads to a further change in *Time spent exercising* – and so on around the loop. IDs do not have polarities assigned to influence links.

The team can then use the collection of individual diagrams to explore similarities and differences in their thinking about (mental models of) the system (Newell & Proust, 2018).

Overall, system dynamics can support a wide spectrum of activities. At the systems thinking end of the spectrum, the collaborative development of IDs or CLDs can help *any* multi-disciplinary team co-develop hypotheses concerning system structure and behaviour (Newell & Proust, 2012; 2018). The systems thinking principles listed in Box 2.2 summarise a typical system dynamics perspective.

At the system modelling end of the spectrum, working stock-and-flow models can support exploration of the dynamics of various complex system structures. In practice, policy development needs to begin at the systems thinking end of the spectrum with a broad investigation of potentially relevant variables and interactions. How far the team can then progress toward quantitative modelling (and the desirability of attempting to do so) depends on many factors, including the nature of the system of interest, the availability of reliable historical data and the team members' skills and experience.

The use of system dynamics can provide a coherent way to facilitate iterative problem exploration and framing. This helps ensure that governance problems are addressed at the right level. It also supports co-production of new knowledge by a multi-disciplinary team, a process that leads to better policies. It is important to note, however, that system dynamics and system models are not a panacea for health systems improvement. The utility of any diagrams or models will be limited by the team's knowledge of the system of interest.

Box 2.2 Systems thinking principles for health system improvement

1. **The Feedback Principle:** Feedback effects are dominant drivers of behaviour in any health system.
2. **The Holistic Principle:** The behaviour of a health system emerges from the feedback interactions between its parts and therefore cannot be optimised by optimising the behaviour of its parts individually.
3. **The Inertia Principle:** The filling and draining of stocks is a pervasive process in health systems. The presence of stocks causes delayed responses, thereby giving rise to system inertia.
4. **The Surprise Principle:** Any action taken in a health system will have multiple outcomes, some expected and some unexpected. The expected outcomes might occur — unexpected outcomes will always occur. The unexpected outcomes are usually unwanted and delayed — the delays make it difficult to identify the triggering actions.
5. **The History Principle:** Knowledge of past activities and patterns of behaviour is essential in any attempt to understand how a health system works.
6. **The Myopia Principle:** No one person can see the whole of a health system.
7. **The Collaboration Principle:** The boundaries of a health system cut across the boundaries of traditional disciplines, organisations, governance sectors and sub-cultures. An effective systems approach therefore requires deep collaboration between people with different backgrounds, worldviews, values and allegiances.

Adapted from Newell and Proust (2018), Box 5.1.

2.3 Application of the Systems Dynamics Approach in This Publication

Using the Malaysian health system as an example, this book illustrates the use of a systems dynamics approach in health systems analysis. We address the two challenges identified above, namely, engaging non-systems experts and creating a useful system model of the health system. In doing this we also address the learning goals described in Chapter 1.

This book is a product of collaboration between experts across government policy, the private sector, health experts and academics. The process involved sustained engagement and collaboration between health experts and systems thinkers through discussion, debate and iteration towards a genuinely co-produced and co-owned product with capacity-building as a further by-product. We suggest that this approach could be considered for use as a model for endeavours in this field (see Sterman, 2000, chapter 3).

Section II discusses the development of the Malaysian health system. Chapter 3 provides an overview of the larger historical context for the Malaysian health system, followed by an analysis of the individual building blocks of the health system (Chapters 4–12). The service delivery building block is divided into four thematic areas: primary care, secondary and tertiary care, disease control, and environmental health.

Two collaborative approaches between health experts and systems thinkers were taken in applying systems thinking in Section II. The first was used to examine the development of the overall health system building blocks. Each of the health system building block chapters begins with an overview of the development of that building block. The documentation of the development of the Malaysian health system and the lessons learned were led by health experts, who undertook a process of document review and interviews in consultation with the editorial team.

Examining the development of the health system building blocks over the past 60 years was a substantial challenge. Documentation of many important events in the earlier development of the Malaysian health system was scarce and located largely in the grey literature. Thus the health experts and the editorial team relied on individuals with knowledge of the grey literature and with first-hand experience of the key events. These histories are thus selective due to methodological limitations, but also because of space constraints. Nonetheless, they are critical for identifying trends and patterns that provide systemic insights into the development of the health system. In describing the development of each building block, emphasis was placed on linkages with other building blocks and with important drivers, enablers and obstacles outside the health system. The systems thinkers then reviewed these findings to derive systemic observations from the histories.

The second approach was used in the case studies that address significant systemic interventions, problems or events within individual building blocks. Here, the health experts and systems thinkers undertook a more in-depth co-production process for developing the case studies, using the methodology described by Tan et al. (2019). While we endeavoured to have at least one case study for each health system building block, case study selection was largely driven by the availability of health experts willing to engage in the process and the extent of their expertise. Accordingly, the case studies are not an attempt to provide a comprehensive overview of issues in health systems or in systems thinking.

An iterative sense-making process was used to determine the system of interest in each case study; it involved: (1) narrative problem framing by the health experts; (2) interrogation of the narrative by the systems thinkers to discover interrelations, causal links, feedback and emergence; and (3) development of CLDs by the systems thinkers to represent the narrative developed by the health experts. The preliminary CLDs often served as a mirror that helped the health experts refine or revise their problem framing. When this process was complete, the feedback structures in the CLDs were analysed to improve understanding of the systemic issues, problems and enablers seen in the case studies.

The choice of approaches maximised the goals of the publication within the time and resource constraints. The case studies provided a sufficiently well-defined problem space for the health experts and systems thinkers to engage in meaningful co-production within a limited timeframe. The different levels of systems insights from the two approaches provide an example of what can be achieved at varying levels of investment into system analysis. The case studies illustrate how a problem-based approach works – regardless of the level of the problem.

To obtain a full range of perspectives, including both the historical development of the building blocks and the case studies, a series of stakeholder meetings was convened for comments and critique. Several of these meetings revealed very different perspectives concerning some issues. These differences were shaped by differences in experience and understanding that reflected the position from which individual stakeholders had engaged the issue. The input from these meetings led to further investigation of disputed data and iteration of system analysis.

Section III of this book consolidates the learnings from the investigations reported in Section II. Chapter 13 synthesises key health system development lessons from experience generated within the Malaysian health system. These lessons should be relevant to health systems worldwide, especially those in LMICs. Chapter 14 reflects on lessons concerning the application of systems thinking to health systems. There, we attempt to derive a broad, systemic model of health systems that connects the system models developed in the tightly defined problems of the case studies. By combining a whole-systems approach with detailed case studies, we hope to provide multiple examples of how systems methodologies can be applied at all levels of health systems strengthening to produce outputs and understandings that are accessible to all.

References

Adam, T. (2014). Advancing the application of systems thinking in health. *Health Research Policy and Systems*, 12, 50. DOI: https://doi.org/10.1186/1478-4505-12-50

Baugh Littlejohns, L., Baum, F., Lawless, A. and Freeman, T. (2018). The value of a causal loop diagram in exploring the complex interplay of factors that influence health promotion in a multisectoral health system in Australia. *Health Research Policy and Systems*, 16(1), 126. DOI: https://doi.org/10.1186/s12961-018-0394-x

Boyden, S. (1986). An integrative approach to the study of human ecology. In R. J. Boyden, J. Jacobs and G. L. Young, eds., *Human Ecology: A Gathering of Perspectives*. College Park, MD: Society for Human Ecology, pp. 3–25.

Carey, G., Malbon, E., Carey, N., Joyce, A., Crammond, B. and Carey, A. (2015). Systems science and systems thinking for public health: a systematic review of the field. *BMJ Open*, 5(12), e009002. DOI: https://doi.org/10.1136/bmjopen-2015-009002

Chughtai, S. and Blanchet, K. (2017). Systems thinking in public health: a bibliographic contribution to a meta-narrative review. *Health Policy and Planning*, 32(4), 585–94. DOI: https://doi.org/10.1093/heapol/czw159

de Savigny, D. and Adam, T. (eds.). (2009). *Systems Thinking for Health Systems Strengthening*. Geneva: World Health Organization.

de Savigny, D., Blanchet, K. and Adam, T. (2017). *Applied Systems Thinking for Health Systems Research: A Methodological Handbook*. Online publication. http://researchonline.lshtm.ac.uk/4646083

El-Jardali, F., Adam, T., Ataya, N., Jamal, D. and Jaafar, M. (2014). Constraints to applying systems thinking concepts in health systems: a regional perspective from surveying stakeholders in Eastern Mediterranean countries. *International Journal of Health Policy and Management*, 3(7), 399–407. DOI: https://doi.org/10.15171/ijhpm.2014.124

Forrester, J. W. (1961). *Industrial Dynamics*. Portland, OR: Productivity Press.

Forrester, J. W. (1968). *Principles of Systems*, 2nd ed. Portland, OR: Productivity Press.

Forrester, J. W. (1969). *Urban Dynamics*. Waltham, MA: Pegasus Communications.

Forrester, J. W. (1990). *Systems Dynamics as a Foundation for Pre-college Education*. Cambridge, MA: Systems Dynamics Group, Massachusetts Institute of Technology.

Johnson, J. A., Anderson, D. E. and Rossow, C. C. (2019). *Health Systems Thinking: A Primer*. Online publication. www.jblearning.com/catalog/9781284167146

Lakoff, G. and Johnson, M. (2003). *Metaphors We Live By*. Chicago, IL: University of Chicago Press.

Meadows, D. H. (2009). *Thinking in Systems: A Primer*. London: Earthscan.

Mutale, W., Ayles, H., Bond, V., Chintu, N., Chilengi, R., Tembo Mwanamwenge, M. et al. (2017). Application of systems thinking: 12-month postintervention evaluation of a complex health system intervention in Zambia: the case of the BHOMA. *Journal of Evaluation in Clinical Practice*, 23(2), 439–52. DOI: https://doi.org/10.1111/jep.12354

Newell, B. (2012). Simple models, powerful ideas: towards effective integrative practice. *Global Environmental Change*, 22, 776–83.

Newell, B. (2015). Towards a shared theoretical framework. In R. Dyball and B. Newell, eds., *Understanding Human Ecology: A Systems Approach to Sustainability*. London: Earthscan/Routledge, pp. 111–36.

Newell, B. and Proust, K. (2012). *Introduction to Collaborative Conceptual Modelling*. Working Paper, ANU Open Access Research. Online paper. https:/digitalcollections.anu.edu.au/handle/1885/9386

Newell, B. and Proust, K. (2018). Escaping the complexity dilemma. In A. König, ed., *Sustainability Science: Key Issues*. London: Earthscan/Routledge. Online publication.

Richardson, G. P. (1991). *Feedback Thought in Social Science and Systems Theory*. Waltham, MA: Pegasus.

Sautkina, E., Goodwin, D., Jones, A., Ogilvie, D., Petticrew, M., White, M. and Cummins, S. (2014). Lost in translation? Theory, policy and practice in systems-based environmental approaches to obesity prevention in the Healthy Towns programme in England. *Health & Place*, 29, 60–66. DOI: https://doi.org/10.1016/j.healthplace.2014.05.006

Sterman, J. D. (2000). *Business Dynamics: Systems Thinking and Modeling for a Complex World*. Boston, MA: Irwin McGraw-Hill.

Tan, D. T., Siri, J. G., Gong, Y., Ong, B., Lim, S. C., MacGillivray, B. H. et al. (2019). Systems approaches for localising the SDGs: co-production of place-based case studies. *Global Health*, 15, 85. DOI: https://doi.org/10.1186/s12992-019-0527-1

Wilkinson, J., Goff, M., Rusoja, E., Hanson, C. and Swanson, R. C. (2018). The application of systems thinking concepts, methods, and tools to global health practices: an analysis of case studies. *Journal of Evaluation in Clinical Practice*, 24(3), 607–18. DOI: https://doi.org/10.1111/jep.12842

SECTION II

3 *Malaysia's Health and Socio-economic Transformation*

JO. M. MARTINS

3.1 Human Development and Health

Malaysia's health development has been part of the wider process of human and other socio-economic progression. This chapter provides the broader context to the Malaysian health system through a brief analysis of socio-economic development and its impact on health risks and conditions. There were also associated health improvements that in turn fostered human development. This analysis provides a macro and concise framework for the more detailed examination in other chapters of the development of the Malaysian health system in terms of its service delivery, related inputs and more detailed outcomes.

Malaysians have made noteworthy socio-economic progress since the country's independence in 1957, in view of the advantages and challenges of their physical and equatorial environment. As a result of these efforts, Malaysia is now among the countries that have achieved very high human development according to the United Nations Development Programme (UNDP), based on attained life expectancy, education and income per capita (United Nations Development Programme, 2018). Malaysia is also among the group of high- to middle-income countries with a gross national income per capita of \$26,190 in 2015 (purchasing power parities, 2015), compared with the substantially lower average of \$15,627 for countries in the same income group (World Bank, 2017), and is on the pathway to joining the high-income group of nations.

Malaysia is a good example of a comprehensive approach to development. Since independence, government policies have been progressively articulated in five-year development plans in a holistic manner that deals not only with the economic elements but also other social elements of human development, including health. Thus health interventions are planned and implemented in the context of a range of complementary activities in socio-economic development. They reflect priorities set across the board, including labour force and financial resource constraints, and the steps taken to address them. Therefore, it is essential to examine health advances in conjunction with concurrent socio-economic development that affects the way people live and where, and what they do, with an impact on social organisation, as well as geographical and financial factors that have a bearing on relative access to health services and living conditions.

The progress made in human development in Malaysia has been substantial in terms of the three measures used by the UNDP in its index of human development: life expectancy, education and gross domestic product (GDP) per capita. Using 1970 as a basis, life expectancy had increased by 11 years to 75.6 years in 2015, secondary education enrolment more than doubled to 85%, and GDP per capita increased by more than five times to 35,100 Malaysian Ringgit (Table 3.1).

Three major phases can be identified in human development since independence. Their expression in health development is as follows:

- The first phase, during the 1960s and 1970s, emphasised rural development and capacity building of the health system.
- The second phase, in the 1980s and 1990s, was one of consolidating socio-economic transformation and the health system, from a rural

Table 3.1 *Human development, Malaysia, 1970–2015*

	Human development measures		
Year	Life expectancy (years)[1]	Education: secondary school enrolment (%)[2]	GDP per capita constant prices (MYR 000s)[3]
1970	64.4	39.2	6.2
2015	75.1	85.0	35.1
2015/1970	1.17	2.17	5.66

Sources: World Bank (2019a; 2019b; 2019c). Calculations made by the author.
[1] The average number of years lived from birth.
[2] The percentage of children of relevant age attending secondary school.
[3] The average gross domestic product (GDP) per capita at constant prices in thousand Malaysian Ringgit (MYR).

setting to rising employment in secondary industries, urbanisation with migration from rural to urban centres and growing health system capacity.

- The third phase, in the 2000s and 2010s, has the characteristics of a more developed socio-economic configuration, with growing urbanisation and sustained employment in manufacturing but a larger proportion of people employed in services. Conditions have continued to improve, but growing affluence and more sedentary occupational and recreational activities have led to lifestyles that compromise the rate of health enhancements.

Health status has been closely associated with poverty, and in turn, health services provision has contributed to poverty alleviation (Hammer et al., 1995). In addition to socio-economic factors in development during the above three phases, four variables will be used in the analysis to examine the evolution that affected health status in Malaysia: poverty prevalence for social and economic security affecting health status; urban/rural residence for the manner of social organisation and geographical access to health services; rate of safe deliveries for access to and coverage by basic health services; and infant mortality rates as a marker of health status in a relatively young society, even today.[1]

3.2 Reaching the Poor in Rural Malaysia and Increasing Capacity (1960s and 1970s)

At independence in 1957, about three-quarters of Malaysians lived in rural areas (74%), and close to half of the labour force worked in agriculture (47%), mostly in rubber plantations and rice cultivation. The unemployment rate was estimated at 13%, but it was posited that there was considerable additional disguised unemployment (Fernandez et al., 1975; Jones, n.d.; Supplementary Table 3.J). Poverty was pervasive, with 51% living below the poverty line on average and 60% living in rural areas (Roslan, 2001; Supplementary Table 3.D). This was associated with a high population growth rate (almost 3% per year) driven by a high fertility rate of more than 5 live births per woman, which led to a large proportion of the population being under 15 years of age (44%) and a dependency rate of 82% on the working-age population but a relatively low proportion of people aged 65 years and over (3%). However, the high rate of infant mortality (75/1,000 live births) contributed to low life expectancy at birth of only 57 years at that time (Fernandez et al., 1975; Supplementary Tables 3.E, 3.H and 3.I). In addition, poor health due to the high incidence of malaria, tuberculosis and other communicable diseases (Roemer, 1976) affected the productivity of human capital. There is also evidence of malnutrition in children from poor rural areas (McKay et al., 1971; Chong et al., 1984). The low level of education was another dimension of the quality of human capital: in 1957, more than half the population aged over 14 years (53%) were illiterate in any language (Ministry of Education Malaysia, 1967), with implications for female fertility and maternal and child health associated with the level of education of women.

Few doctors and nurses were concentrated in urban centres in relation to the population (Supplementary Tables 3.K and 3.L) to address the large burden of disease and mortality. There was significant reliance on traditional healers, with services provided by *bomohs* (healers) and *kampong bidans* (village midwives) in the Malay tradition. *Sinsehs* (Chinese physicians) provided herbs and other traditional Chinese medicines, supplemented on occasion by Western-type medicines. There were also a few Ayurvedic practitioners from India. It was not uncommon for care to be sought interchangeably regardless of ethnicity. Although there were reservations about the effectiveness of traditional practices, the household expenditure survey for 1957/1958 indicated that households spent almost as much on traditional medicines with a lower price as they did on more costly Western ones (Roemer, 1976).

It was in this context that various Malaya and Malaysian[2] plans were formulated to address both economic and social development during this first phase. Rural development became a major policy objective in the 1950s and 1960s to address the productivity, income and living conditions of most people in Malaysia. Government development expenditure rose from 3.6% of the GDP in 1956–1960 to 6.8% in 1966–1970 and government revenue from the export of oil rose to 12.6% of the GDP in 1976–1980 (Lee & Chew-Ging, 2017). During 1956–1980, about a third of development expenditure was for infrastructure such as roads, power and communication that enhanced rural and regional transport and communication, and about one-quarter was for agriculture to improve productivity and the income of poor rural populations engaged in rice cultivation, reforming rubber plantations and developing palm oil cultivation in small holdings with improved productivity. A substantial development expenditure that included security (due in part to internal emergency and confrontation with Indonesia over the sovereignty of Sabah and Sarawak) absorbed some 16% of the total government development expenditure during this period. Development expenditure on education and health (which tends to be less than that on security, transport and public works) amounted respectively to about 8% and 2% of the total during this period (Peacock, 1981; Fong, 1985; Aslam & Hassan, 2003).

The importance of health services reaching the poor in rural areas was expressed in the priority given to the following complementary activities (Suleiman & Jegathesan, n.d.):

- Training of health personnel and recruitment in rural areas.
- Provision of rural health services, including safe water and sanitation.
- Prevention and management of communicable diseases.
- Improved hospital capacity to support primary care.
- Family planning and nutrition supplementation.

This reflected the considerable regional differences in infant mortality that prevailed through the 1960s and 1970s, which were associated with the proportion of people living in rural areas and with levels of household poverty. Accordingly, the state of Terengganu, with 68% of households living in poverty and 73% of its population in rural areas, had an infant mortality rate of 54 per 1,000 live births; Selangor, including Kuala Lumpur (Malaysia's large urban capital), had a lower proportion of rural population (55%), a lower level of poverty (43%) and a substantially lower infant mortality rate of 30 per 1,000 live births (Hasan, 1986).

The efforts made to improve economic productivity resulted in an average GDP annual growth rate of 7.1% in the 20-year period of 1960–1980. However, the large population growth reduced it to a still-helpful rate of 3.7% per head of population (Supplementary Tables 3.A and 3.E). Even though primary industries continued to constitute a large proportion of the GDP (31%) in 1980, the proportion of secondary production almost doubled to 25% of the GDP, with little change in the proportion of services (44%) (Supplementary Table 3.B). Employment saw a substantial decline in the proportion of the population employed in primary industries, mostly in rural areas, from 50% to 39% during the 20-year period and an increase in the proportion of those employed in services from 30% to 40% (Supplementary Table 3.C). Although the majority of the population continued to live in rural areas, greater urbanisation took place, and the proportion of the population living in urban areas increased from 26% in 1960 to 42% in 1980 (Supplementary Table 3.J), with consequences for the mode of living, type of work and conditions and relative ease of access to health services. Further, substantial gains were made in education. By 1967, enrolment among children of relevant age in primary education had risen to 94% and to 52% in lower secondary education, with considerable progress in the education levels of women (Ministry of Education Malaysia, 1967), which is associated with fertility and maternal and child health (Hasan, 1986). This was coupled with the increase in the female labour force participation rate from 37% in 1970 to 44% in 1980 and the observed substantial decline in fertility, which was also enhanced by the family planning programme in 1965 (Fernandez et al., 1975; World Bank, 2019d; Supplementary Table 3.G).

Development in terms of personnel and rural health facilities made substantial progress during this phase. The number of people per nurse declined about four-fold and that per doctor declined by about half during the 20-year period of 1960–1980 (Supplementary Tables 3.K and 3.L; Chapter 8). Public hospital services were upgraded without an increase in the number of beds per head of population, but their use rose by 43% during the same period (Chapter 5). The proportion of the population served by sewerage rose by about 89% and that with access to safe water increased by about 82% in the 10-year period 1970–1980 (World Bank, n.d.; Chapter 7). The impact on health of the various preventive and management interventions is illustrated by the 29% decline in the incidence of malaria and 96% decrease in the incidence rate of diphtheria in the 4-year period of 1976–1980 (Chapter 6). This progress was achieved with a relatively low total health expenditure. Estimates for 1973 indicated that total health expenditure amounted to only about 2% of the GDP, and that 65% of it was spent in the public sector (Roemer, 1985; Chapter 8).

During 1960–1980, socio-economic development and changed employment opportunities increased the proportion of the urban population from 26% to 42% in 1980, and poverty levels declined from 49% in 1970 to 37% in 1980. Easier access to health services and increased

Table 3.2 ***Changes in poverty, urbanisation, safe deliveries and infant mortality, Malaysia, 1960–1980***

Year	Households in poverty (%)	Urban population (%)	Safe deliveries[1] (%)	Infant mortality rate[2]
1960	n.a.	25.6	41.3[3]	68.9[3]
1970	49.3	33.5	67.1[3]	38.5[3]
1980	37.4	42.0	85.4[3]	23.8
Change 1960–1980	-11.9[4]	+16.4	+44.1	-45.1

Sources: Supplementary Tables 3.D, 3.J and 3.G; Ministry of Health Malaysia (1982).
[1] Those performed by professionally trained health personnel.
[2] The ratio of the number of deaths of those aged under 1 year per 1,000 live births.
[3] Peninsular Malaysia.
[4] Change from 1970 to 1980.
n.a. – not available

service provision in rural areas led to greater health services coverage. In Peninsular Malaysia, safe deliveries by professionally trained health personnel rose from 41% to 85% during this 20-year period; as a proxy measure of health improvement in a young population, the infant mortality rate declined by more than half from 69 per 1,000 live births in 1960 to 24 in 1980 (Table 3.2). Life expectancy at birth rose by 8 years to 68 years in that period (Supplementary Table 3.G).

3.3 Transition and Consolidation (1980s and 1990s)

The core development objectives in the 1980s and 1990s were the eradication of poverty, the re-structuring of society and more balanced regional development (Prime Minister's Department, 1989). The related health policy goals set out in the Fourth to Seventh Malaysia Development Plans were (Suleiman & Jegathesan, n.d.):

- Training of health personnel and their engagement to serve the growing population and a better mix of human resources to provide needed services.
- Reduction in the disparity of health status among different population groups and areas.
- Control of preventable infectious diseases.

- Promotion of healthy living environment.
- Collaboration in health promotion between the public and private sectors and among agencies.
- Improvement in productivity and quality of services.

A major transition took place in Malaysia during these two decades. The population almost doubled from about 14 million to 23 million (Supplementary Table 3.E) in spite of a decline in the average fertility from four to three children per woman (Supplementary Table 3.G). Consequently, the proportion of children aged under 15 years decreased, with a compensating increase in the proportion of working-age people (15–64 years), which reduced child dependency on working-age people from about 70% to 53%, but the proportion of older people aged over 64 years remained low at 4% (Supplementary Tables 3.H and 3.I). The growth in working-age people was accompanied by a major shift in economic activity from agriculture to manufacturing and related employment. Accordingly, employment in primary industries, mostly agriculture, declined from 39% in 1980 to 16% in 2000, and the proportion of people employed in secondary industries (manufacturing and construction) rose from 21% to 36% (Supplementary Table 3.C). The economic transformation provided a wider range of employment opportunities, and the unemployment rate, which had risen to 8% in 1987 (Department of Statistics Malaysia, 1989), fell to 3% in 2000 (Department of Statistics Malaysia, 2001a). Income rose faster than the large growth in population and led to a substantial increase in GDP per head of population at an average annual rate of 3.7% during that period (Supplementary Table 3.A).

However, the rate of progress was upset by the oil crisis in 1979, which affected government revenue and led to fiscal constraints in the 1980s and an economic recession in 1985–1986. Government development expenditure that was still substantially high at 11% of the GDP in 1981–1985 dropped to 6% by 1996–2000 (Lee & Chew-Ging, 2017). As the emphasis on development moved to manufacturing, government development expenditure on agriculture was reduced by about half to 12% of the total in 1981–2000, while investments in infrastructure for roads, communication and power generation continued to receive about one-third (34%) of the total, and investments in industry increased somewhat from 14% to 17%. Government recognition of the importance of the continual improvement of human capital for both economic and social purposes was shown in the rise of development expenditure on education from 8% to 12% and that on health from 2% to 3% (Aslam & Hassan, 2003). Primary education enrolments became almost universal (97%); secondary school enrolments rose to 65% and that in tertiary education to 26%, with female enrolments, of particular importance to health, being at least on a par with that of men (United Nations Educational, Scientific and Cultural Organization, 2011).

Another aspect of the socio-economic transformation was internal migration to urban areas with employment opportunities. A study carried out in 1989–1990 (Department of Statistics Malaysia, n.d.) indicated that the more rural states lost some of their population due to internal migration, while the more industrialised states gained population that way. As might be expected, internal migrants, both male and female, were younger, and with a higher level of secondary and tertiary education. The majority were Malays from rural areas. By 2000, most people lived in urban areas (Supplementary Table 3.J).

These major socio-economic shifts involved a number of inter-related features that affected population composition and altered health risks. The larger urban population employed in manufacturing and services and the greater participation of better-educated women in the labour force were associated with lower fertility and a rise in the proportion of people of working age, with lower levels of unemployment, higher household income and less poverty. However, occupations required less physical activity, while food intake was enhanced by higher household income and less poverty. As the socio-economic transformation took hold, demographic and epidemiological transitions took place. The epidemiological transition was expressed in terms of a decline in the burden of disease from infectious diseases because of the success of related health interventions, but non-communicable diseases increased with occupational and leisure activities and greater affluence, with an effect on health risks, health conditions and mortality (Table 3.3).

Access to medical services improved during the two decades of 1980–2000 as the number of people per doctor declined by more than half (Supplementary Table 3.K; Chapter 8). The number of nurses and midwives rose in relation to the population, but the number of assistant nurses declined (Supplementary Table 3.L; Chapter 8). Vaccination of infants for a range of communicable diseases reached over 90% coverage in most cases (Chapter 4). Rural household sanitation rose to 98% and access to safe water to 94% (Ministry of Health Malaysia, 2002; Chapter

Table 3.3 *Epidemiological transition and causes of death, peninsular Malaysia, 1982–1990*

	Age-specific death rates Percentage change for 1982–1990 in age group (years)						
Cause of death	<1	1–14	15–29	30–44	45–59	60–64	>64
Infectious diseases and fever	−65.1	−60.3	−46.1	−46.1	−57.7	−59.4	
Accidents, poisoning and violence	−1.4	−27.1	−10.3	−0.4	−4.0	−11.4	
Cancer	−14.9	+20.0	+2.7	+17.3	+29.3	+28.9	
Heart attack	+62.5	−23.6	−1.2	+18.2	−23.6	+37.5	
Unknown and other	−25.8	−33.0	−8.2	−7.8	−15.1	−31.6	
Old age (aged over 64 years)							−2.7
All causes	−36.3	−37.4	−14.9	−8.8	−11.3	−17.7	−2.7

Source: Suleiman & Jegathesan, n.d.

7). The rise in urbanisation and higher household incomes made access to private health services easier. This was associated with an increase in the proportion of doctors in the private sector (46%) (Ministry of Health Malaysia, 2002) and almost double the number of people employed in private hospitals and maternity homes (Department of Statistics Malaysia, 2001b). This meant that the rate of both outpatient visits and inpatient admissions to public hospitals per head of population either stayed about the same or declined slightly (Ministry of Health Malaysia, 1992; 2002). The transition is reflected in the estimated proportion of visits to doctors that might have been about equal between the public and private sectors in the 1980s but might have been higher in the private sector in the 1990s (Health Policy Research Associates et al., 2013). The rising use of the private sector had an impact on the level of health expenditure in relation to the GDP. A study of health financing indicated that total health expenditure in 1983 amounted to 2.8% of the GDP and that 76% was related to services provided by the public sector (Westinghouse Health Systems, 1985), while estimates for 2000 show that total health expenditure was 3.3% of the GDP and that 54% was financed by the public sector (Ministry of Health Malaysia, 2017; Chapter 8). This indicates that the rise in total health expenditure in relation to the GDP in that period might have been mostly from the growth in the private sector.

The socio-economic transformation during 1980–2000, with increasing employment opportunities and migration to urban areas, resulted in most people living in urban areas. It also led to a dramatic drop in the proportion of households living in poverty, from 37% in 1980 to 9% in 2000. Empirical evidence shows that, in addition to its direct impact on health status, the provision of health services by the public sector had considerable distributional effects on alleviating poverty in Malaysia (Hammer et al., 1995). Greater coverage of and access to healthcare was facilitated by urbanisation and services rendered by both the public and private sector and the greater use of preventive and other services in the public sector. This was reflected in the increase in the proportion of safe deliveries by health professionals to 97% in 2000. Infant mortality at 7 per 1,000 live births in 2000 had declined to about one-third of that in 1980 (Table 3.4); life expectancy continued to rise by 5 years to 73 years in 2000 (Supplementary Table 3.G).

Progress was also made in narrowing the differences between regions, although the differences prevailed. Kelantan, with a high proportion of its population living in rural areas (66%), had the highest

Table 3.4 *Changes in poverty, urbanisation, safe deliveries and infant mortality, Malaysia, 1980–2000*

Year	Households in poverty (%)	Urban population (%)	Safe deliveries[1] (%)	Infant mortality rate[2]
1980	37.4	42.0	85.4[3]	23.8
1990	16.5	49.8	95.1	13.1
2000	8.5[4]	62.0	96.6	6.8
Change 1980–2000	–28.9	+20.0	+11.2	–17.0

Sources: Supplementary Tables 3.D, 3.G and 3.J; Ministry of Health Malaysia, 1982; 1992; 2002.

[1] Those performed by professionally trained health personnel.

[2] The ratio of the number of deaths of those aged under 1 year per 1,000 live births.

[3] Peninsular Malaysia.

[4] The poverty rate is for 1999.

infant mortality rate in Peninsular Malaysia, being about twice that of Selangor in 2000 (Table 3.5). However, the difference had been almost three times higher in 1980 (Suleiman & Jegathesan, n.d.).

3.4 Health in a More Affluent and Urban Society (2000s and 2010s)

The steered socio-economic transformation of Malaysia has led to a more affluent and increasingly urban society. Globalisation of the economy is nothing new to Malaysians. At independence, Malaysia was substantially dependent on rubber and tin production for global markets. Its economy evolved as global markets for different commodities changed to the production of palm oil and crude oil and the manufacture of electronic components and products, again mostly for global markets. Thus Malaysia felt the effects of both the Asian financial crisis in the late 1990s and the impact of the global financial crisis in the mid-2000s. Economic growth that faltered in the late 1990s to the mid-2000s regained its strength after 2010, and the GDP per head of population grew at an annual rate of 3.5% in 2010–2017 compared with 2.6% in 2000–2010 (Supplementary Table 3.A).

Table 3.5 *Infant mortality, poverty and rural living, Malaysia, 2000*

State	Infant mortality rate[1]		Households in poverty (%)		Rural population (%)	
	2000[2]	Change 1980[3]	1999[2]	Change 1980[3]	2000[2]	Change 1980[3]
Kelantan	10.5	-20.4	18.5	-36.5	65.8	-6.1
Perlis	8.6	-15.6	13.3	-49.8	65.8	-25.3
Pahang	8.5	-18.9	5.5	-21.4	58.0	-15.9
Kedah	7.8	-20.5	13.5	-40.3	60.7	-24.9
Melaka	7.5	-12.1	5.7	-14.7	32.8	-43.8
Terengganu	6.9	-24.1	14.9	-38.2	51.3	-5.8
Kuala Lumpur	6.5	-4.9	2.3	[4]	0	0
Perak	6.4	-18.5	9.5	-21.0	41.3	-26.5
Johor	6.2	-18.6	2.5	-15.7	34.8	-30.0
Penang	5.7	-14.4	2.7	-17.0	19.9	-32.6
Negeri Sembilan	5.5	-17.0	2.5	-23.8	46.6	-20.8
Selangor	5.3	-14.3	2.0	[4]	12.4	-53.4
Labuan	20.4	n.a.	[5]	[5]	22.3	[5]
Sabah	6.8[6]	-16.0	20.1[5]	-38.2[5]	52.0	-27.4
Sarawak	5.7[6]	-13.8	6.7	-49.8	51.9	-30.1
Malaysia	6.8	-17.0	7.5	-34.9	38.0	-27.8

Sources: Department of Statistics Malaysia, 1992; 2003a; Abbas, 1997); Suleiman & Jegathesan, n.d.; Hatta and Ali, 2013.

[1] The ratio of deaths of those aged under 1 year per 1,000 live births for 2000.

[2] The infant mortality rate and percentage of rural population are for 2000 whereas the percentage of households in poverty is for 1999.

[3] Represents the change in the rate from 1980 to 2000 or from 1980 to 1999.

[4] Changes for Selangor and Kuala Lumpur could not be estimated because of aggregation of the two in 1980.

[5] Labuan was aggregated with Sabah for 1980 and 1999.

[6] Birth and infant mortality recorded, especially in Sabah, were of questionable reliability.

n.a. – not available

The Malaysian economy has the features of more developed countries, with a decline in the proportion of the GDP from primary industries, a continuing large contribution from secondary industries and more than half of total production from services (Martins et al., 2018), with similar employment patterns. By 2017, 62% of people employed worked in services, 26% worked in manufacturing and construction and 12% worked in primary industries, mostly in agriculture (Supplementary Tables 3.B and 3.C). The larger proportion of employment in secondary and tertiary industries and the decline in agriculture were associated with the growth of urbanisation to 75% in 2017 (Supplementary Table 3.J).

The importance of training and education to economic activity is reflected in the high level of education of people employed in 2016: no formal education, 3%; primary education, 15%; secondary education, 55%; and tertiary education, 27% (Department of Statistics Malaysia, 2017a). In 2017, the net enrolment of people of relevant age in primary education was 99% (female, 99%); secondary education, 75% (female, 78%); and tertiary education, 75% (female, 78%) (Ministry of Education, 2018). The labour force participation rate of working-age people increased to 68% in 2017, with female participation rising to 55% (Department of Statistics Malaysia, 2017a; 2018a). The unemployment rate rose only slightly from 3.1% in 2000 to 3.4% in 2017 (Department of Statistics Malaysia, 2003b; 2018a).

The greater urbanisation, higher education levels and greater female participation in the labour force were associated with a substantial fall in fertility from above replacement level (2.8 children per woman) in 2000 to below replacement level (1.9 children per woman) in 2017. Population growth continued to be high due to the large proportion of young people of reproductive age, but the rate of growth was reduced by half from an annual average of 2.6% in 2000 to 1.3% in 2017 (Supplementary Table 3.E). A feature of this continuing population growth was the increase in the proportion of people other than those identified as ethnic Bumiputra, Chinese or Indian[3] from less than 1% (0.5%) of the population in 1980 to 11% in 2017, which indicated a substantial growth in immigration (Supplementary Table 3.F).

The decline in fertility led to a demographic bonus in terms of the rise in the proportion of working-age people from 63% in 2000 to 70% in 2017 and a more productive young population. In the same period, the proportion of children dropped from 33% to a still-high percentage of 24%, while the proportion of older people increased somewhat from

4% to 6% (Supplementary Table 3.H). This meant a fall in the child dependency rate on the working population from 53% in 2000 to 35%, and old age dependency rose from 6% to a still-low 9% during the same period (Supplementary Table 3.I).

Among other priorities, health priorities identified in the three Malaysia Plans covering 2001–2015 were concerned with (Economic Planning Unit, 2001; Ministry of Health Malaysia, n.d.):

- Improving accessibility to affordable and quality care and addressing inequalities.
- Expanding wellness programmes aimed at improving quality of life.
- Promoting co-ordination and collaboration between the public and private providers of healthcare.
- Increasing the supply of healthcare human resources.
- Addressing efficiency issues in healthcare delivery.
- Strengthening regulatory and enforcement function to administer the health sector.

The concern with human resources in the provision of health services was met by a substantial increase in the availability of the two major professional resources. The number of people per doctor was about halved from 2000 to 632 in 2016 (Supplementary Table 3.K), and the number of people per nurse more than halved to 308 (Supplementary Table 3.L). By 2016, an increasing proportion of the larger number of doctors were in the public sector (65% in 2015), and even more so in the case of nurses (76% in 2015) (Ministry of Health Malaysia, 2018a; Chapter 8).

Prevention of infectious diseases remained a major objective, and child vaccination coverage continued to be high (Ministry of Health Malaysia, 2018a; Chapter 4). The same was true for access to safe water and sanitation, and the incidence of malaria continued to be low (Ministry of Health Malaysia, 2018a; Chapters 6 and 7). Another achievement was the eradication of polio. However, the incidence of dengue, often associated with growing urban centres, increased considerably, but better management of those affected resulted in a decline in case fatality rates. A major concern during this period was the threat of HIV/AIDS, which reached its incidence peak in 2002. Prevention efforts led to a fall in incidence by about half in 2016. However, HIV/AIDS affected efforts to control the incidence of tuberculosis, which increased to some extent (Ministry of Health Malaysia, 2018b; Chapters 4 and 6).

Urbanisation, sedentary occupations and greater affluence are associated with a rise in health risks related to non-communicable diseases, such as obesity (Ministry of Health Malaysia, 2018b). A study of diet, physical activity and smoking, which have an impact on health risks, such as diabetes, circulatory diseases and lung cancer, indicated that cultural differences resulted in varying behaviours among ethnic groups, and the authors proposed that a more culturally targeted approach was needed for these health risks. It is noteworthy that the study found that access to healthcare also made a difference (Botabara-Yap et al., 2017). The increasing burden of non-communicable diseases was reflected in the increasing proportion of heart and cerebrovascular diseases from 18% to 21% of all deaths from 2001 to 2017 (Department of Statistics Malaysia, 2007; 2018b). It is also manifested in the prevalence of diabetes, which increased from 12% to 15% in the 5-year period from 2006 to 2011 (Ministry of Health Malaysia, 2013; Chapter 6).

Public hospital outpatient visits increased, but their number per head of population declined, and visits to other public health clinics rose (Ministry of Health Malaysia, 2018a; Chapters 4 and 5). Evidence from household surveys indicated that the number of visits to doctors in the private sector might have been larger than the number of visits to doctors in the public sector (Health Policy Research Associates et al., 2013). Nevertheless, public sector health services remained the highest provider of both preventive and medical care. The number of people employed in private hospitals continued to grow by more than two-fold in 1999–2015 (Department of Statistics Malaysia, 2001b; 2017b), and the use of private inpatient care increased. However, admissions to public hospitals also rose substantially (Ministry of Health Malaysia, 2002; 2018a; Chapter 5). Despite the rise in private sector provision, the public sector continued to be the largest provider of inpatient as well as preventive and ambulatory medical services. It has been estimated that the above-mentioned considerably higher proportion of both preventive and curative services supplied by the public sector was financed by the public sector at only 51% of total health expenditure in 2015. The private sector, with a considerably lower proportional provision, was financed by 49% of the total health expenditure (Ministry of Health Malaysia, 2017; Chapter 9). A possible implication of this, all other things being equal, would be a considerable rise in health expenditure as a proportion of the GDP (4.6% in 2015) if all health services provided were at the expenditure per unit of service prevailing in the private sector.

Continuing economic development and employment opportunities in secondary industries, but especially in services in urban areas, continued to fuel the growth in urbanisation, which rose from 62% in 2000 to 75% in 2016. It was also associated with high levels of employment that improved social and income security further, which helped to alleviate poverty and its associated health conditions. The household poverty rate declined from 8.5% to 0.4% in 2000–2016 (Table 3.6). Although the substantial decline in poverty is not questioned, the actual levels and methodology have been queried in more recent times in view of alternative estimates (Ravallion, 2019). Despite caveats regarding the measurement of poverty, it is apparent that poverty has continued to decline since 1999. Infant mortality was highest in Sabah, which had the highest rate of poverty and a large proportion of its population still living in rural areas, and was lowest in urban Kuala Lumpur, which had one of the lowest levels of poverty in Malaysia (Nair and Sagaran, 2015; Department of Statistics Malaysia, 2013; 2016a).

As a measure of essential health service coverage and provision in a still relatively young population, safe birth deliveries by professional personnel were almost universal (99.5%) by 2016. Although fertility declined substantially, the momentum from the high proportion of people of reproductive age kept the birth rate at 16 per

Table 3.6 ***Changes in poverty, urbanisation, safe deliveries and infant mortality, Malaysia, 2000–2016***

Year	Households in poverty (%)	Urban population (%)	Safe deliveries[1] (%)	Infant mortality rate[2]
2000	8.5[3]	62.0	96.6	6.8
2010	3.8[4]	70.9	98.6	6.9
2016	0.4	74.8	99.5	6.7
Change 2000–2016	-8.1	+12.8	+2.9	-0.1

Sources: Supplementary Tables 3.D, 3.G and 3.J; Ministry of Health Malaysia, 2002; 2012; 2018b.

[1] Those performed by professionally trained health personnel.

[2] The ratio of the number of deaths of those aged under 1 year per 1,000 live births.

[3] Poverty rate is for 1999.

[4] Poverty rate is for 2009.

1,000 people. A reflection of the need to support the larger number of childbirths is that about a third of admissions (32%) to public hospitals, which provided the most obstetric care in 2015, were related to childbirth and related conditions (Department of Statistics Malaysia, 2017a).

In contrast to previous periods, the infant mortality rate did not improve to any significant extent, remaining at about 7 per 1,000 live births during 2000–2016 (Table 3.6). This lack of improvement was also observed for maternal mortality, which remained at around 24 per 100,000 live births during the same period (Ministry of Health Malaysia, 2018b). Although not reflected in formal records of infant mortality (Department of Statistics Malaysia, 2003a; 2016a), analysis of the location of the growing number of non-citizens (10% of the total population in 2017) (Department of Statistics Malaysia, 2017c) shows that states that experienced continued improvements in infant mortality, such as Kelantan, tended to have a lower proportion of non-citizens in the population, while those with a higher proportion, such as Johor, experienced either a standstill or a worsening (Department of Statistics Malaysia, 2003a; 2016a). This raises the question of potential inaccuracies in the registration of infant deaths of non-citizens.

Notwithstanding the stagnation in the recorded trend towards lower infant and maternal mortality, an achievement was the increase in life expectancy since 1999, in spite of the threat of HIV/AIDS and risks from more sedentary occupations and affluent lifestyles: life expectancy rose by more than 2 years between 1999 and 2017 (Table 3.7).

The potential for further improvements in health status and life expectancy is suggested by studies of *avoidable deaths* (Ministry of Health Malaysia & Harvard T. H. Chan School of Public Health, 2016) and *potential years of life lost* due to premature mortality and disability (Institute of Public Health, 2017).

These studies point to the potential gains from improvements in occupations and lifestyles that affect mortality and disability from non-communicable diseases, as well as better identification and management. Injury from traffic accidents and other causes is another major area for potential gains. The importance of mental health is also apparent. The research also indicates the continuing importance of preventing and managing infectious diseases (Table 3.8).

Table 3.7 ***Life expectancy by sex and years of age, Malaysia, 1999 and 2017***

	Life expectancy (years)				Change in years 2017–1999	
	1999		2017			
Age (years)	Female	Male	Female	Male	Female	Male
At birth	74.9	69.9	77.4	72.7	2.5	2.8
1	74.4	69.6	76.8	72.1	2.4	2.5
5	70.6	65.8	72.9	68.2	2.3	2.4
20	56.0	51.4	58.2	53.7	2.2	2.3
40	36.7	33.1	38.8	34.9	2.1	1.8
55	23.0	20.2	25.2	22.2	2.2	2.0
60	18.9	16.5	21.0	18.4	2.1	1.9

Sources: Department of Statistics Malaysia, 2000; 2017c.

3.5 Progress and Challenges

This chapter provides a concise and macro analysis that places salient features of health development in its socio-economic framework as a basis for the following chapters, which address the various components of the health system and their complementary contributions to health outcomes.

Health has been an integral and important part of Malaysia's socio-economic and human development that has aimed at alleviating poverty, enriching human capital, improving living conditions and enhancing health status.

Strategies have been articulated in five-year development plans in which health development has played a vital role in conjunction with education, employment and living conditions. These strategies have evolved as the success of rural development has taken hold and economic development has provided employment opportunities in secondary industries, with growing urbanisation and an increase in related living conditions. The health system's success in preventing and managing communicable diseases has led to an epidemiological transition that has improved health status but that has made it more dependent on the control of the non-communicable diseases characteristic of more developed, urban and affluent societies. Accordingly, progress has improved health, but it has also created new challenges to continued

Table 3.8 *Burden of disease and injury, Malaysia, 2014*

	DALY[1]	YLL[2]	YLD[3]
Cause/disease	Percentage of total		
Cardiovascular and circulatory diseases	20.8	28.5	8.3
Unintentional injuries	11.9	15.8	5.5
Malignant neoplasm	9.4	14.9	0.4
Diabetes mellitus	7.8	5.2	12.2
Mental and behavioural disorders	7.2	0.1	18.8
Respiratory diseases	6.5	5.0	9.0
Respiratory infections	5.5	7.4	2.6
Infectious diseases	5.1	5.0	5.3
Other	25.6	18.1	38.0
All causes/diseases	100.0	100.0	100.0
Number of years lost	4,993,000	3,099,000	1,894,000

Source: Institute of Public Health, 2017.
[1] The combined potential years of life lost from premature mortality and disability.
[2] The number of potential years of life lost due to premature mortality.
[3] The number of years of life lost due to disability.

success in addressing the risks of infectious diseases while strategies and means of tackling the threats posed to wellbeing by the burden of non-communicable diseases are being developed.

3.6 Key Messages from Malaysia's Experience

3.6.1 *What Went Well?*

- The provision of healthcare can be an important factor not only for the improvement of health status but also for the quality of human capital, its productivity and the alleviation of poverty.
- Poor people cannot afford to pay for health services; for them, services need to be free of charge.
- Market mechanisms did not meet the health needs of most of the population, especially those in rural areas, and public intervention was required.
- Social change, urbanisation and economic development alleviate some health problems but give rise to others.

3.6.2 *What Did Not Go So Well?*

- Fragmentation of responsibility between various agencies significantly impacted health. Recognition and management of fragmentation varied.
- The health system is constrained in its ability to deal with some politically charged issues, such as undocumented migrant groups.

3.6.3 *Trends and Challenges?*

The continued growth of the private health sector and rising health expenditure will be a challenge for the future development of healthcare.

References

Abbas, F. A. (1997). *Poverty Reduction in Malaysia, 1970–1995: Major Features*. Kuala Lumpur: Economic Planning Unit.

Ahmad, N. (2007). *Overview of Poverty Eradication in Malaysia*. Putrajaya: Economic Planning Unit. Online report. www.ssig.gov.my/wp.content/uploads/2013/07/10985.pdf

Aslam, M. and Hassan, A. S. (2003). Development planning and regional imbalances in Malaysia. FEA Working Paper No. 2003-5. Presented at the 9th International Planning History Conference. 20–23 August 2000. Helsinki University of Technology, Finland.

Botobara-Yap, M. J., Razon-Estrada, M. and Balila, E. (2017). The influence of culture and access to health care delivery and predictors of health behaviours among Malaysians of different cultural backgrounds. *International Forum*, 20(2), 57–74.

Chong, Y. H., Tee, E. S., Ng, T. K. W., Kandiah, M., Hussein, R. H., Teo, P. H. and Shahid, M. (1984). Status of community nutrition in poverty kampungs. In *Institute of Medical Research Malaysia Bulletin No. 22*. Kuala Lumpur: Institute of Medical Research, pp. 1–64.

Department of Statistics Malaysia. (n.d.). *Internal Migration in Peninsular Malaysia 1989–1990*. Kuala Lumpur: Department of Statistics Malaysia.

Department of Statistics Malaysia. (1989). *Yearbook of Statistics Malaysia 1988*. Kuala Lumpur: Department of Statistics Malaysia.

Department of Statistics Malaysia. (1991). *Vital Statistics Time Series, Peninsular Malaysia 1911–1985*. Kuala Lumpur: Department of Statistics Malaysia.

Department of Statistics Malaysia. (1992). *Yearbook of Statistics Malaysia 1991*. Kuala Lumpur: Department of Statistics Malaysia.

Department of Statistics Malaysia. (2000). *Yearbook of Statistics Malaysia 2000*. Kuala Lumpur: Department of Statistics Malaysia.

Department of Statistics Malaysia. (2001a). *Yearbook of Statistics Malaysia 2001*. Putrajaya: Department of Statistics Malaysia.

Department of Statistics Malaysia. (2001b). *Censuses of Professional and Institutional Establishments: Private Sector*. Putrajaya: Department of Statistics Malaysia.

Department of Statistics Malaysia. (2003a). *Vital Statistics Malaysia 2003*. Putrajaya: Department of Statistics Malaysia.

Department of Statistics Malaysia. (2003b). *Yearbook of Statistics Malaysia 2003*. Putrajaya: Department of Statistics Malaysia.

Department of Statistics Malaysia. (2007). *Social Statistics Bulletin Malaysia 2007*. Putrajaya: Department of Statistics Malaysia.

Department of Statistics Malaysia. (2010). *Yearbook of Statistics Malaysia 2009*. Putrajaya: Department of Statistics Malaysia.

Department of Statistics Malaysia. (2013). *Statistics Yearbook Malaysia 2012*. Putrajaya: Department of Statistics Malaysia.

Department of Statistics Malaysia. (2016a). *Vital Statistics Malaysia 2015*. Putrajaya: Department of Statistics Malaysia.

Department of Statistics Malaysia. (2016b). *Population (000s) 1891–2015, Malaysia*. Putrajaya: Department of Statistics Malaysia. Online report. www.data.stats.gov.my/download_bppd.php?cat=3&id=1

Department of Statistics Malaysia. (2017a). *Statistics Yearbook Malaysia 2016*. Putrajaya: Department of Statistics Malaysia.

Department of Statistics Malaysia. (2017b). *Health and Social Work Services: Economic Census 2016*. Putrajaya: Department of Statistics Malaysia.

Department of Statistics Malaysia. (2017c). *Abridged Life Tables, Malaysia, 2015–2017*. Putrajaya: Department of Statistics Malaysia.

Department of Statistics Malaysia. (2017d). *Social Statistics Bulletin Malaysia 2017*. Putrajaya: Department of Statistics Malaysia.

Department of Statistics Malaysia. (2018a). *Labour Force Survey Report, Malaysia 2017*. Putrajaya: Department of Statistics Malaysia.

Department of Statistics Malaysia. (2018b). Statistics on Causes of Death, Malaysia, 2018. Putrajaya: Department of Statistics Malaysia. Online report. www.dosm.gov.my/v1/index.php?

Department of Statistics Malaysia. (2018c). *Current Population Estimates, Malaysia, 2018*. Putrajaya: Department of Statistics Malaysia.

Department of Statistics Malaysia. (2019). Vital Statistics Malaysia 2017. Putrajaya: Department of Statistics Malaysia. Online report. www.dosm.gov.my/v1/index.php?

Economic Planning Unit. (1996). *Seventh Malaysia Plan 1996–2000*. Kuala Lumpur: Economic Planning Unit.

Economic Planning Unit. (2001). *Eighth Malaysia Plan 2001–2005*. Putrajaya: Economic Planning Unit.

Economic Planning Unit. (2015). *Eleventh Malaysia Plan 2016–2020: Anchoring Growth on People*. Putrajaya: Economic Planning Unit.

Economic Planning Unit. (2016). *The Malaysian Economy in Figures, 2016*. Putrajaya:Economic Planning Unit.

Fernandez, D. Z., Hawley, A. H. and Predeza, S. (1975). *The Population of Malaysia*. Paris: Committee for International Research in Demography.

Fong, C. O. (1985). Integrated population-development program performance: the Malaysian FELDA experience. *Journal of Development Areas*, 19(2), 149–70.

Hammer, J. S., Nabi, I. and Cercone, J. (1995). Distributional effects of social sector expenditures in Malaysia, 1974 to 1989. In D. van de Walle and K. Nead (eds.), *Public Spending and the Poor: Theory and Evidence*. Washington, DC: World Bank, pp. 521–54.

Hasan, A. R. (1986). *Changes in the Level and Pattern of Mortality Rates in Peninsular Malaysia, 1971–1983*. Canberra: Australian National University.

Hatta, Z. A. and Ali, I. (2013). Poverty reduction policies in Malaysia: trends, strategies and challenges. *Asian Culture and History*, 5(2), 48–52.

Health Policy Research Associates (HPRA), Institute for Health Systems Research (IHSR) and Institute for Health Policy (IHP). (2013).*Malaysia Health Care Demand Analysis: Inequalities in Healthcare Demand and Simulation of Trends and Impact of Potential Changes in Healthcare Spending*. Putrajaya: Ministry of Health Malaysia.

Institute of Public Health. (2017). *Malaysian Burden of Disease and Injury Study 2009–2014*. Shah Alam: National Institutes of Health.

Jones, G. W. (n.d.). *The Growth of Malaysia's Labour Force*. Canberra: Australian National University.

Lee, C. and Chew-Ging, L. (2017). The evolution of development planning in Malaysia. *Journal of Southeast Asian Economies*, 34(3), 436–57.

Mahari, Z., Wan, R. O., Khalili, M., Esa, S. and Miskiman, N. (2011). Demographic Transition in Malaysia: The Changing Roles of Women. Conference paper, 15th Conference of Commonwealth Statisticians, New Delhi, February 2011.

Martins, J. M., Guo, F. and Swanson, D. (2018). *Global Population in Transition*. Cham: Springer International.

McKay, D. A., Lim, R. K. H., Notaney, K. H. and Dugdale, A. E. (1971). Nutritional assessment by comparative growth achievement in Malay children below school age. *Bulletin of the World Health Organization*, 45, 233–42.

Ministry of Education Malaysia. (1967). *Educational Statistics of Malaysia 1938 to 1967*. Kuala Lumpur: Ministry of Education Malaysia.

Ministry of Education Malaysia. (2018). *Malaysia Educational Statistics: Quick Facts 2018*. Putrajaya: Ministry of Education Malaysia.

Ministry of Health Malaysia. (n.d.). *Country Health Plan 2011–2015*. Putrajaya: Ministry of Health Malaysia.

Ministry of Health Malaysia. (1982). *Annual Report Ministry of Health Malaysia 1980*. Kuala Lumpur: Ministry of Health Malaysia.

Ministry of Health Malaysia. (1992). *Annual Report Ministry of Health Malaysia 1990*. Kuala Lumpur: Ministry of Health Malaysia.

Ministry of Health Malaysia. (2002). *Annual Report Ministry of Health Malaysia 2000*. Putrajaya: Ministry of Health Malaysia.

Ministry of Health Malaysia. (2012). *Annual Report Ministry of Health Malaysia 2010*. Putrajaya: Ministry of Health Malaysia.

Ministry of Health Malaysia. (2013). *National Diabetes Registry Report 2009–2012*. Putrajaya: Ministry of Health Malaysia.

Ministry of Health Malaysia. (2017). *Malaysia National Health Accounts: Health Expenditure Report 1997–2015*. Putrajaya: Ministry of Health Malaysia.

Ministry of Health Malaysia. (2018a). *Health Facts 2018*. Putrajaya: Ministry of Health Malaysia.

Ministry of Health Malaysia. (2018b). *Annual Report Ministry of Health 2016*. Putrajaya: Ministry of Health Malaysia.

Ministry of Health Malaysia and Harvard T. H. Chan School of Public Health. (2016). *Malaysian Health Systems Research Volume 1: Contextual Analysis of the Malaysian Health System March 2016*. Putrajaya: Ministry of Health Malaysia.

Nair, S. and Sagaran, S. (2015). Poverty in Malaysia: need for a new paradigm shift. *Institutions and Economics*, 7(3), 95–123.

Peacock, F. (1981). Rural poverty and development in west Malaysia. *Journal of Development Areas*, 15(4), 639–54.

Prime Minister's Department. (1965). *First Malaysia Plan 1966–1970*. Kuala Lumpur: Prime Minister's Department.

Prime Minister's Department. (1971). *Second Malaysia Plan 1971–1975*. Kuala Lumpur: Prime Minister's Department.

Prime Minister's Department. (1989). *Mid-Term Review of the Fifth Malaysia Plan 1986–1990*. Kuala Lumpur: Prime Minister's Department.

Prime Minister's Department. (1991a). *The Second Outline Perspective Plan 1991–2000*. Kuala Lumpur: Prime Minister's Department.

Prime Minister's Department. (1991b). *Sixth Malaysia Plan 1991–1995*. Kuala Lumpur: Prime Minister's Department.

Ravallion, M. (2019). *Has Malaysia Virtually Eliminated Poverty?* Online article. Retrieved from https://economicsandpoverty.com/2019/01/21/ha-malaysia-virtually-eliminated-poverty

Roemer, M. I. (1976). *Health Care Systems in World Perspective*. Ann Arbor, MI: Health Administration Press.

Roemer, M. I. (1985). *National Strategies for Health Care Organization*. Ann Arbor, MI: Health Administration Press.

Roslan, A. H. (2001). *Income Inequality, Poverty and Development Policy in Malaysia*. Paris: UNESCO.

Suleiman, A. B. and Jegathesan, M. (eds.). (n.d.). *Health in Malaysia: Achievements and Challenges*. Ministry of Health Malaysia.

United Nations Development Programme (UNDP). (2018). *Human Development Indices and Indicators: 2018 Statistical Update*. New York: UNDP.

United Nations Education, Scientific and Cultural Organization (UNESCO). (2011). *Secondary Education Regional Information Base: Country Profile – Malaysia*. Bangkok.

Westinghouse Health Systems. (1985). *Malaysia Health Services Financing Study*. Kuala Lumpur: Asian Development Bank/Westinghouse Overseas Service Corp.

World Bank. (n.d.). *Malaysia Data Book*. Washington, DC: World Bank.

World Bank. (2017). *World Development Indicators 2017*. Washington, DC: World Bank.

World Bank. (2019a). *Life Expectancy at Birth, Total (Years)*. Online report. www.data.worldbank.org

World Bank. (2019b). *School Enrolment, Secondary (% Gross)*. Online report. www.data.worldbank.org

World Bank. (2019c). *GDP per Capita (Constant LCU)*. Online report. www.data.worldbank.org

World Bank. (2019d). *Labor Force Participation Rate, Female (% of Female Population Ages 15+)*. Online report. www.data.worldbank.org

World Bank. (2019e). *Gross Domestic Product at Constant 2010 Dollars*. Online report. www.data.worldbank.org

World Bank. (2019f). *Fertility Rate, Total (Births per Woman)*. Online report. www.data.worldbank.org

World Bank. (2019g). *Urban Population (% of Total) Malaysia*. Online report. www.data.worldbank.org

Young, K., Bussink, W. C. F. and Hasan, P. (1980). *Malaysia Growth with Equity in a Multiracial Society*. Baltimore, MD: Johns Hopkins University Press.

Supplementary Table 3.A *Gross domestic product growth, Malaysia, 1960–2017*

	Average growth rate per year as percentage			
Period	GDP[1]		GDP per capita	
1960–1970	6.3		3.5	
1970–1980	7.9	7.1[2]	5.5	4.5[2]
1980–1990	5.8		3.1	
1990–1995	9.1		6.5	
1995–2000	4.7	6.3	2.2	3.7
2000–2005	4.6		2.6	
2005–2010	4.4		2.6	
2010–2015	5.2		3.4	
2015–2017	4.9	4.8	3.5	2.9
Average 1960–2017	6.1		3.8	

Source: World Bank, 2019e. Calculations made by the author.

[1] Gross domestic product (GDP) growth rate is based on GDP and GDP per capita at 2010 constant prices.

[2] The growth rates to the right of each column are for the intervening period, e.g. 1960–1980: 7.1 and 4.5.

Supplementary Table 3.B *Gross domestic product by industry, Malaysia, 1961–2017*

	Industry as percentage[1] of gross domestic product		
Year	Primary[2]	Secondary[2]	Tertiary[2]
1961	45	13	42
1970	38	17	45
1980	31	25	44
1990	28	30	42
1995	21	36	43
2000	19	35	46
2005	17	33	50
2010	21	27	52
2015	18	28	54
2017	17	27	56
Change 2015–1961	–28	+14	+14

Sources: Young et al., 1980; Prime Minister's Department, 1991a; 1991b; Economic Planning Unit, 1996; 2015; Department of Statistics Malaysia, 2003b; 2010; 2018c.

[1] Estimated from a variety of sources and indicative of trends, rather than precise.

[2] Primary includes agriculture, fisheries, forestry and mining; secondary includes manufacturing and construction; tertiary includes all services and utilities.

Supplementary Table 3.C ***Employment by industry, Malaysia, 1970–2017***

Year	Employment by industry as percentage		
	Primary[1]	Secondary[1]	Tertiary[1]
1970	50	20	30
1980	39	21	40
1990	27	26	47
2000	15	36	49
2011	12	27	61
2015	12	27	61
2016	12	26	62
Change 2016–1970	–38	+6	+32

Sources: Young et al., 1980; Prime Minister's Department, 1991a; 1991b; Department of Statistics Malaysia, 1989; 2003b; 2010; 2013; 2017a; Economic Planning Unit, 1996; 2001; 2015.

[1] Primary includes agriculture, fisheries, forestry and mining; secondary includes manufacturing and construction; tertiary includes all services and utilities.

Supplementary Table 3.D ***Poverty in Malaysia, 1970–2016***

Year	Percentage of households		
	All	Rural	Urban
1957	51.2	59.6	29.7
1970[1]	49.3	58.6	24.6
1980	37.4	45.8	17.5
1990	16.5	21.1	7.1
1999[2]	8.5	14.8	3.3
2004	5.7	11.9	2.5
2009	3.8	8.4	1.7
2014	0.6	1.6	0.3
2016	0.4	1.0	0.2
Change 1970–2014	-48.9	-57.6	-24.4

Sources: Roslan, 2001; Ahmad, 2007; Economic Planning Unit, 2016; Department of Statistics Malaysia, 2017a.

[1] Peninsular Malaysia only.

[2] Change in methodology increased the overall rate in 1999 from 8.1% to 8.5%.

Supplementary Table 3.E *Population growth, Malaysia, 1960–2017*

Year	Population (000s)	Average annual population growth rate (%)[1]
1960	8,118.0[2]	2.9
1970	10,881.8	2.4
1980	13,879.2	2.7
1990	18,102.4	2.6
2000	23,494.9	2.0
2010	28,588.6[3]	1.7
2015	31,186.1	1.3
2017	32,022.6	
Change 1960–2017	+23,904.6	2.4

Source: Department of Statistics Malaysia, 2016b; 2018c. Calculations made by the author.

[1] The average annual population growth rates are for 10-year periods, except for 2010–2015 and 2015–2017.

[2] The population of Peninsular Malaysia was 6.9 million in 1960 before Sabah and Sarawak joined the federation.

[3] At the time of the population census in 2010, there was an estimated 28.5 million people in Malaysia: 22.7 million in Peninsular Malaysia, 3.3 million in Sabah and the federal territory of Labuan, and 2.5 million in Sarawak.

Supplementary Table 3.F *Population by ethnic group, Malaysia, 1957–2010*

	Ethnic group as percentage of total population				
Year	Malay and other Bumiputra[1]	Chinese	Indian	Other[2]	All[3]
1957[4]	49.8	37.2	11.3	1.8	100.0
1970	56.0	34.1	9.0	0.8	100.0
1980	58.8	32.1	8.5	0.5	100.0
1991	57.9	26.9	7.6	7.6	100.0
2000	61.2	24.5	7.2	7.1	100.0
2010	61.8	22.6	6.7	8.9	100.0
2017	61.8	20.8	6.2	11.2	100.0
Change 1957–2017	+12.0	−16.4	−5.1	+9.4	

Sources: Department of Statistics Malaysia, 1989; 1991; 1992; 2003b; 2010; 2013; 2017a; 2018c.

[1] Includes Malays and other indigenous groups in Sabah and Sarawak.

[2] Includes non-Malaysian citizens.

[3] Percentages may not add up due to rounding.

[4] The proportions for 1957 are for Peninsular Malaysia.

Supplementary Table 3.G ***Fertility and life expectancy, Malaysia, 1960–2017***

Year	Total fertility rate[1] (number of children)	Life expectancy[2] (years)	Infant mortality rate[3]
1960	6.45	59.5	69.8
1970	5.01	64.4	38.5
1980	4.07	68.0	23.8
1990	3.55	70.7	13.1
2000	2.78	72.8	6.8
2010	2.15	74.2	6.7
2015	2.01	74.6	6.9
2017	1.90	74.8	6.7
Change 1960–2017	-4.55	+15.3	-63.1

Sources: Department of Statistics Malaysia, 1992; 2003a; 2016a; 2017c; 2019; World Bank, 2019f.

[1] The average number of children a woman has during her lifetime.

[2] The average number of years lived after birth.

[3] The number of deaths of those aged under 1 year per 1,000 live births.

Supplementary Table 3.H ***Age distribution of the population of Malaysia, 1957–2017***

	Age group as proportion of total population (years)			
Year	0–14	15–64	65 and over	All
1957	43.8	53.4	2.8	100.0
1970	44.9	52.0	3.1	100.0
1980	39.6	56.8	3.6	100.0
1991	36.5	59.8	3.7	100.0
2000	33.3	62.8	3.9	100.0
2010	27.6	67.3	5.0	100.0
2015	24.9	69.2	5.8	100.0
2017	24.1	69.6	6.3	100.0
Change 1957–2017	-19.7	+16.2	+3.5	

Sources: Mahari et al., 2011; Department of Statistics Malaysia, 2013; 2017a; 2018c.

Supplementary Table 3.I *Dependency rates, Malaysia, 1957–2017*

	Dependency rate (percentage)		
Year	Child[1]	Old[2]	Total[3]
1957	82.1	5.2	87.3
1970	86.2	5.9	92.1
1980	69.6	6.4	76.0
1991	61.0	6.2	67.2
2000	53.0	6.2	59.2
2010	41.0	7.4	48.4
2015	36.0	8.4	44.4
2017	34.6	9.1	43.7
Change 1957–2017	–47.5	+3.9	–43.6

Sources: Mahari et al., 2011; Department of Statistics Malaysia, 2013; 2017a; 2018c. Calculations made by the author.

[1] The ratio of the population aged 0–14 years to that of working age of 15–64 years.

[2] The ratio of the population aged 65 years and over to that of working age of 15–64 years.

[3] The ratio of child and old populations to that of working age.

Supplementary Table 3.J *Urban population, Malaysia, 1960–2017*

Year	Urban population as percentage of total
1960	25.6
1970	33.5
1980	42.0
1990	49.8
2000	62.0
2010	70.9
2015	74.2
2017	75.4
Change 1960–2017	+49.8

Source: World Bank, 2019g.

Supplementary Table 3.K ***Number of people per doctor, Malaysia, 1964–2016***

Year	Peninsular Malaysia	Sabah	Sarawak	Malaysia
	Number of people per doctor[1]			
1964	6,000	13,100	14,000	7,145
1970	4,100	7,900	11,100	4,691
1980	3,284	7,170	6,571	3,563
1990	2,294	5,053	4,781	2,532
2000	1,318	3,354	2,719	1,490
2010	851	1,851	1,491	859
2016	581	1,155	765	632

Sources: Prime Minister's Department, 1965; 1971; Department of Statistics Malaysia, 1992; 2003b; 2013; 2017a.

[1] Approximations that show the degree of magnitude and trends, as different sources tend to yield slightly different ratios over time.

Supplementary Table 3.L ***Number of people per nursing personnel, Malaysia, 1964–2016***

Year	Peninsular Malaysia	Sabah	Sarawak	Malaysia
	Number of people per nursing personnel[1],[2]			
1964	2,500	1,500	3,000	2,488
1970	1,900	1,100	2,200	1,879
1980	517	825	1,620	570
1990[3]	438	628	1,379	481
2000[3]	771	830	1,144	801
2010	611	662	781	629
2016	288	452	394	308

Sources: Prime Minister's Department, 1965; 1971; Department of Statistics Malaysia, 1992; 2003b; 2013; 2017b.

[1] Includes midwives, nurses and assistant nurses.

[2] Approximations that show the degree of magnitude and trends, as different sources tend to yield slightly different ratios over time. The ratios are the average number of people per individual nurse.

[3] While the number of nurses counted increased, the number of assistant nurses fell considerably, hence the rise in the number of people per nursing personnel from 1990 to 2000.

Notes

1. Some might query the relevance of using safe deliveries and infant mortality as indicators in later periods. Their relevance is sustained by the 2015 continuing high birth rate of Malaysia of 17 live births per 1,000 population, which is 50% higher than that of Canada in the same year (11/1,000) and about double that of Italy (8/1,000). Further, the importance of these indicators is reflected, among other things, by the fact that about one-third of hospital admissions in Malaysia are still related to childbirth.
2. Malaya became Malaysia in 1963 with the unification of Peninsular Malaysia with Sabah and Sarawak in North Borneo.
3. The three major ethnic groups in Malaysia are Bumiputra (a political and ethnic grouping of the indigenous and Malay populations), Chinese and Indian (Supplementary Table 3.F).

4 Health Service Delivery

Primary Health Care

SHIANG CHENG LIM, INDRA PATHMANATHAN AND SAFURAH JAAFAR

4.1 Introduction

The term 'primary health care' (PHC) has been operationalised in a variety of ways since it was first coined as part of the historic Alma Ata Declaration (Box 4.1). In this chapter, we operationally define PHC to cover the 'first level of contact of individuals, the family and community with the national health system' and 'reflect(s) and evolve(s) from the economic conditions and sociocultural and political characteristics of the country'. The elements of PHC we will focus on include 'education concerning prevailing health problems, ... maternal and child health care including family planning and immunization, and appropriate treatment of common diseases and injuries'. Other aspects of PHC, such as safe water and basic sanitation, prevention and control of locally endemic diseases, and provision of essential drugs, are covered in other chapters.

This chapter explores the development of PHC during the 60-year period after Malaysia achieved independence (1957–2018). The development process is viewed in the context of the interaction of various components of the health system, as well as the interactions with other sectors and the influence of international movements. Two distinct phases of development are evident, as described in Sections 4.2 and 4.3.

4.2 The First Phase of PHC Development (1960s–1990s)

4.2.1 *Drivers and Contexts*

At independence, about 75% of the population lived in rural areas, and almost half the population lived in poverty (Mohd Ashad & Shamsudin, 1997). The ethnic composition reflected the urban–rural divide, with ethnic Malays being largely rural, ethnic Chinese largely

Box 4.1 Excerpts from the Declaration of the Alma Ata International Conference on Primary Health Care, September 1978

- Primary health care is essential health care ... made universally accessible to individuals and families in the community through their full participation and at a cost that the community and country can afford.
- It is the first level of contact of individuals, the family and community with the national health system ... and constitutes the first element of a continuing health care process.
- Involves, in addition to the health sector, all related sectors and aspects of national and community development, in particular agriculture, animal husbandry, food, industry, education, housing, public works, communications and other sectors; ... and demands the co-ordinated efforts of all those sectors.
- Sustained by integrated, functional and mutually supportive referral systems, leading to the progressive improvement of comprehensive health care.

(www.who.int/social_determinants/tools/multimedia/alma_ata/en, accessed September 2019.)

urban and ethnic Indians largely in the rubber estates. Maternal and child mortality was high, nutritional status was poor and the incidence of infectious diseases was high. Table 4.1 provides a glimpse of Malaysia's health status at independence and its evolving status during the subsequent 30 years.

The PHC system developed for Malaysia was built on the healthcare system inherited from the British colonial system. It consisted of outpatient clinics attached to hospitals, a few dispensaries and infant welfare centres provided by the government, and private sector clinics operated by doctors (general practitioners, or GPs). Almost all of these services were in urban areas. This healthcare system evolved from the requirements of the expatriate governing staff, that is, the more educated and affluent urban population.

The predominantly rural population depended on practitioners of traditional medicine, while workers in the larger rubber estates

Table 4.1 *Health indicators in Malaysia, 1957–1990*

	1957	1970	1980	1990
Life expectancy at birth, male (years)	55.8	61.6	66.4	68.9
Life expectancy at birth, female (years)	58.2	65.6	70.5	73.5
Maternal mortality ratio per 1,000 live births	2.8[1]	1.6[2]	0.6	0.2
Infant mortality rate per 1,000 live births	73.0[1]	43.8[2]	23.8	13.1
Toddler mortality rate per 1,000 population aged 1–4 years old	8.9[1]	5.0[2]	2.1	1.0

Source: Suleiman and Jegathesan, n.d..
[1] 1956–1960
[2] 1966–1970

depended on estate clinics provided by employers. However, four years prior to independence, the country introduced a service to serve the rural population, which evolved into the Rural Health Service (RHS) in 1956, just before Malaysia gained independence (Rudner, 1972; Ismail, 1974; J. H. W. Wong et al., 2019).

Independence brought into power an elected coalition of ethnically based political parties, led by the ethnic Malay political party. Unsurprisingly, the political focus shifted to prioritise rural communities to reflect the location of strong Malay support. The major thrust of development was to achieve socio-economic transformation by developing the country's basic rural infrastructure, modernising agricultural production in rural areas and improving education and health (Federation of Malaya, 1960; Rudner, 1972; Lee & Lee, 2017). Infrastructure development was an integrated approach that included rural roads, drainage and irrigation, schools and clinics (Mohd Ashad & Shamsudin, 1997). Planning and development was co-ordinated by the Economic Planning Unit in the Prime Minister's Department, and the progress of all elements within each administrative district was monitored in an integrated fashion through a 'Red Book' that commanded the attention of politicians and civil service administrators at national, state and district levels. The RHS was a major component of this integrated development, such that a district would receive an integrated package that increased physical access to basic education and healthcare, while parallel initiatives addressed its economic needs.

4.2.2 The Rural Health Service

The RHS was government funded. A basic RHS unit served 50,000 population. It consisted of a main health centre (MHC), 4 sub-centres (HSC) and 20 satellite midwife clinics, each with an attached residential facility for the midwife (MCQ). This basic unit was designed to provide 'integrated curative and preventive health services' (Jayasuria, 1967). Table 4.2 illustrates the services and notional staffing pattern of the basic RHS unit. The number of rural health facilities increased significantly between 1960 and 1980 (Table 4.3).

During the first 10 years, the major challenges included difficulty in matching the rate of facility construction with that of population growth, inadequately trained staff for facilities that had been completed, and prevailing cultural beliefs and taboos that hindered service utilisation. After 15 years of development, by 1975, the facility-to-population ratios showed that only 50% of population coverage targets had been achieved. A community survey showed that 24% of the rural villages in the survey areas were 'underserved' (Noordin, 1978). To increase access, the static facility-based services were supplemented with mobile clinics-cum-dispensaries that travelled by road or river, and dental clinics funded by the government, all providing free access to the population (Ismail, 1974; Tate Abdullah et al., 2005). These teams visited remote villages and provided a PHC package consisting mainly of curative, MCH and immunisation services periodically.

4.2.3 The Influence of the Alma Ata Declaration on the RHS: Community Mobilisation, Enhanced Intersectoral Co-ordination, Referral Systems

By the time of the Alma Ata Declaration (1978), Malaysia had already adopted many of the basic concepts of the Declaration. The serving Director-General of Health, Dr Raja Ahmad Noordin, stated: 'Malaysia viewed PHC as an extension to its existing health care services' (Noordin, 1978). The major contribution of Alma Ata was to provide a fillip for the conceptual enhancement of PHC services by spurring the introduction of community mobilisation, enhancing intersectoral co-ordination and strengthening referrals to and support from hospitals (secondary healthcare) (Box 4.2).

Table 4.2 ***Rural Health Services and notional staffing pattern***

Facility	Services	Notional staffing pattern
Main health centre (designed for 50,000 population)	1. Outpatient care with essential drug list, maternal and child health (MCH), domiciliary midwifery, immunisation, family planning, nutrition education, school health services	Doctor, medical assistant, dispenser Nurses (public health, staff, assistant) and midwives
	2. Sanitation and safe water supply	Public health overseer and public health inspector
	3. Dental care	Dental nurse
Health sub-centre (HSC, 10,000 population)	Outpatient care	Medical assistant (with visiting doctor)
	MCH and family planning, and midwifery	Nurses and midwives (with supervisory nurses from MHC)
Midwife clinic and quarters (2,000 population)	Domiciliary midwifery	Midwives (with supervisory nurses from MHC or HSC)

Source: J. H. W. Wong et al., 2019.

Table 4.3 *Number of rural health facilities in Peninsular Malaysia*

	Main health centres	Sub-health centres	Midwife clinics
1960	8	8	26
1965	39	122	643
1970	44	180	943
1975	73	246	1282[1]
1980	77	252	1465[1]

Sources: Prime Minister's Department, 1971; 1976; 1981; Ismail, 1974.
[1] Including clinics already converted to community clinics (*klinik desa*).

Box 4.2 Key strategies that advanced PHC in Malaysia

- **Use of trained allied health personnel** (particularly nurses and midwives) instead of reliance on doctors. Infrastructure development quickly outstripped the availability of human resources. Rapid but strictly regulated training of nurses and midwives, with registration, defined roles with relevant competencies, and appropriate deployment was a success (see also Chapter 8).
- **Partnerships with traditional birth attendants (TBAs).** In the Malay communities, TBAs (*bidan kampung*) were influential. In 1967, about 3,000 TBAs conducted an estimated 47% of the 174,000 deliveries (Peng, 1979). In some areas, the percentage could reach 80% due to both the shortage of midwives and the belief system of the community (Ali & Howden-Chapman, 2007). Recognising the key position of TBAs in rural communities, the Ministry of Health introduced a training programme for TBAs in 1965 (Suleiman and Jegathesan, n.d.) to change their role. They would recognise the danger signs of pregnancy and childbirth, avoid harmful practices and conduct home visits to encourage women to utilise midwife clinics and health centres for antenatal and postnatal care. They also provided support to certified government midwives during home deliveries. The TBAs were allowed to continue to perform harmless traditional practices such as postnatal massage.
- **Community mobilisation.** Several parallel thrusts mobilised community support. Health officials took advantage of the system of village development committees established by the rural development programmes to mobilise the support of the *penghulu* (village headman) and his committee for various health issues

(Pathmanathan et al., 2003). Women's development programmes provided entry points to raising awareness and providing practical avenues for better child-rearing and nutrition. The school health programme provided the vehicle for mobilising school children not only to understand and improve their own lifestyle but also to influence their parents' health behaviour.

- **Partnerships with other public sector agencies with grassroots presence.** Police posts in rural villages had the function of issuing birth certificates and burial permits. Midwives and nurses obtained data on births and deaths in their districts from the police. Similarly, police communications systems (radios) provided the means for front-line health staff to call for ambulances and assistance during medical emergencies.

Dr Noordin spearheaded community mobilisation to make it an integral complement to expanding health services. Additionally, facility expansion was accelerated such that the RHS configuration was modified to extend the coverage of the basic unit to serve a population of 20,000. Staffing profiles changed accordingly. Emulating the successful experience in one state (Sarawak), midwives were upgraded to become rural (community) nurses and given a wider scope of responsibility (Chapter 8). Accelerated training of nurses and midwives enabled rapid upgrading of the quality of services. Simultaneously, community mobilisation took several forms, with active efforts to encourage communities and families to promote health, prevent illness and utilise health services appropriately. Health staff became focal points for organised community efforts, as exemplified in the rural sanitation programme (Chapter 7). Nursing and midwifery staff gained entry to male-dominated village development committees by working in partnership with sanitation staff. This approach enabled them to promote safe childbirth by sensitising communities to the danger signs in childbirth and pregnancy and encouraging the acceptance of prompt medical intervention to save the lives of mothers and babies. Pregnancy care included supervision of childbirth at home by trained, certified midwives, followed by 10 days of daily postnatal home visits that enabled the visiting health staff to build a rapport with the family and the community while establishing breastfeeding and healthy nutritional habits (Pathmanathan et al., 2003).

Inter-sectoral co-ordination became a part of service delivery as well as infrastructure development. Child health included growth monitoring, oral re-hydration techniques, breastfeeding, immunisations, food supplementation, female literacy and family planning. Partnership with rural women's development programmes enabled health staff to raise awareness of hygiene and nutrition. Health topics were integrated into school curricula through interagency co-ordination between the Health and the Education Ministries, and school visits by nurses and dental nurse teams brought basic screening, referral and simple treatment to the doorstep of the expanding school-enrolled population. Partnership with traditional birth attendants (TBAs) reduced unsafe childbirth while giving the TBAs a continuing role in supporting birthing women (Pathmanathan et al., 2003). Nutrition demonstration sessions by nurses in rural clinics gained popularity. The Applied Food and Nutrition Programme, implemented in districts with high levels of malnutrition, is an example of a partnership with the agriculture, rural development and women's empowerment initiatives.

Regional disparities in social status and poverty led to targeted poverty reduction programmes. These programmes included initiatives for better access to healthcare and for addressing childhood malnutrition in disadvantaged areas. The prevalence of childhood malnutrition was used as a surveillance tool, while the prevalence of undernourished children was a criterion for identifying low-income families to receive food supplementation as well as assistance with education, housing and employment (Economic Planning Unit, 2004).

Another influence of Alma Ata was to highlight the health needs of remote populations, including the indigenous people (*Orang Asli*), who had limited access to transport to and communication with healthcare facilities. Mobile teams had to travel over unsealed roads, by river and on foot to serve these communities periodically.

The effectiveness of these measures, in combination with the broader socio-economic development issues discussed in Chapter 3, is evident, for example, in the rising levels of childbirth attended by skilled birth attendants, immunisation coverage and declining maternal and child mortality (Table 4.4) (Suleiman & Jegathesan, n.d.). The proportion of deliveries by trained personnel increased from 77.2% (Peninsular Malaysia) in 1975 to 95.2% (Malaysia) in 1996 (Suleiman & Jegathesan, n.d.). Referral systems were established particularly for maternity and for infectious diseases such as malaria and tuberculosis (TB). When nurses based in rural

Table 4.4 ***Percentage of institutional deliveries and immunisation coverage, 1970–1990***

	1970	1980	1990
Place of delivery			
Government hospitals	30.0[1]	43.9[1]	59.1
Other medical institutions	11.4[1]	10.7[1]	16.1
Home deliveries	58.6[1]	45.4[1]	24.8
Immunisation coverage			
Bacille Calmette-Guerin (BCG) (infant)	46.6	88.2	98.7
Diphtheria, pertussis and tetanus (DPT) (3rd dose)	15.0	67.0	92.0
Polio (3rd dose)	15.0	72.0	91.5
Measles (infant)	10.0	20.0	69.6

Source: Suleiman and Jegathesan, n.d..

[1] Peninsular Malaysia only.

clinics referred patients with obstetric problems to hospitals, these patients were given priority and prompt attention. Pregnant women and young children carried personal health cards displaying their pregnancy and healthcare information, thereby facilitating information exchange between PHC and secondary levels of care (United Nations Development Programme, 2005; Awin, 2011). The major communicable disease control programmes established similar referral systems (Chapter 6). The parallel development of rural roads and the provision of ambulances stationed at the MHCs facilitated the movement of referred patients, thereby supporting the referral system. This service delivery system in turn enhanced the credibility and acceptability of health services for the rural population. Senior obstetricians who served in public sector hospitals during that period freely attributed the decline in maternal death to the sterling efforts of rural-based nurses and midwives in identifying complications of pregnancy and childbirth and getting patients to hospital in time for effective interventions (Pathmanathan et al., 2003).

4.2.4 PHC in Urban Areas

Public sector. During the first three decades after independence, the ambulatory health service component of PHC in urban areas was provided by a combination of government-funded public services, the private sector (funded through out-of-pocket expenditure by users) and non-governmental organisation (NGO) services supported by civil society and government grants. There was very little co-ordination across these sectors. However, these services are collectively credited with raising awareness and acceptance of allopathic medical interventions, particularly among those who had relied mainly on traditional remedies and were steeped in cultural beliefs that were obstacles to the use of effective healthcare.

The public sector hospitals each had outpatient (ambulatory) services that provided walk-in care mostly geared to acute episodes of illness, as well as accident and emergency (A&E) services that were available 24 hours a day. In the larger hospitals, doctors aided by hospital assistants (later re-named medical assistants) were backed by pharmaceutical services (Suleiman & Jegathesan, n.d.). These services provided referrals for admission and specialist care when needed. Almost all of these hospital-based outpatient services were confined to curative care, except for pregnancy, for which antenatal and postnatal clinics provided counselling and services, including that for family planning. Additionally, in the larger urban configurations, the local authority (such as the city council) provided maternal and child health services through a network of clinics. These services predated independence and were the prototype that was later used by the RHS for maternal and child health services. All of these services were provided for nominal or no fees, and utilisation rates in ambulatory facilities were very high, resulting in queues and long waiting times. During the third decade post-independence (the 1980s), the state of the overcrowded, understaffed services began to cause concerns about the quality of care. This contributed to the genesis of the Quality Assurance initiative (see later in this chapter and Chapter 5).

Private sector. The private sector complemented the public sector in urban areas. Medical doctors (GPs) owned and provided healthcare, including dispensing medication through small clinics that operated from modest premises. Most were in 'shop houses', that is, two- or three-storeyed premises with the clinic on the ground floor. The higher floors sometimes served as short-stay hospitals for patients and came to be known as nursing homes or as private hospitals. Such premises were flanked by other shops. Most patients paid a fee for the service, which was generally very low, affordable and popular with the urban population. They received 'one-stop' care by the doctor, sometimes assisted by trained nurses or medical assistants; medication was dispensed on the spot, and minor surgery was performed on the premises.

Non-governmental organisations (NGOs). NGOs played a small but very significant role in the development of PHC in urban areas. Some NGOs, such as St John Ambulance and Red Crescent, filled gaps in the services provided by the public sector. Others, such as the family planning associations (FPAs) (Box 4.3) and several associations related to special needs, such as impaired hearing, vision and disabilities arising from illness (e.g. leprosy) or genetics, provided small-scale models of care and strong advocacy that served to mobilise civil society to recognise unmet needs. They established partnerships with the public sector, which provided financial grants. For example, the FPAs received an annual grant of RM 200,000 from the government from 1962 until the early 1980s (Tey, 2007). In later years, when capacity grew, the public sector took over many of these services and used the care models developed earlier by the NGOs.

Box 4.3 The role of NGOs in a health system dominated by the public sector

The FPAs (now known as the Federation of Reproductive Health Associations, Malaysia, or FRHAM) were largely led by prominent obstetricians and personalities active in civil society. They had the ear of policymakers, although the services they provided were limited mainly to small clinics situated in urban MCH clinics and hospital postnatal wards. The uptake of contraceptives was not impressive. The West Malaysia Family Survey conducted in 1966 found that the contraceptive prevalence rate was only 8.8% (Ahmad et al., 2010). Advocacy and the service models used by the FPAs contributed to the establishment of the National Family Planning Program under the First Malaysia Plan in 1966 to improve families' health and welfare and promote national economic development. The programme was expanded and integrated into RHS in the mid-1970s to serve rural and remote communities. The rapid expansion of the MCH and FP services have been a major factor in lowering the infant mortality rate across the country (Pathmanathan et al., 2003).

Traditional and complementary medicine (TCM). Although traditional practitioners were and continue to be widely available, there is little information about them. They were not registered, and their practice was not regulated. More recently, there has been stronger oversight of the products they use, and this is discussed in Chapter 11.

4.3 The Second Phase: The Continuing Journey towards Integrated PHC Services (1990–2017)

4.3.1 Drivers of Change

Economic growth continued over the following 30 years, although there were a number of setbacks, including the Asian financial crisis. The population became increasingly urban, reaching almost 70%, and the proportion of teens and young adults increased, followed by an increase in the number of elderly people (Chapter 3). Lifestyles and health-related behaviour, particularly around food and physical activity, began to change. For example, during the 1990s, tobacco smoking and drug addiction were major concerns, while in the 2000s, the obesity epidemic took centre stage (Suleiman & Jegathesan, n.d.). As people became increasingly well-connected with the world through media and travel, public expectations of healthcare increased.

Rising healthcare costs competed with other priorities in the national budget and increased pressure on the health sector to consider alternate approaches for healthcare financing (Chapter 9) and cost containment. The voices of civil society became stronger, with a growing dichotomy between conservative and liberal value systems. This generated debates and tension on many health-related issues, such as reproductive health and HIV/AIDS. Additionally, international pressures, first towards achieving Millennium Development Goals (MDGs) and subsequently re-aligning towards Sustainable Development Goals (SDGs), influenced national health goals (Chapter 6, Case Study 6.1).

All of these interacting forces were drivers that influenced health policy and the evolution of PHC, first towards the provision of a greater range of services to cater for new and emerging needs; second towards better integration between services. Integration and co-ordination were needed to remove institutional barriers between the multiple healthcare services that catered to any particular family and to focus on providing health services to meet the needs of people within their families and communities. The rapid urbanisation also required different modalities from rural settings for the provision of integrated PHC.

The Seventh Malaysia Plan (1996–2000) marked a change for PHC with the establishment of a new PHC division in the Ministry of Health (MoH) (Economic Planning Unit, 1996). The evolving PHC services during this period had two major characteristics. First, in the public sector (mainly MoH services), there was convergence of the hitherto separate services for promotional-cum-preventive health provided at health centres and the curative outpatient services provided by MoH hospitals and health centres. Second, in the private sector, serious stresses emerged in services provided by GPs, associated with issues of financing and competition from public-sector clinics and by specialist practitioners who also provided primary care (Chapter 4, Case Study 4.2).

4.3.2 PHC Services in the Public Sector

The overarching goal of the public sector was to achieve equitable access to more comprehensive primary care. Three threads of interlinked thrusts towards this goal are discernible, namely:

- Expanding the scope of PHC services to encompass additional age groups and health needs.
- Integrating preventive-cum-promotional services with curative services to address segmentation and compartmentalisation and provide seamless care for individuals, families and communities.
- Improving the quality of services to respond better to expectations in the community and professional groups.

4.3.2.1 Expanded Scope of Preventive PHC Services in the Public Sector

During the 1990s, responding to demographic and morbidity trends, the preventive and health promotional services provided by health centres expanded to include additional age groups (adolescents, adults, women's and workers' health, the elderly, children with special needs) and health problems, such as mental health and screening for iodine deficiency and glucose-6-phosphate dehydrogenase (G6PD) deficiency, while the national childhood immunisation programme expanded to include measles, mumps and diphtheria, and *Haemophilus influenzae* (Suleiman & Jegathesan, n.d.).

The clinic-based services were complemented by community-based programmes. The nutritional surveillance of children and pregnant women conducted in 1988 provided valuable input to the national poverty reduction initiatives and rehabilitation efforts (National Coordinating Committee on Food and Nutrition, 2006). The Food Basket Programme (also known as the rehabilitation programme for malnourished children) for children with poor nutritional gain continued to reach out to poor communities (National Coordinating Committee on Food and Nutrition, 2006). Clinic-cum-community services were also initiated to support anti-tobacco smoking efforts, which included smoking cessation clinics. The health clinic advisory panels (*panel penasihat*), with local community representatives, worked with health staff on four major areas: healthy ageing, advocacy for immunisation, dengue control, and diabetes and overweight management (Mustapha et al., 2014).

Simultaneously, the hitherto rural health services gradually increased their coverage to include urban areas in response to demands from local authorities that had little interest in providing services that did not generate revenue. This required organisational re-structuring, including the transfer of authority, staff and some physical facilities from the local authority to the national MoH, particularly in the metropolitan cities of Penang, Melaka and Kuala Lumpur. It also paved the way subsequently for easier integration of preventive and curative services.

Gaps in and limitations to expansion. Financial and human resources constraints limited some of the service expansion. For example, cervical cancer screening had already been planned to incrementally cover larger sections of the target age group, but laboratories could not cope, and the turnaround time was slow. Screening reached only 6% of eligible women (aged 20–65 years) between 1996 and 2003 (Figure 4.1) (Ministry of Health Malaysia, 2005), and follow-up call services were inadequate (L. P. Wong et al., 2008). Also, other components of the health system interacted with PHC services in the public sector to initiate, facilitate or limit the expansion of PHC services. Examples are summarised in Box 4.4.

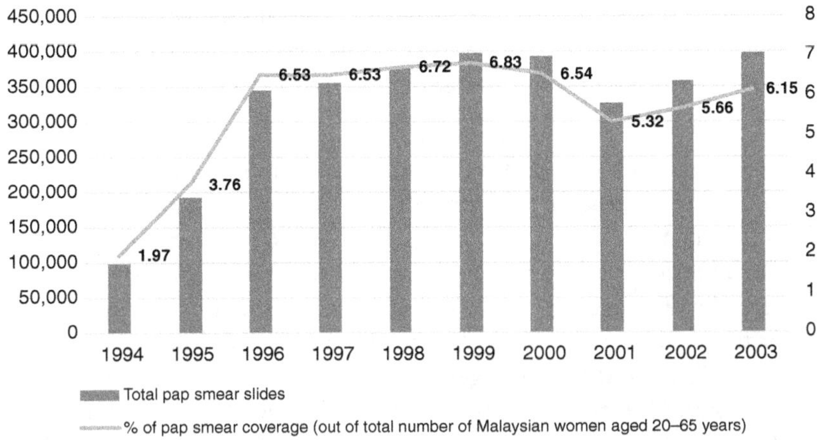

Figure 4.1 Pap smear slides taken and coverage in Malaysia, 1994–2003. Source: Ministry of Health Malaysia, 2005.

Box 4.4 Influence of other health system components on PHC: summary of illustrative examples

Examples of Limiting Factors

Finance: Dictated the speed and influenced the scope of expansion. While new programmes were added, some existing programmes, such as family planning and cervical cancer and breast cancer screening programmes, failed to gain traction.

Workforce: Upgrading the competencies and recruitment of new categories with different competencies needed, such as finance, training and managerial support. For example, the lack of trained staff hampered the ability to provide rehabilitation, occupational therapy, home visits and home care nursing services for the elderly.

Examples of Enabling Factors

Medical products and technology: Additional affordable vaccines (measles, mumps and rubella (MMR), hepatitis B, human papillomavirus (HPV)) and the availability of simple field tests (G6PD and hypothyroidism screening) enabled the expansion of services. Staff training and financial support enabled this expansion.

Health information: Nutritional surveillance identified anaemic pregnant women and malnourished children and enabled the provision of food baskets for them as part of multi-sectoral poverty reduction; Teleprimary Care enabled better management of diabetes and hypertension by providing data for targeted monitoring and follow-up.

Governance: Community mobilisation and inter-sectoral co-ordination supported strategies for reducing disease risk factors. Grants were allocated for promotion, prevention, early screening and rehabilitation care. Illustrative examples are the mobilisation of teens through peer-to-peer counselling within school communities for targeted purposes such as tobacco smoking and drug use (PROSTAR) and for more general behaviour change purposes such as healthier lifestyles (Doktor Muda) (Ministry of Health Malaysia, 2005). New legislation established standards for care, including care of older people in private healthcare facilities, and also mandated the sale of iodised salts in districts with high risk of iodine deficiency disorders.

Sources: Government of Malaysia, 1998; 2012; 2018; Ministry of Health Malaysia, 2003; 2007; 2012; 2013.

4.3.2.2 Integration of Preventive and Curative Services in the Public Sector

Prior to the mid-1990s, curative PHC services were provided by:

- Outpatient departments (OPDs) of public sector hospitals and some satellite clinics for free or for a nominal charge.
- Public sector health centres and dispensaries, also free or for a nominal charge.

During the 1990s and early 2000s, two related organisational changes within the MoH led to better integration of preventive and curative services. First, the implementation of a policy decision to move OPDs out of hospitals and into health centres began in the late 1990s and continued incrementally over the next decade. Second, this move was followed by the re-organisation of services in the health centres to better serve the goal of developing people-centred PHC.

Transfer of OPDs. Historically, hospital OPDs primarily catered for acute episodes of illness, rarely providing health prevention or promotion,

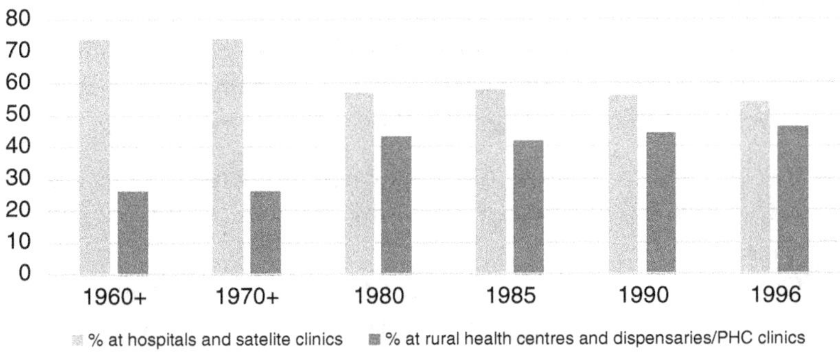

Figure 4.2 Trends in the utilisation pattern of OPDs.
Source: Suleiman and Jegathesan, n.d.

and were not geared for the continuity of care essential for non-communicable disease (NCDs). Conversely, health centres had separate arms – the family health arm had good competence for providing preventive and health promotional services for family health aimed at clients in various phases of the life cycle (pregnancy, childhood, adolescence, old age), including individuals, families and communities on a long-term basis. However, the outpatient arm of the health centres mainly provided for walk-in patients. The utilisation of OPD services evolved, with the health centres gradually overtaking the hospital OPDs in terms of volume of utilisation (Figure 4.2).

Additionally, by the late 1990s, the proportion of patients with illnesses such as hypertension and diabetes, which require long-term management, was increasing. Meanwhile, public sector hospitals had difficulties managing outpatient services (OPDs), as their focus was mainly on secondary and tertiary care. Therefore, a policy decision was implemented to transfer OPDs from hospitals to health centres.

Re-organisation of health services. The outpatient services in health centres were re-vamped to cater to the integration of preventive and health promotional services with illness management (Economic Planning Unit, 1996). The health centres adopted a new approach that integrated basic PHC concepts in addressing the continually expanding initiatives required to deal with NCDs. Box 4.5 summarises the concepts involved, and the illustrative case study on REAP-WISE (Reviewed Approach: Wellness, Illness, Support Services, Emergency Information) elaborates on the initiative. Imaging, laboratory and

Box 4.5 The journey towards integration

The health centre services renewed the PHC concept with a new approach to accommodating its additional services, namely:

1. Preventing and reducing disease burden by treating the ill, managing those with risks and preventing the onset of preventable risks.
2. Enhancing healthcare delivery for fast access to safe and high-quality services with greater comfort in a hassle-free environment.

The wellness focus

covers the life-course from antenatal to child and geriatric age for early identification of and management of medical conditions. All new activities for wellness are mapped against age group needs. Teams oversee policy development for the collective activities for each age group in order to integrate workflow processes, accounting for monitoring indicators, quantity and quality of human resources required, the diagnostic equipment, pharmaceutical requirements, and physical space for these activities. These workflow processes are then phased in at clinics nationwide. (Jaafar et al., 2007)

pharmacy facilities were upgraded progressively as staff and physical infrastructure became available (Economic Planning Unit, 1996; 2001). Communication between primary, secondary and tertiary care was strengthened, and information systems were upgraded to include electronic personal medical records that facilitated the integration of information from the various services that catered to each patient and family (Economic Planning Unit, 2001).

Gaps and limitations to the integration and re-organisation. This re-organisation process required the re-allocation of budget and human resources between hospitals and health centres, and it also required re-engineering health information systems to provide real-time access to patient information for care providers at primary and secondary level. Table 4.5 illustrates the gaps and challenges in integration and re-organisation as well as the action taken to address such challenges.

Table 4.5 *Gaps and challenges and action taken in integrating preventive and curative services*

	Gaps and challenges	Action taken
Finance	Limited	Transfer of OPDs was done incrementally over a period of more than a decade
Health workforce	Rapid turnover of staff, particularly junior doctors who needed rotational postings as part of career development	• Family medicine specialists (FMSs) were placed at health centres to oversee and manage patient care teams • Multi-disciplinary team approach rather than individual doctors to serve clients from specified geographic zones
Medical products	Hospitals and health centres have separate budgets for pharmaceuticals – it was difficult to estimate the portion of hospital pharmacy budget needed for OPD as separate from inpatient care	State-level pharmacy departments took over budget management for pharmaceuticals for both health and hospital services
Service delivery	• Existing building spaces and facilities could not accommodate the expanded functions • Staff who had hitherto provided either curative or preventive/promotional services needed guidance on how to merge both components of care	• New building designs for health centres were created for integrated services • Laboratories and imaging services had to be updated to support the upgraded clinical services • Practice guidelines were implemented for the newly expanded team of FMS, medical officer, medical assistant and nurses

Sources: Economic Planning Unit, 1996; Awin, 2003; 2004.

4.3.2.3 Focus on Improving Quality of Care

During the late 1980s, the rising expectations of the public, as well as the strong commitment of professional leaders to quality of care, led to the introduction of a variety of quality improvement initiatives in the MoH (Suleiman & Jegathesan, n.d.). The scope of quality improvement was defined as including technical quality of care, client satisfaction and resource utilisation. This compares well with the statement 30 years later by the Organisation for Economic Co-operation and Development (OECD), the World Health Organization (WHO) and the World Bank defining the 'measurable characteristics of quality as effectiveness, safety, people-centeredness, timeliness, equity, integration of care and efficiency' (OECD et al., 2018). The key initiatives included raising the levels of competence in the PHC workforce and introducing systematic monitoring of quality followed by measures to identify and address systemic weaknesses that contributed to inadequate quality.

Higher levels of competence in the PHC workforce. Medical officers, who were the front-line providers of care for illness episodes in health centres and OPDs, had no post-graduate or vocational training and had limited ability to manage more complex and chronic conditions, such as NCDs and mental illness. Years of effort by professional leaders (Rajakumar, 1984) culminated in universities offering a new post-graduate training programme of Family Medicines, while the MoH created a new cadre of specialist: the family medicine specialist (FMS). This new category of FMS was expected to provide leadership in upgrading the quality of primary care services that included a more holistic approach of seamless care for health promotion, disease prevention, illness management and rehabilitation for individuals and families (Awin, 2004).

In tandem, the competencies of nurses and medical assistants were upgraded. The local production of allied health professionals, such as diagnostic radiographers, medical laboratory technologists, physiotherapists and dieticians, was stepped up with a higher level of qualifications and was modernised through integrated training approaches. Previously, the services of these allied health personnel were available only in hospitals, but now they were added to PHC teams (Ministry of Health Malaysia, 2006).

Box 4.6 Dimensions of quality that were monitored and improved

- Workforce skill levels and competence
- Outcomes of prevention and management of illness
- Client satisfaction
- Resource utilisation

Quality monitoring and improvement strategies. Hitherto focused on monitoring and improving ethnic and regional disparities in equitable access to care and health outcomes, PHC services added new dimensions to their performance monitoring (Box 4.6). Table 4.6 shows illustrative examples. The conglomerate of activities created a 'bottom–up' quality culture within the organisation.

4.3.3 PHC Services in the Private Sector

In the private sector, doctors (GPs) provide ambulatory non-specialist curative services on a fee-for-service basis. In the 1980s and 1990s, as rural to urban migration increased and the economy improved, the size and utilisation of the private sector increased rapidly (Figure 4.3).

Box 4.7 summarises the characteristics of GPs, who provide about half of ambulatory care in Malaysia. Despite their importance in the health sector, governance and financing arrangements result in GPs having few incentives to provide prevention and promotion services. Their fee schedule is per visit and has not been adjusted for inflation over the past 15 years (Maharajah, 2018). It is not geared to reward the time and effort spent on health promotion. For many GPs, the fee is so low that it is not financially sustainable, and they rely on the sale of medications to maintain financial viability. Patients are free to move between doctors; doctor-hopping is frequent and therefore continuity of care could be compromised, and it can be difficult to build a trusting and long-standing relationship between providers and clients and their families. Additionally, there is no restriction on patients seeking primary care from doctors who practise as specialists in any discipline in the private sector. Therefore, specialist doctors are in direct competition with GPs.

Table 4.6 *Quality monitoring and improvement: examples of experiences in primary care*

Approaches to quality improvement	Examples	Benefits derived from the initiative
MoH Quality Assurance Programme adopted the approach of: Nationwide monitoring of selected indicators of system failure, for: • Identification of outlier units in relation to agreed expected standards • Analysis of root causes and implementation of remedial action	During the early stages of the programme, indicators were: • Eclampsia of pregnancy • Puerperal sepsis • Severe neonatal jaundice During later stages, indicators included: • Appropriate management of asthma • Appropriate management of diabetes • Appropriate admission to medical wards	• Improved health information: – Accuracy and timeliness of data – Use of data in problem-solving • Increased appreciation of quality and its relationship to clinical outcomes, resource utilisation and patient satisfaction
Participation in nationwide quality improvement strategies by health districts, health centres, hospital OPDs, laboratories and pharmacies	• Quality control circles (waiting times, counter services) • Client charter • Work culture • MS ISO 9000 certification	• Improved managerial competence at local level • Improved resource utilisation • Improved client satisfaction

Sources: Suleiman and Jegathesan, n.d.; Ministry of Health Malaysia, 2004.

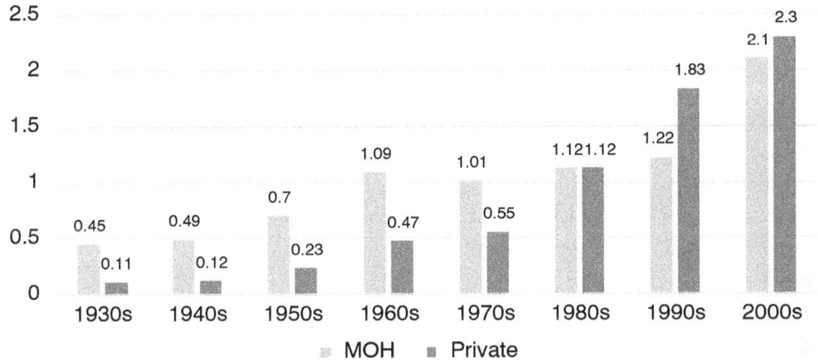

Figure 4.3 Estimated outpatient visits to clinics per capita per annum, Malaysia, 1930s–2000s.
Note: Private outpatient refers to outpatient visits to both hospitals and clinics.
Source: Health Policy Research Associates et al., 2013.

Box 4.7 What are GPs?

- GPs are medical doctors.
- Few have any specialist or vocational training to function as providers of comprehensive PHC such as the requirements for GPs in the United Kingdom or Australia.
- Most GP clinics are urban and semi-urban, with fewer than six staff members. They use private laboratory and imaging services.
- GPs prescribe and dispense medicines.
- The public utilises GP services largely for acute illness episodes while largely visiting public PHC clinics for more chronic and complex conditions (Table 4.7).

A Quality and Costs of Primary Care (QUALICOPC) study showed that three-quarters of the patients who visited private clinics reported that they did not have a primary doctor to follow up on their condition (Sivasampu et al., 2016). Health information systems are underdeveloped. Few patients' medical records are computerised and there are no incentives for recall and follow-up of patients who require long-term management. There is no systematic monitoring of the quality of care (Sivasampu et al., 2016). In contrast, for example, in Australia, there

Table 4.7 *Top three reasons for encounters in public and private clinics*

	Rate per 100 encounters
Public sector primary care clinics	
Hypertension	31.3
Diabetes	22.5
Lipid disorder	18.5
Private sector clinics	
Fever	28.3
Cough	26.5
Runny nose/rhinorrhea	19.4

Source: Clinical Research Centre, 2014.

Box 4.8 System observations: when systems outcomes diverge from stated goals

The policy environment in which private clinics currently operate presents obstacles to preventative and chronic care. This shows how stated goals, such as the aim of the MoH to increase integration and comprehensiveness of primary care, may differ from systems outcomes. Policies and resources for public clinics have enabled significant advances toward these goals. However, private clinics operate under fee structures, lack of integrated information systems and other policy obstacles that create barriers to preventative and chronic care. Private GPs have persisted in health promotion despite these obstacles (Table 4.9). The MoH needs to invest in an enabling system for private GPs to sustain and maximise their contribution to comprehensive primary care.

are targeted incentives for private sector primary care providers to support immunisation and cervical smear testing and for installing information technology (Khoo, 2002).

Additionally, GPs face serious economic challenges arising from the introduction of third-party administrators (see Case Study 4.2). On top of that, medical insurance schemes generally do not cover ambulatory care. In a recent survey, 70% of GPs interviewed cited as serious threats market competition from community pharmacies, and 55% cited market competition from the public sector 1Malaysia clinics (Kenny, 2017).

4.3.4 Traditional and Complementary Medicine

TCM is responsible for about 6% of expenditure on ambulatory care. For the first 50 years after independence, the allopathic healthcare system adopted an attitude of peaceful co-existence with TCM, responding only to curb practices that were known to be dangerous to health. This chapter is hampered because there is little empirical evidence of TCM practices or their outcomes. During the last 10 years, initial efforts were directed at establishing a database of practitioners and practices and developing regulations to set standards for practitioners (Mahmud et al., 2009; Division of Traditional and Complementary Medicine, 2017). These were the first steps in integrating TCM into the country's PHC system. Case Study 11.1 provides insights into some of the challenges.

4.3.5 Outcomes of PHC in the Public and Private Sectors

Access, satisfaction, quality and continuity of care. A QUALICOPC study showed that patients generally did not perceive barriers to access (physical and financial) to care and were satisfied with the care they received at both public and private clinics (Table 4.8) (Sivasampu et al., 2015; 2016).

The large majority of doctors in both public and private clinics were reportedly involved in health promotion as part of their normal patient contact, though not in group sessions (Table 4.9).

Referral linkages with secondary and tertiary care were not strong (Table 4.10), particularly in terms of feedback from secondary to primary care level and in horizontal communication between primary care providers.

As the doctor-shopping phenomenon was observed and there was a lack of longitudinal continuity at private primary care clinics (Sivasampu et al., 2016), it is not surprising that significant differences were noted in aggregated performance indicators of quality of care

Table 4.8 *Access to and satisfaction with primary care*

Patients' perceptions of accessibility of primary care and satisfaction with care	% of patients interviewed	
	Public clinic	Private clinic
Clinic not too far away	77.5	85.4
Opening hours not restricted	59.2	73.3
Able to get a home visit	43	18.9
Out-of-office hours	58.3	68.1
Never postponed or abstained from a visit when needed	80	85
Satisfied with the duration of the consultation	96.7	96

Sources: Sivasampu et al., 2015; 2016.

Table 4.9 *Doctors reporting involvement in health promotion during routine patient encounters*

	Proportion (%)	
	Public clinic	Private clinic
Smoking	88	95
Diet	92.8	97.9
Problematic use of alcohol	52.9	66.5
Physical exercise	85.5	98.7

Sources: Sivasampu et al., 2015; 2016.

between public and private sector primary care, with the public sector surpassing the private sector (Table 4.11).

4.4 Summary of the Malaysian Experience

Although the PHC services predated the Alma Ata Declaration of 1978, the guiding principles used in Malaysia were akin to those formulated in Alma Ata. Over 60 years, these services evolved in incremental stages in response to population dynamics and behaviour, changing disease patterns and economic pressures, taking advantage of local opportunities and recognising constraints. The government

Table 4.10 ***Referral experiences reported by doctors***

	Proportion (%) of doctors stating:					
	Usually/always		Occasionally		Seldom/never	
	Public clinic	Private clinic	Public clinic	Private clinic	Public clinic	Private clinic
Received patient records from previous doctor	36.2	7	51.6	39	12.2	54
Used referral letters	99	91				
Obtained feedback from specialists	19	19	30.8	31	50.2	50
Obtained discharge report from hospital	27[1]	22[1]	13.7[2]	29[2]	58.4	49

Sources: Sivasampu et al., 2015; 2016.
[1] Within 1–14 days.
[2] Delayed by >14 days.

Table 4.11 ***Clinical outcomes for the management of diabetes and hypertension***

Percentage of:	Public	Private
Controlled diabetics[1]	38.1	35.5
Hypertension management[2]	44.1	39
Hypertension management[3]	50	n.a.

Source: Ministry of Health Malaysia & Harvard T. H. Chan School of Public Health, 2016.
[1] MHSR (Malaysia Health Systems Research) analysis using NHMS (National Health and Morbidity Survey) 2015 data. Fasting blood glucose of 4.0–6.1 mmol/L or non-fasting blood glucose of 4.4–8.0 mmol/L.
[2] MHSR analysis using NHMS 2015 data. Target blood pressure of ≤140/90 mmHg.
[3] MHSR analysis using Teleprimary Care data, which relates only to care at MoH clinics.
n.a. – not available

assumed responsibility for free public sector services that led the way and dominated the subsequent evolution of PHC in the country. Achieving equitable access for a wide range of 'essential services', including PHC services, has remained a cornerstone of the evolution. These services included preventive and health promotional services, including nutrition, as well as curative services provided at hospital OPDs and by the private sector.

PHC services retained the focus on people throughout the evolution – variously reaching out to communities to mobilise them in improving or sustaining health. The process of evolution saw a progressive expansion of the range of preventive and promotional services – beginning with pregnancy, childbirth and infancy and progressing through each age group to old age while simultaneously addressing specific localised concerns, such as iodine deficiency and mental health, as they arose. The parallel evolution of ambulatory curative services saw a progression from managing acute illness episodes to dealing with illnesses that require long-term care, such as hypertension and diabetes. The evolutionary process recognised the benefits of merging the parallel development of preventive/promotional services with the curative stream, and the system was able to accomplish rather complex organisational restructuring to achieve such merging.

The other cornerstone of the evolution was the continuing thrust to improve quality. The features of the success in Malaysia are: strong and sustained leadership and commitment to quality; adherence to basic principles of quality improvement, including monitoring; and improvement that originated from the service providers themselves, thereby reducing the fear of punitive repercussions and increasing accountability and transparency.

Several challenges surfaced from time to time. As elaborated on in Chapter 8, some were addressed successfully, while others continue to haunt the evolutionary process. For example, the evolving profile of a workforce with higher qualifications has created demands for higher remuneration and better career paths. The workforce in the public sector PHC service is part of the larger civil service in the country. Hence, change is fraught with repercussions. Meanwhile, the private sector is reluctant to absorb higher-paid categories and prefers task-shifting, for example, using nurse assistants in place of trained nurses.

In the past, the private sector has complemented the public sector by providing care for those who were able to pay out of pocket for prompt and convenient care. The last couple of decades has seen publicly funded primary care growing faster than the private sector. While the public sector moves closer to comprehensive primary care and keeps an

Box 4.9 System observations: overcoming limits to growth

The development of PHC clearly illustrates the systems concept *limits to growth*, in which a previously successful strategy runs into a new limitation that requires a new approach. We see in this chapter the rapid expansion of maternal and child health clinics to improve coverage, followed by the expansion of services, which in turn led to the development of multi-disciplinary teams. Each of these developments came about as the prior strategy encountered limitations in improving population health, and they required substantial re-alignment of clinic organisation, practices and personnel. The growing challenges of chronic care and health promotion in urban settings will probably require similar experiments and paradigm shifts among public primary health clinics.

eye on quality and responsiveness, the private sector is struggling with issues of governance, financing, skills in the workforce and disincentives to move towards comprehensive care. There is a risk that public perceptions of public and private services will change. Wealthier sections of the population might change their health-seeking behaviour accordingly and drift towards the highly subsidised public sector despite being able to afford private services. This would have a negative impact on PHC by overburdening the government budget. Efforts to establish a more collaborative model of operation have been repeatedly frustrated by political pressures and priorities.

4.5 Key Messages from Malaysia's Experience

4.5.1 What Went Well?

- PHC is part of rural development; PHC benefits from the development of education and communication and contributes to rural development.
- The cornerstone of PHC is equitable access to services; close linkages with secondary care and community mobilisation are key; urban settings require different modalities from rural settings in the provision of integrated PHC.

- Appropriately trained and supervised allied health workers provide low-cost, high-impact PHC.
- Systematic monitoring, focused on identifying and resolving systems issues rather than creating a blame culture, improved quality of care.

4.5.2 What Did Not Go So Well?

- The dichotomy between the public and private sectors in terms of financing and governance continually generates challenges that have not been addressed adequately.
- The rigid structure of the civil service (including the public sector health services) and the fee-for-service mechanisms of the private sector continue to be major constraints in the development of PHC.

4.5.3 Trends and Challenges

Epidemiologic, demographic and technological trends will require flexible adaptive responses from PHC.

References

Ahmad, N., Tey, N., Kamarul Zaman, K., Muhd Sapri, N., Abdul Manaf, M. and Yeoh, Y. (2010). Status of family planning in Malaysia. UNFPA – ICOMP Regional Consultation: Family Planning in Asia and the Pacific – Addressing the Challenges. Bangkok, Thailand.

Ali, A. and Howden-Chapman, P. (2007). Maternity services and the role of the traditional birth attendant, bidan kampung, in rural Malaysia. *Journal of Public Health Management and Practice*, 13(3), 278–86. Online article. https://journals.lww.com/jphmp/Fulltext/2007/05000/Maternity_Services_and_the_Role_of_the_Traditional.8.aspx

Awin, N. (2003). Review of PHC in Malaysia. In *Public Health: A Multifaceted Discipline in Medicine – Primary Health Care: Health for All Starts at the Community*. Kuala Lumpur: Malaysian Public Health Physicians' Association, pp. 251–73.

Awin, N. (2004). Family medicine specialist in the future health system. In *Public Health: A Multifaceted Discipline in Medicine – Volume 3 (Primary Health Care: Health for All Starts at the Community)*. Kuala Lumpur: Malaysian Public Health Physicians' Association, pp. 47–68.

Awin, N. (2011). *Public Health: A Multifaceted Discipline in Medicine*. Kuala Lumpur: Malaysian Public Health Physicians' Association.

Clinical Research Centre. (2014). *National Medical Care Survey*. Putrajaya: Ministry of Health Malaysia.

Division of Traditional and Complementary Medicine. (2017). *Annual Report 2017*. Putrajaya: Ministry of Health Malaysia.

Economic Planning Unit. (1996). *Seventh Malaysia Plan 1996–2000*. Kuala Lumpur: Economic Planning Unit.

Economic Planning Unit. (2001). *Eighth Malaysia Plan 2001–2005*. Putrajaya: Economic Planning Unit.

Economic Planning Unit. (2004). *Malaysia: 30 Years of Poverty Reduction, Growth and Racial Harmony. A Case Study from Scaling Up Poverty Reduction*. Washington, DC: World Bank.

Family Health Development Division. (2015). *Operating Policy Guide for Health Clinics*. Putrajaya: Ministry of Health Malaysia.

Federation of Malaya. (1960). *Second Five-Year Plan, 1961–1965*. Kuala Lumpur: Government of Malaya.

Government of Malaysia. (1998). *Private Healthcare Facilities and Services Act 1998 (Act 586)*. Kuala Lumpur: Percetakan Nasional Malaysia Bhd.

Government of Malaysia. (2012). *Act 281: Food Act 1983 and Food Regulations 1985*. Kuala Lumpur: Percetakan Nasional Malaysia Bhd.

Government of Malaysia. (2018). *Act 802: Private Aged Healthcare Facilities and Services Act 2018*. Kuala Lumpur: Percetakan Nasional Malaysia Bhd.

Health Policy Research Associates (HPRA), Institute for Health Systems Research (IHSR) and Institute for Health Policy (IHP). (2013). *Malaysia Health Care Demand Analysis: Inequalities in Healthcare Demand and Simulation of Trends and Impact of Potential Changes in Healthcare Spending*. Putrajaya: Institute for Health Systems Research, Ministry of Health Malaysia.

Ismail, H. A. M. (1974). The history of early medical and health services in Malaysia. *Malaysia in History*, 17(2), 6–15.

Jaafar, S., Suhaili, M. R., Mohd Noh, K., Zainal Ehsan, F. and Lee, F. S. (2007). *Primary Health Care: Key to Intersectoral Action for Health and Equity*. Geneva: World Health Organization.

Jayasuria, L. W. (1967). *Organisation and Administration of Rural Health Services*. Setia Alam: Institute for Public Health.

Kenny, K. (2017). A study on the health economics of general practitioners in Malaysia: trends, challenges and moving forward. *International Journal of Public Health Research*, 7(1), 765–73.

Khoo, E. M. (2002). Primary health care and general practice: a comparison between Australia and Malaysia. *Asia-Pacific Journal of Public Health*, 14 (2), 59–63.

Lee, C. and Lee, C. G. (2017). The evolution of development planning in Malaysia. *Journal of Southeast Asian Economies*, 34(3), 436–61.

Maharajah, R. K. (29 August 2018). No increase in consultation fees. *The Sun Daily*. Online article. www.thesundaily.my/archive/no-increase-consultation-fees-EUARCH575040

Ministry of Health Malaysia. (2003). *Annual Report*. Kuala Lumpur: Ministry of Health Malaysia.

Ministry of Health Malaysia. (2004). *Annual Report*. Putrajaya: Ministry of Health Malaysia.

Ministry of Health Malaysia. (2005). *Annual Report 2003*. Putrajaya: Ministry of Health Malaysia.

Ministry of Health Malaysia. (2006). *Annual Report 2004*. Putrajaya: Ministry of Health Malaysia.

Ministry of Health Malaysia. (2007). *Annual Report 2005*. Putrajaya: Ministry of Health Malaysia.

Ministry of Health Malaysia. (2009). *Annual Report 2007*. Putrajaya: Ministry of Health Malaysia.

Ministry of Health Malaysia. (2012). *Annual Report 2010*. Putrajaya: Ministry of Health Malaysia.

Ministry of Health Malaysia. (2013). *Annual Report 2011*. Putrajaya: Ministry of Health Malaysia.

Ministry of Health Malaysia. (2016). *Annual Report 2016*. Putrajaya: Ministry of Health Malaysia.

Ministry of Health Malaysia and Harvard T. H. Chan School of Public Health. (2016). *Malaysian Health Systems Research Volume 1: Contextual Analysis of the Malaysian Health System March 2016*. Putrajaya: Ministry of Health Malaysia.

Mohd Ashad, F. and Shamsudin, M. N. (1997). *Rural Development Model in Malaysia*. Serdang: Universiti Putra Malaysia.

Mustapha, F. I., Omar, Z. A., Mihat, O., Noh, K. M., Hassan, N., Abu Bakar, R. et al. (2014). Addressing non-communicable diseases in Malaysia: an integrative process of systems and community. *BMC Public Health*, 14(Supplement2), S4.

National Coordinating Committee on Food and Nutrition. (2006). *National Plan of Action for Nutrition of Malaysia (2006–2015)*. Putrajaya: Ministry of Health Malaysia.

Noordin, R. A. (1978). *Primary Health Care Approaches in the Underserved Areas with Special Reference to Malaysia*. Kuala Lumpur: Ministry of Health Malaysia and World Health Organization.

OECD, World Health Organization and World Bank Group. (2018). *Delivering Quality Health Services: A Global Imperative*. Geneva: World Health Organization. DOI: https://doi.org/10.1787/9789264300309-en

Pathmanathan, I., Liljestrand, J., Martins, J. M., Rajapaksa, L., Lissner, C., de Silva, A. et al. (2003). *Investing in Maternal Health: Learning from Malaysia and Sri Lanka*. Washington, DC: World Bank.

Peng, J. (1979). The role of traditional birth attendants in family planning programs in Southeast Asia. *International Journal of Gynecology & Obstetrics*, 17(2), 108–13.

Prime Minister's Department. (1971). *Second Malaysia Plan 1971–1975*. Kuala Lumpur: Office of the Prime Minister.

Prime Minister's Department. (1976). *Third Malaysia Plan 1976–1980*. Kuala Lumpur: Office of the Prime Minister.

Prime Minister's Department. (1981). *Fourth Malaysia Plan 1981–1985*. Kuala Lumpur: Office of the Prime Minister.

Rajakumar, M. K. (1984). A proposal for the training of physicians in primary care for the rural areas of Malaysia. *Family Practitioner*, 7(1), 58–61.

Rudner, M. (1972). The draft development plan of the Federation of Malaya 1950–55. *Journal of Southeast Asian Studies*, 3(1), 63–96.

Mahmud, S. Z., Tahir, A., Ida Farah, A., Ami Fazlin, S. M., Sondi, S., Azman, A. H. et al. (2009). Use of traditional and complementary medicine in Malaysia: a baseline study. *Complementary Therapies in Medicine*, 17(5–6), 292–9.

Sivasampu, S., Mohamad Noh, K. and Chin, M. C. (2015). *Quality and Costs of Primary Care (QUALICOPC) Malaysia: Phase 1 – Public Clinics*. Putrajaya: Ministry of Health Malaysia and Harvard T. H. Chan School of Public Health, Harvard University.

Sivasampu, S., Mohamad Noh, K., Husin, M., Wong, X. C. and Ismail, S. A. (2016). *Quality and Costs of Primary Care (QUALICOPC) Malaysia: Phase II – Private Clinics*. Putrajaya: Ministry of Health Malaysia and Harvard T. H. Chan School of Public Health, Harvard University.

Suleiman, A. B. (1999). *Keynote Address: Developing an Integrated Health System*. Putrajaya: Ministry of Health Malaysia.

Suleiman, A. B. and Jegathesan, M. (eds.). (n.d.). *Health in Malaysia: Achievements and Challenges*. Ministry of Health, Malaysia.

Tate Abdullah, M., Khoo, K. and Gabriel, S. (2005). *The History of Medicine in Malaysia: The Foundation Years*. Kuala Lumpur: Academy of Medicine of Malaysia.

Tey, N. P. (2007). The family planning program in Peninsular Malaysia. In W. C. Robinson and J. A. Ross, eds., *The Global Family Planning Revolution: Three Decades of Population Policies and Programs*. Washington, DC: World Bank, pp. 257–76.

United Nations Development Programme. (2005). *Malaysia: Achieving the Millennium Development Goals – Successes and Challenges*. Kuala Lumpur: United Nations Country Team, Malaysia.

Wong, J. H., Ng, C. and Su, T. (2019). Malaysia's rural health development: foundation of universal health coverage. *Jurnal Sains Kesihatan Malaysia*, 17(1), 31–41.

Wong, L., Wong, Y., Low, W., Khoo, E. and Shuib, R. (2008). Cervical cancer screening attitudes and beliefs of Malaysian women who have never had a pap smear: a qualitative study. *International Journal of Behavioral Medicine*, 15, 289–92.

SYSTEM ANALYSIS CASE STUDY 4.1: REAP-WISE: MALAYSIA'S EXPERIENCE IN INTEGRATED PRIMARY HEALTH CARE SERVICES

Shiang Cheng Lim, Safurah Jaafar and David T. Tan

Expansion of PHC Services Creates Integration Needs

PHC services in Malaysia were initially targeted at maternal and child health. As significant gains were made, the scope of services offered in primary health centres expanded, beginning in the 1980s (Figure 4-A), towards comprehensive primary health, targeting additional population age groups, namely adolescents, adults and the elderly. An unintended consequence of this expansion was the proliferation of parallel

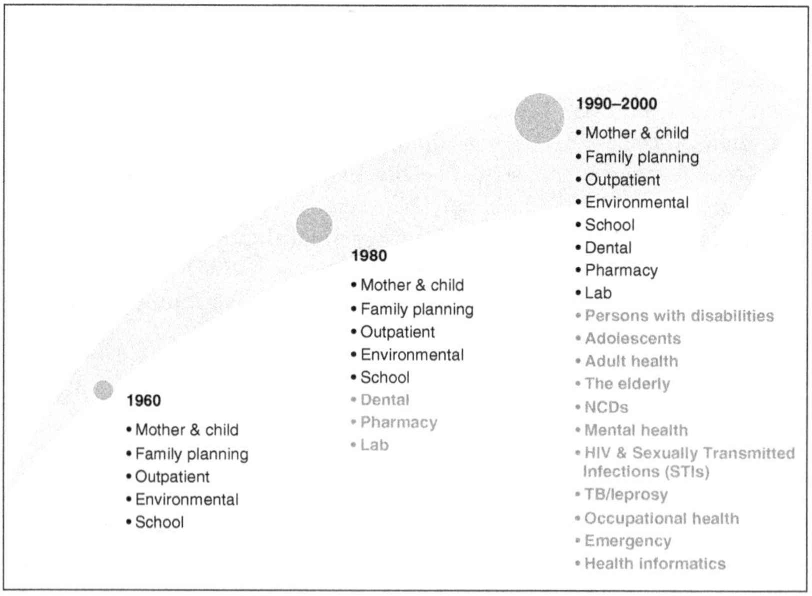

Figure 4-A Expansion of scope in PHC services.

clinics operating independently of each other and altering the ecosystems of PHC clinics. Monitoring indicators for these clinics were limited to the number of cases seen or managed, such that the impact on the overall function of PHC clinics was not monitored.

Forward-looking leaders in the MoH saw the need to integrate healthcare services to achieve continuous and co-ordinated care. The keynote address delivered by Tan Sri Dato' Dr Abu Bakar Suleiman, then MoH Director-General, at the Directors' Conference in 1999 emphasised that *'the successful health system of the future must be an* ***integrated system of networks*** *that share information and resources, and that is* ***responsive to social needs*** *as well as to advances in technology. There will be an emphasis on equity and the two key concepts would be* ***universal coverage*** *and* ***care according to needs****, consistent with available resources'* (Suleiman, 1999).

Reviewed Approach: Wellness, Illness, Support Services, Emergency Information (REAP-WISE) and Its Transitions

In response, the Reviewed Approach (REAP) of PHC, with a focus on Wellness, Illness, Support, Emergency and Information (WISE), was introduced under the Ninth Malaysia Plan (Jaafar et al., 2007). The goal of REAP-WISE was to integrate PHC clinics' operations to deliver comprehensive and continuous care and strengthen the focus on population-based outcomes (Box 4-A). Achieving this would require major disruptions to the existing operations of PHC clinics. While the silos created by the parallel clinics approach were unintentional and suboptimal, institutions, culture and practices in primary health centres had developed around the existing practice (Figure 4-B). This included: (1) locus of financing and decision-making, (2) scope and alignment of healthcare staff responsibilities, (3) professional development pathways, and (4) set-up of facilities and operations. These created an ecosystem that reinforced the status quo, requiring an ecosystems overhaul of these feedback loops to achieve the desired changes (Figure 4-C). Each of these four changes is described in the following sections.

Re-orientation of Policies on Delivery of Care (R1a and R2a)

Before REAP-WISE, MoH officers in the federal-level MoH programme, such as control of non-communicable diseases (NCD), who

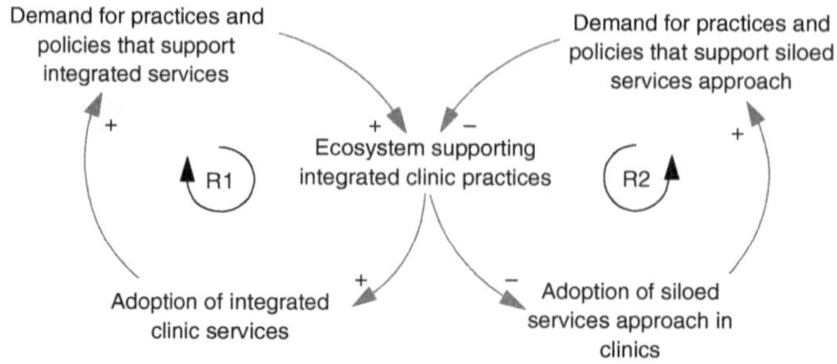

Figure 4-B Approaches to healthcare require supportive practices and systems, which in turn create an ecosystem that is aligned to and facilitates that approach. Shifting a healthcare approach requires comprehensive changes to the healthcare ecosystem.

were responsible for implementing new health initiatives had the direct authority to direct PHC clinics to implement these activities. While each new programme and clinic had funding and possibly staffing segregated from the PHC clinics' operations, they nonetheless competed for the clinics' resources and services, including funding, human resources, laboratory services, etc. This competition and lack of co-ordination led to duplication of efforts, inefficiency in care delivery and fragmentation of the system. An unintended consequence of this approach was the creation of 'little clinics' within a PHC clinic, such as an occupational health clinic, hypertension clinic, diabetes clinic, adolescent clinic, elderly clinic and more. Furthermore, these new initiatives were often not sustainable, creating further disruptions when they ended.

WISE addressed this by placing the Family Health Development Division (FHDD) in the federal-level MoH as the co-ordinator for the new initiatives and programmes and providing an overarching framework (Box 4-A) to rationalise the integration of new activities. All aspects of programmes carried out in PHC clinics, including funding, staffing, monitoring and reporting, were integrated into the existing primary care plan and framework and co-ordinated by the FHDD. This shift in implementation authority ensured that healthcare providers at the PHC clinics could deliver healthcare services seamlessly according to patients' needs and not merely to satisfy a particular programme target (Figure 4-C, R1a and R1b).

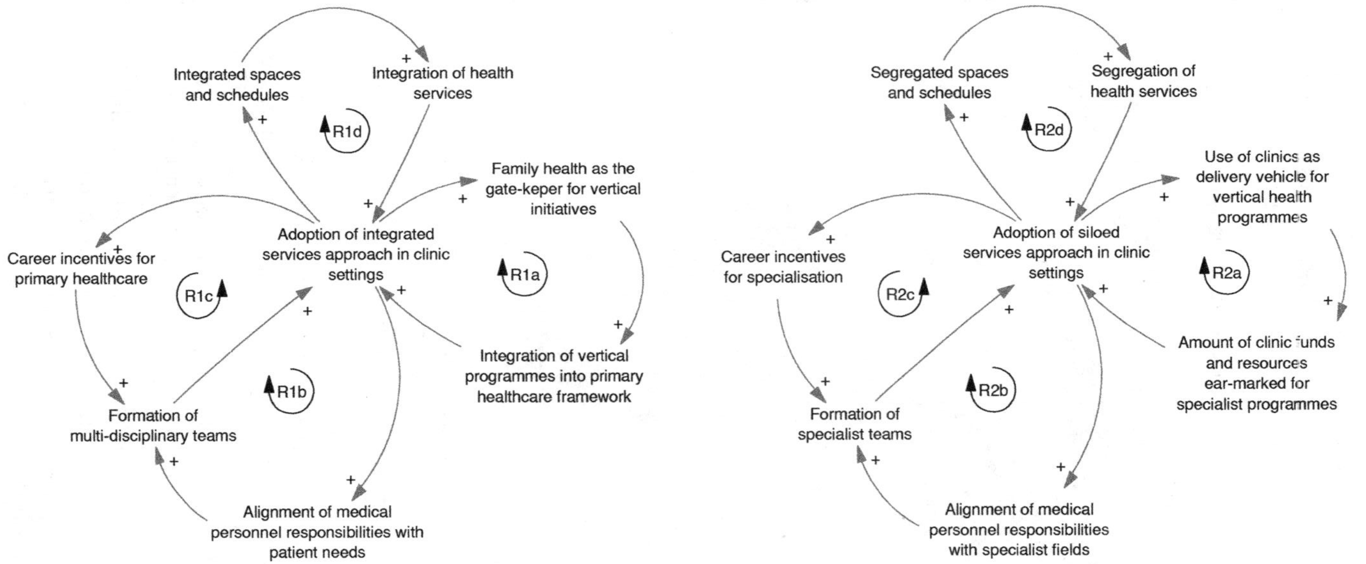

Figure 4-C Four changes to the PHC clinics' setting were critical to the ecosystem change: locus of financing and decision-making, scope and alignment of healthcare staff responsibilities, professional development pathways, and facilities and operations.

Box 4-A Reviewed approach of PHC: wellness, illness, support services and emergency information (REAP-WISE).

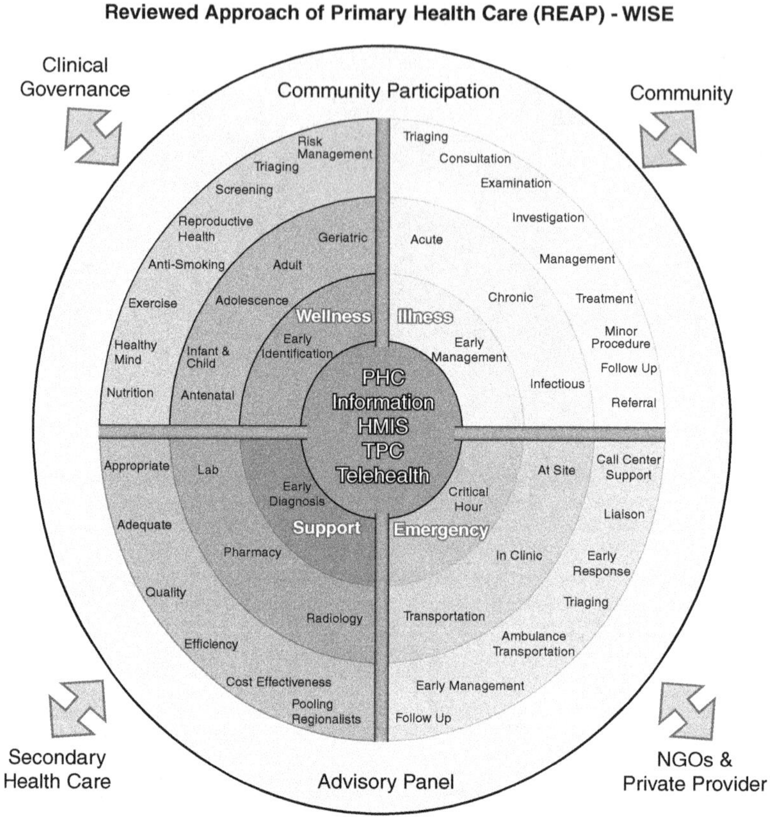

Figure 4-D Reviewed approach of primary healthcare (REAP-WISE). Source: Fadzil et al., 2018.

REAP-WISE is a framework for facilitating integrated service in the delivery of PHC. Central to the operation of the framework is the PHC information system, which includes the health management information system (HMIS) and Teleprimary Care (TPC) electronic system, which provides a monitoring mechanism that tracks achievements and gaps in service delivery.

Wellness covers the life course from antenatal through childhood and geriatric age for the early identification and management of medical conditions. All new activities that support wellness are mapped against age group needs. Teams oversee policy development for the collective activities for each age group to integrate workflow processes, accounting for monitoring indicators, quantity and quality of human resources required, diagnostic equipment, pharmaceutical requirements and physical space for these activities. These workflow processes are then phased in at clinics nationwide.

Illness covers early management of the acute, chronic and infectious conditions patients present with at clinics, as well as those in the community. Infectious diseases are assigned a separate patient workflow. Different processes for acute cases and chronic conditions were established to improve the utilisation of resources, waiting times and patient outcomes.

Support covers the three main diagnostic support arms (lab, pharmacy and radiology) in PHC. The level of support services has been reviewed to make it commensurate with the expansion and integration of PHC.

Emergency covers cases on site, in the clinic or during transportation to or from the clinic and hospitals, and it addresses the critical hour of management. Services have been expanded from stabilisation and referral to hospitals only to more extensive treatment services.

The framework is supported by strong community participation and the collaboration of an advisory panel. The relationship with the community, NGOs and private providers, secondary healthcare providers and strong clinical governance provide a robust foundation for strengthening PHC (Jaafar et al., 2007).

Alignment of Healthcare Providers' Responsibilities and Introduction of Multi-disciplinary Team (R1b and R2b) and Career Pathway Creation (R1c and R2c)

At the implementation level in health centres, REAP-WISE required the re-distribution of work and responsibilities among healthcare providers. The previous method of implementing new medical services and activities had created dedicated healthcare teams trained to deliver task-specific services, such as MCH services or specific clinical examinations or procedures. The implementation of REAP-WISE required the re-distribution of work among healthcare providers' responsibilities, equipping healthcare personnel to perform a much wider range of tasks, and the creation of multi-disciplinary teams to replace the previous specific-services-based setup. The multi-disciplinary teams include the FMS, medical officer, pharmacist, nutrition science officer, health education officer, counsellor officer, medical social worker, dietetic officer, dental officer, assistant medical officer, nurse, environmental health officer and radiographer (Family Health Development Division, 2015). The multi-disciplinary team shares the responsibility to provide comprehensive healthcare to the patient and family rather than focusing on specific ailments or types of service.

The creation of a workforce capable of handling the increased scope of services required a new level of qualifications. One such change was the adoption and rapid increase of allied health personnel with diplomas and degrees in primary health centre settings. Previously, many categories of allied health personnel, such as dietitians, nutritionists, etc., provided services only in hospital settings. Now, they provide services in health centres as well. Not only has the overall number of posts in each category increased in line with service expansion, but additional promotional posts and new categories of professional staff have also been created to increase the stature of primary healthcare careers.

On the other hand, for medical officers, practice in PHC clinics was seen as less desirable. Career incentives led to medical officers preferring to pursue specialist pathways leading to hospital practice. This created a situation where medical officers in PHC clinics were mainly those who were less experienced and less qualified and had high rates of turnover. To address this situation, a new category of specialist doctors with post-graduate training in Family Medicine (FMSs) was introduced in 1997 for PHC clinics. They were expected to improve the quality of PHC services by overseeing and managing patient care teams. The FMSs are given the same recognition and remuneration as hospital-based clinical specialists so as to retain their presence in the public PHC clinics.

Concerns that the new FMS category of specialists would overlap in function with other existing specialists led to initial resistance. However, a clear definition of the roles expected of them within the REAP-WISE strategy in PHC clinics managed to establish firmly the need for specialist doctors working at primary care level. FMSs are expected to provide leadership and set standards for clinical practice, encourage teamwork, emphasise integration of health screening and facilitate long-term treatment of chronic conditions. The creation of this cadre provided a career development pathway aimed at retaining experienced doctors in the primary care setting.

Two major constraints affect the implementation of this approach. First, the rate of production of FMSs is relatively slow (Ministry of Health Malaysia, 2007). In 2016, almost 20 years after the cadre was created, only about one-third of public sector primary health centres had an FMS (Ministry of Health Malaysia, 2016). Second, many FMSs, being trained by doctors from other specialities, lack the generalist approach required at primary care level.

Re-arrangement of Space and Scheduling (R1d and R2d)

The PHC clinics that were built during the previous three decades were no longer suitable, in terms of size or layout, for the increasing complexity of the new scope of services. PHC clinics had been taking over outpatient services from hospitals, and the rise of NCDs requiring long-term treatment, continuity of care, and preventative and health-promotional services made PHC clinics the appropriate locus for outpatient services. Indeed, this shift contributed significantly to the proliferation of health services and activities that necessitated the integrated framework provided through REAP-WISE. Apart from increased patient numbers, the rapidly increased scope of services required additional and more complex equipment, along with the space to house it.

The physical layout of PHC clinics posed a challenge to the goal of REAP-WISE. For historical reasons, maternal and child healthcare was frequently physically segregated from other outpatient care and integrated services, often having separate registration counters and even buildings, and were managed by a separate team. Furthermore, to achieve human resources efficiency, a 'clinic day' concept was adopted, in which specific days of the week were allocated for a particular population, health condition or service. Re-allocation of space and scheduling was necessary to achieve service integration and multidisciplinary teams.

Substantial resources were also invested in re-designing the physical spaces of PHC clinics to accommodate the new functions and workflows. An Operation Policy for Health Clinics (*Polisi Operasi Klinik*

Kesihatan) was developed as a guide for PHC clinics to implement REAP-WISE (Family Health Development Division, 2015). The 'daily clinic concept' was adopted, and individuals or patients with any condition can now access the services they need on any day of the week. Central and integrated registration and triage systems were put in place to support the holistic treatment of the patient.

Outcomes of the Transition

The PHC services in Malaysia have been evolving over the years. The initiation and adoption of REAP-WISE demonstrated the strong commitment of the MoH to improving the quality of care at PHC clinics by integrating preventive and health-promotional services with illness management. While there is a lack of evidence, such as impact evaluation, for outcomes of REAP-WISE, the QUALICOPC study showed that almost all health centres have services for early detection and health promotion as an integral component of cliniczal management, and user satisfaction is high (Sivasampu et al., 2015). Nonetheless, there are gaps in continuity of care (due to fast turnover of doctors), while the referral and counter-referral systems between primary and secondary/tertiary care need to be strengthened to ensure optimal patient outcomes.

Systems Lessons

Systems analysis identifies complex structural changes that are required for the successful implementation of apparently straightforward and rational changes in service provision. The transformation from silo-oriented service provision towards integrated, people-centred care required a fundamental change in mindset from healthcare providers that had to be supported by systemic change of the healthcare structure. Four categories of structural changes are discernible. First, re-alignment of managerial authority and responsibility to integrate initiatives aimed at different disease entities or population groups, re-designing of workflows, and development of explicit standards and operational guidelines. Second, human resources development, including definition of roles and re-distribution of workload, upgrading competencies, and creation of career paths. Third, re-design of the physical configurations of clinic spaces. Fourth, several of these required additional financial support, and this has been a limiting factor in the speed at which the full scope of transformation can be implemented nationwide.

References

Fadzil, F., Jaafar, S. and Ismail, R. (2020). 40 years of Alma Ata Malaysia: targeting equitable access through organisational and physical adaptations in the delivery of public sector primary care. *Primary Health Care Research & Development*, 21(e4), 1–8. DOI: http://10.1017/S146342362000002X

Family Health Development Division. (2015). *Operating Policy Guide for Health Clinics*. Putrajaya: Ministry of Health Malaysia.

Jaafar, S., Suhaili, M. R., Mohd Noh, K., Zainal Ehsan, F. and Lee, F. S. (2007). *Primary Health Care – Key to Intersectoral Action for Health and Equity*. Geneva: World Health Organization.

Ministry of Health Malaysia. (2007). *Annual Report 2007*. Putrajaya: Ministry of Health Malaysia.

Ministry of Health Malaysia. (2016). *Annual Report 2016*. Putrajaya: Ministry of Health Malaysia.

Sivasampu, S., Mohamad Noh, K. and Chin, M. C. (2015). *Quality and Costs of Primary Care (QUALICORP) Malaysia: Phase 1 – Public Clinics*. Putrajaya: Ministry of Health and Harvard T. H. Chan School of Public Health, Harvard University.

Suleiman, A. B. (1999). Developing an integrated health system. Keynote address, Ministry of Health Malaysia, pp. 27–34.

System Analysis Case Study 4.2: Managed Care Organisations as Intermediaries in the Provision of Healthcare by GPs to Private Sector Employees

Kuan Joo Lim, Milton Lum, Indra Pathmanathan and David T. Tan

Medical Care for Private Sector Employees

Private sector employers provide health and medical benefits to their employees as a job perk rather than as a means to achieve comprehensive medical coverage. No law requires them to provide benefits.[1] As such, the extent of healthcare benefits provided to private sector employees is dependent on the desire of employers to attract and retain

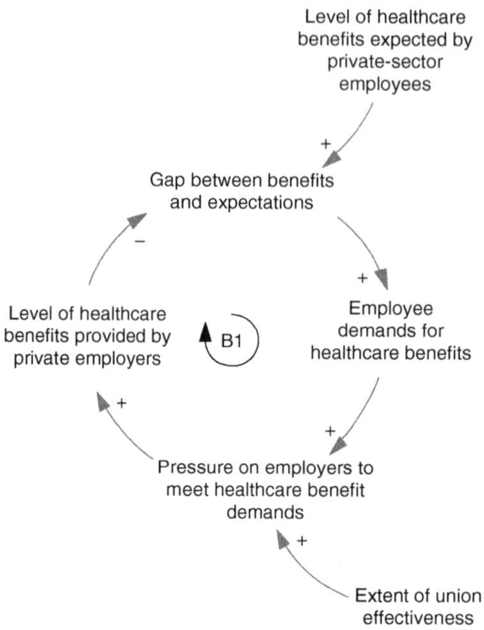

Figure 4-a Employee expectations and unionisation determine the effectiveness of their demands of employers for healthcare benefits.

employees and on employees' ability to unionise and make demands of employers (B1 loop) (Figure 4-a).

Before the advent of third-party administrators (TPAs), employers either appointed selected private GPs or private hospitals to medical panels to treat employees or purchased medical insurance policies that covered employees and dependents. Both approaches paid fees for services, with negotiated discount rates. The employers' human resources departments monitored and controlled utilisation, which was burdensome to the employer and in some cases very weak or absent. Consequently, the system was open to abuse, including the provision of services unrelated to the condition of the patient or the supply of non-therapeutic items. Some employers perceived that this could increase the costs to employers.

Third-Party Administrators (TPAs)

Consequently, TPAs, commonly known in Malaysia as managed care organisations (MCOs), have emerged and rapidly increased in number.

MCOs enter into contracts with employers to manage medical benefits on behalf of employees and charge the employer an administrative fee.[2] Their services include the selection of care providers, monitoring and managing utilisation, and providing recommendations to the employer on reimbursement to care providers. As they provide services to multiple employers, MCOs pool administrative and monitoring costs. MCOs surmised that they would be able to reduce the medical care costs for employers by negotiating with care providers. They reckoned that they would have strong bargaining positions, as each MCO would represent several employers, not an individual employer, while most GPs were individuals or small-group practitioners and were increasingly dependent on appointment to employer panels.

MCOs control progressively larger proportions of the patient market; currently, this is an estimated 10% of private sector employees (Malaysia Productivity Corporation, 2016). Unlike MCOs in the United States and Singapore (Phua, 2000), the contracts signed between MCOs and GPs in Malaysia are based on a fee-per-visit basis, rather than capitation. MCOs introduced practices to limit the pay-out of health benefits. Their high bargaining power enabled them to dictate conditions. The conditions they imposed have shifted hidden portions of the costs of healthcare to GPs and patients and have generated maladaptive responses with negative consequences for patient health.

A prime example is the common practice of capping reimbursement per visit regardless of the condition of the patient (Rauber, n.d.). These rates have often been set at the low end of the legally approved fee schedule, often alleged by GPs to be too low to cover costs, which affects their management of patients (Chan et al., 2016). Struggling to recover costs due to low caps per visit, GPs tend to limit the supply of medicines to a maximum of three days and medical leave to a single day. Thus patients often have to return to the clinic for multiple visits (Figure 4-b).

This passes the burden to the patients. At a minimum, patients suffer the inconvenience and costs of multiple visits for the same episode of illness. More worrying is that some patients are unable or unwilling to make the multiple visits necessary to receive the full scope of care. Patients with chronic illnesses that require long-term care and medication, such as hypertension and diabetes, are especially disadvantaged. As the benefit packages offer very limited benefits, the cost of any

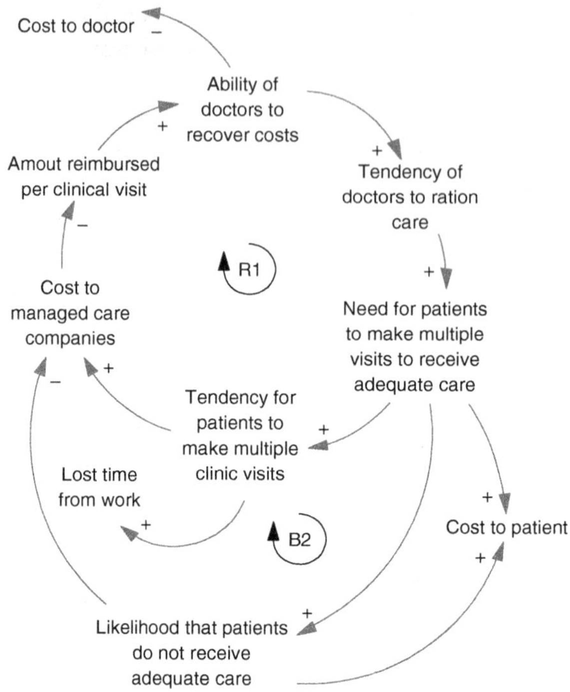

Figure 4-b MCO-imposed caps on per-visit reimbursement generates hidden costs through multiple visits (R1) or inadequate provision of care (B2). These hidden costs are largely borne by GPs, patients and employers instead of the MCOs.

complications arising from inadequate care is not usually passed on to the MCO or employer. Rather, the system shifts the costs (Figure 4-b: R1 loop) to patients in the form of out-of-pocket payments, loss of earnings and/or poor health.

Impact on Healthcare Delivery

MCOs' practices have impacted health benefits and delivery in many other ways. MCOs have attempted to bill doctors with administrative charges, although this move was aborted due to questions of legality. Employees are often not privy to the contract conditions and benefit limits, leading to higher expectations of medical care than the GP is allowed to provide (Chan, 2017). Many MCOs are financially

Supplementary Table 4-a ***Problems encountered by GPs who had contracts with MCOs***

GPs surveyed (n = 1,800)	Proportion of clinics (%)
Contract with MCOs	78
Interfered with choice of treatment and consultant	51
Reimbursement within 60 days	9
Received no reimbursement	69
Received less than invoiced	76

Source: Kenny et al., 2017.

mismanaged, delaying payments from 90 to 360 days, while several have collapsed, with unpaid debts (Malaysia Productivity Corporation, 2016) (Supplementary Table 4-a).

Impact on Employer–Employee Relationships

Apart from the impact on health delivery, the outsourcing of medical benefits to MCOs is likely to make employers less responsive to employee demands for health benefits (B1b loop, Figure 4-c). This is because MCOs have less incentive than employers to take care of employee welfare. Even when employees persuade employers of the need for better healthcare benefits, it takes time for managed care company contracts to be re-negotiated or for companies to switch MCOs (delay arrow in B1b loop). MCOs sell their services by highlighting the reductions in administrative and direct costs to employers, and both parties overlook the hidden costs to employees and employers. Therefore, employers do not have incentives to pressure MCOs into improving healthcare benefits (B3 loop). In the long term, this arrangement encourages employers to think of healthcare benefits only as a cost to the employer. Another predictable outcome is the likelihood that some of the healthcare costs of private sector employees will shift to the subsidised public sector. Patients who develop medical complications requiring expensive long-term management are likely to seek care in the public sector when they exceed the limits of their private sector benefits packages. Adequate management at an earlier stage could prevent such incidents.

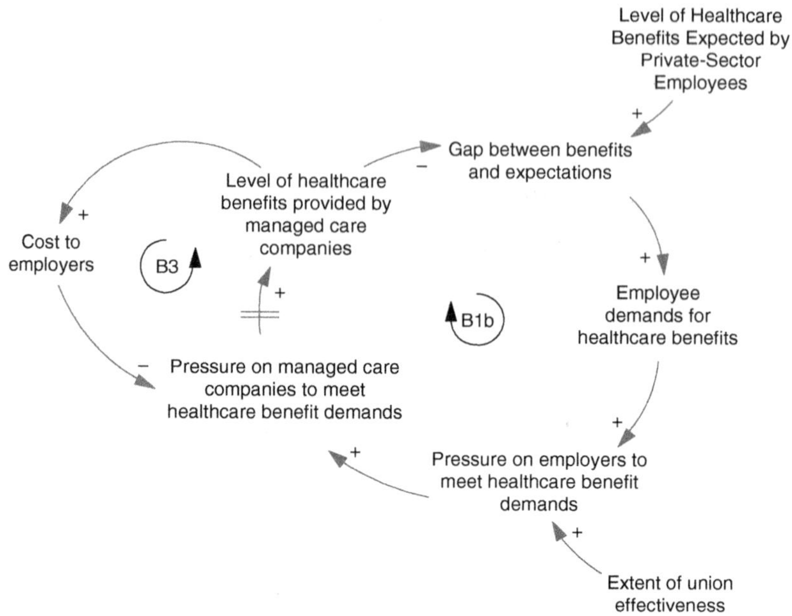

Figure 4-c Impact of MCOs on employer–employee–union dynamics changing the prior system (Figure 4-a) in ways that result in lower health benefits for the workforce.

Governance

Currently, the governance of MCOs is limited or absent. While the MoH assumes responsibility for healthcare providers and the Central Bank (Bank Negara) is responsible for insurance companies, neither is directly responsible for MCOs. The response from the government to the health challenges created by MCOs has been limited.

The MoH has attempted to use the existing Private Healthcare Facilities and Services Act of 1998 to address problems stemming from MCO practices. However, this has been limited to issuing guidelines to healthcare providers, has few enforcement provisions and does not recognise the weak bargaining position of GPs. Thus they are unable to address most of the key problems. Why has the government been reluctant to intervene more vigorously?

Systems analysis of the situation enables us to postulate two factors (Figure 4-d).

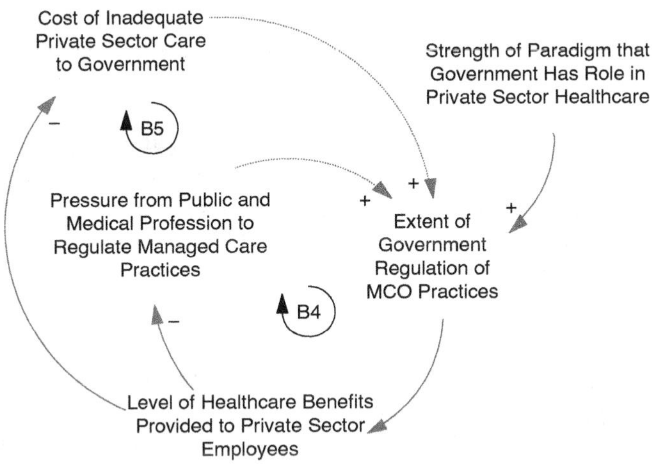

Figure 4-d Pathways toward government regulation of practices related to healthcare benefits are ineffectual due to limited ability of the public and medical professionals to organise (B4 loop) and lack of information on how these practices affect the burden on the public healthcare system (B5 loop).

First, pressure from the medical profession and the public is not sufficient to attract and compel a response from the government (the dotted arrow in B4 loop, Figure 4-d). The medical profession at large has only exerted concerted pressure in response to specific issues that affect daily practice, such as revision of the fee schedule and MCOs' attempts to impose administrative fees. The majority of GPs do not comprehend the full nature and implications of the involvement of third parties. Similarly, patients/the public are even less aware of the issues involved and how they affect their own families. Additionally, they lack the organising mechanisms to lobby for change. Thus political pressure is weak.

The other potential pressure that could energise regulator action is evidence that inadequate patient management due to MCO-imposed conditions results in increased costs to public sector services (the dotted arrow in B5 loop, Figure 4-d). This could happen due to patients choosing public sector care despite having MCO coverage, or after developing costly but avoidable complications as a result of MCO practices. Such information is not being tracked, however, and thus the government has low motivation to act, as it becomes aware of problems only from sporadic complaints either by patients or by doctors.

Systems Lessons

Problems arising from the behaviour and interactions of multiple actors are often perceived from the perspective of one or other of the actors, thereby producing finger pointing and blame games. Systems analysis supports a holistic perspective that re-frames these narratives in light of systemic structural issues. This often reduces points of conflict and increases the likelihood of finding win-win solutions.

References

Chan, H. K. P., Abdul Rasid, S. Z. and Md Husin, M. (2016). The impacts of Malaysian managed care on doctor–patient relationships, ethical practice of medicine, and quality of care: a study on primary care physicians' perception. *International Journal of Healthcare Management*, 9(2), 119–26.

Chan, P. T. (15 May 2017). *The Star Online*. Online letter. www.thestar.com.my/opinion/letters/2017/05/15/urgent-need-to-regulate-managed-care

Federation of Private Medical Practitioners Associations (FFPAM) Malaysia. (n.d.).

Kenny, K., Omar, Z., Kanavathi, E. S. and Madhavan, P. (2017). A study on the health economics of general practitioners in Malaysia: trends, challenges and moving forward. *International Journal of Public Health Research*, 7(1), 765–73.

Lee, S. (31 May 2018). Wrestling with managed health care. *The Star Online*. Online letter. www.thestar.com.my/opinion/letters/2018/05/31/wrestling-with-managed-healthcare

Malaysia Productivity Corporation. (2016). *Reducing Unnecessary Regulatory Burdens on Business: Medical Professional*. Kuala Lumpur: Malaysia Productivity Corporation.

Phua, K. L. (2000). HMOs and managed care in Malaysia: what can we anticipate from the experience of Singapore and the United States? *Journal Kesihatan Masyarakat Isu Khas*, 167–75. https://pdfs.semanticscholar.org/fbb8/61ce5ca77e7c3550e559d228aa866bda49b5.pdf

Rannan-Eliya, R. (2013). *Malaysia Health Care Demand Analysis*. Putrajaya: Ministry of Health Malaysia, Institute of Health Systems Research, Health Policy Research Associates, Institute of Health Policy.

Rauber, C. (n.d.). Managed Care Storms. *Modern Healthcare*. Online article. www.modernhealthcare.com/article/19991115/PREMIUM/911150323/managed-care-storms

Tharmaseelan, N. (6 March 2014). Update* Thank you, but it is still not enough, says MMA. *The Star Online*. Online article. www.theedgemarkets.com/article/update-thank-you-it-still-not-enough-says-mma

Notes

1. Except for the Social Security Act, which applies only to accident-related injuries among employees earning less than RM 2,000 per month.
2. Some MCOs also act as TPAs for insurance companies. They are not included in the scope of this paper.

5 Health Service Delivery

Secondary and Tertiary Care

INDRA PATHMANATHAN, MILTON LUM AND ANUAR ZAINI

5.1 Introduction

Secondary and tertiary care (STC) as discussed in this chapter are services provided in a facility such as a hospital or an ambulatory care setting by a specialist that require more specialised knowledge, skill or equipment than can be provided at the primary care level. The Alma Ata Conference on Primary Health Care (PHC) clearly defined the role of STC within PHC:

> [T]he support of other levels of the health systems is necessary to ensure that people enjoy the benefits of valid and useful technical knowledge that is too complex or costly to apply routinely through primary health care. The rest of the health system, therefore, has to be organised in such a way as to provide support for primary health care. (World Health Organization, 1978)

Mahler, the Director-General of the World Health Organization (WHO) from 1973 to 1988, furthered the concept, for example, by stating in 1980 that 'people in need must have access to skilled surgical care at first-line referral hospitals' (Mahler, 1980). The evolution of STC in the Malaysian health system demonstrates the challenges and achievements in implementing these concepts.

This chapter discusses how access to and quality of STC improved progressively in Malaysia during the 60 years since independence and how the system is currently grappling with the challenge of providing affordable, integrated, seamless care. It discusses the dynamic interactions of various components of the health system and their influence on STC and the influence of the larger Malaysian ecosystem, such as political, socio-economic, demographic and population behaviour.

The appendices provide details of the analysis that underpins the chapter. Appendix I illustrates the application of systems thinking, while Appendix II provides illustrative details of the interactions between components of the health system that are defined in the WHO health system 'building blocks' (see Chapter 1) and also the interaction between the health system and the larger ecosystem.

5.2 The Early Phase (1960s and 1970s): Increasing Access and Reducing Disparity

At independence, Malaysia inherited secondary care services consisting of 10 major hospitals and 56 district hospitals concentrated mainly in urban centres in the West Coast states of Peninsular Malaysia (Box 5.1). Many of them were dilapidated (International Bank for Reconstruction and Development, 1955). Doctors and nurses were in short supply, and specialists were almost entirely expatriate.

Box 5.1 Why were hospitals concentrated in the West Coast states during colonial days?

Pre-independence, specific demands led to the establishment of hospitals.

- The colonial government established hospitals for the healthcare of:
  - Colonial officers and their families
  - Government employees and their families
- Chinese charitable foundations established hospitals that provided a combination of western and traditional Chinese medicine (TCM), basically for the private sector Chinese employees.
- Corporate owners of rubber estates provided small estate clinics with a few beds for their employees, mainly Indians.
- Christian missionaries established a few not-for-profit hospitals, mainly as part of their charitable work.

The respective target populations resided mostly in the urban centres in the West Coast states of Peninsular Malaysia. The largely rural Malay population had limited access to secondary care services (Tate et al., 2005; Tung Shin Hospital, n.d.).

5.2.1 Socio-demographic Pressures and Political Forces

After independence, political and community forces dictated development. Policies aimed to improve health and social services and reduce disparity between regions and ethnic groups (Prime Minister's Department, 1961) (see Chapter 3). For secondary care, these policies translated into measures to increase access to secondary care by upgrading existing hospitals where necessary and providing hospitals in districts that had none. Each hospital provided inpatient as well as outpatient (ambulatory) care. Together with rural health centres and dispensaries that also provided outpatient services (see Chapter 4), outpatient services provided first-contact curative care. A report by the then Director-General of Health credits the 'widespread establishment of outpatient departments and referrals to hospitals' with 'provoking awareness of the rural people of the benefits of modern medical treatment' (Ismail, 1975).

5.2.2 Hospital Services Supported PHC

Even before Mahler's historic 1980 address, the Malaysian district hospitals were first-line referral facilities. They provided support for PHC through secondary care for patients referred from the national disease control programmes, such as those for malaria, tuberculosis (TB) and leprosy (see Chapter 6), and the rural health services, particularly for pregnancy, childbirth and illnesses of childhood (see Chapter 4). The staff of these hospitals were mainly nurses, midwives, medical assistants and junior doctors who were able to address emergencies, minor surgery, childbirth and its simpler complications, and the management of illnesses that required hospitalisation. However, the hospitals had neither the staff and the operating theatres for surgery nor the laboratory and imaging facilities for more complex secondary care. However, the district hospitals did have ambulances that provided free transport links on the one hand between district hospitals and state-level hospitals that had more sophisticated facilities and on the other hand between hospitals and health centres that provided PHC. These ambulances ferried patients, staff and laboratory samples and were crucial in providing the referral link between primary and secondary levels of care.

State-level hospitals provided, at a minimum, specialist care in internal medicine, surgery, obstetrics and gynaecology, paediatrics, and anaesthesia, with appropriate support services (Ismail, 1975). During this period, several existing, dilapidated state-level hospitals were re-built or refurbished. The government highly subsidised medical care in the public sector hospitals and therefore imposed only a nominal charge on patients at the point of care (see Chapter 9).

The development of STC required the production of a sufficient workforce of doctors and nurses. However, the number of doctors produced was small, as there was only one local medical school (later three) (see Chapter 8). Furthermore, there was no local facility for postgraduate specialist training for Malaysian doctors, and very small numbers were sent abroad annually for training, mainly to the United Kingdom. On their return, they slowly replaced the expatriate specialists and provided specialist services and leadership for the different clinical disciplines. However, the rapid production of nurses and assistant nurses (see Chapter 8) facilitated district hospitals in providing selected forms of secondary care services, and this, to some extent, compensated for the much slower production of doctors. Working alone or with doctors, medical assistants provided secondary care for communicable diseases and other common ailments that did not require specialist care. Nurses who had an additional year of midwifery training became nurse-midwives and, assisted by trained midwives, managed uncomplicated childbirth in all hospitals. The number of district hospitals increased, as did hospital beds for TB, leprosy and childbirth. The hospitals also provided support for the rapidly developing primary health care services (Box 5.2).

During the subsequent three decades, advances in medical products and the success of the disease control programmes enabled hospitals to reduce the beds provided for acute communicable diseases (Figure 5.1). Also, improved access to STC for pregnant women contributed to the reduction in maternal deaths and sustained the demand for institutional childbirth. Box 5.3 provides illustrative examples.

The rapid increase in the utilisation of hospitals throughout the country demonstrated the rising demand for STC (Figure 5.2).

Although the availability of hospital services increased, they barely coped with the rate of population increase. Fifteen years after independence, the disparity in the availability of STC between the more

Box 5.2 Secondary care–supported PHC

The hospitals provided support for the evolution of PHC. The key features were:

- Ambulances that provided free transport for patients, staff and laboratory samples between front-line PHC facilities, first-line hospitals and higher-level hospitals.
- Doctors (particularly obstetricians and paediatricians) who worked in state-level hospitals participated in training nurses and medical assistants who subsequently served in district hospitals or PHC facilities.
- This helped establish rapport and trust between staff at PHC and STC level, thereby fostering timely recognition and referrals from peripheral facilities. Such referrals were given priority in the larger hospitals, thereby enhancing the credibility of the staff in the peripheral facilities.

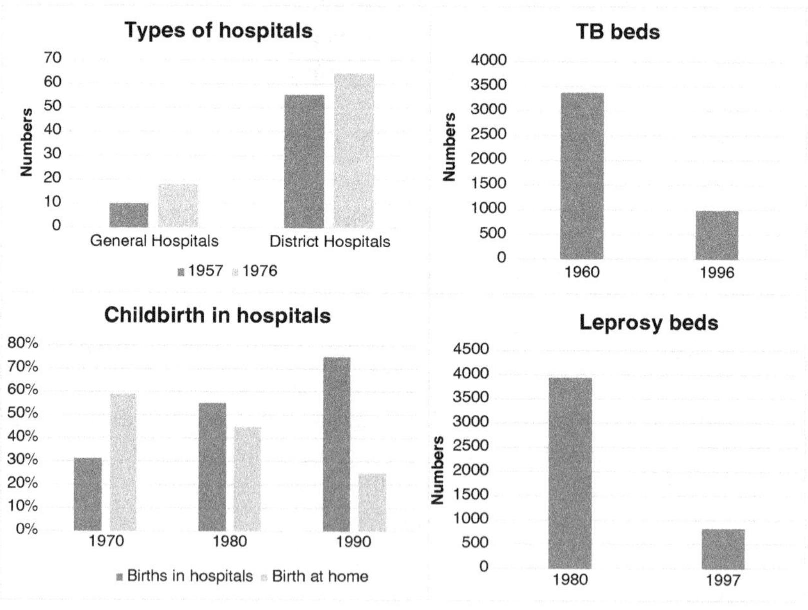

Figure 5.1 Evolving profile of types of hospitals, number of TB and leprosy beds, and childbirth in hospitals.
Source: Calculations by author based on data from Suleiman and Jegathesan (n.d.).

Box 5.3 Illustrative examples: STC-supported public health

Hospital care had a major role in reducing incidence of TB (Suleiman & Jegathesan, n.d.).

- In 1960, beds reserved for TB patients accounted for 25% of hospital beds.
- The aim of hospital management was to treat patients to render them non-infective before sending them back into the community.
- The advent of effective drugs shortened inpatient stay and enabled a reduction in TB beds by 1996.

Maternal deaths declined through an effective and credible system that provided safe childbirth care with timely access to STC (Pathmanathan et al., 2003).

- Essential obstetric care: By 1976, overwhelming demand for childbirth in hospitals resulted in maternity units having extremely high bed occupancy and turnover rates (Institute for Public Health, 1983).
- Emergency and comprehensive obstetric care: Ambulances from rural health centres and district hospitals provided prompt transport for the referral of patients with obstetric complications to hospitals with higher levels of care that included specialist care from obstetricians.[1]

urbanised West Coast states in the Peninsula and the less developed East Coast states[2] remained evident (Table 5.1).

5.2.3 Demand for STC Outstripped Supply

Financial and implementation capacity constraints slowed the progress of building new facilities. In addition, the limited production of doctors led to numerous vacancies in medical officer positions. Meanwhile, societal perceptions were changing. Increased access to hospitals led to a rapid increase in demand for STC. By the mid-1970s, public sector hospitals, particularly the larger ones, faced overwhelming demand, leading to overcrowding. A study of the utilisation of public sector hospitals (Institute for Public Health, 1983) delved into the phenomenon. It

Table 5.1 ***Regional disparity in secondary care in different regions of Malaysia, 1972***

	Acute beds (per 1,000 population)	Admissions (per 1,000 population)
West Coast states	2.16	37.25
East Coast states	1.69	22.50
Peninsular Malaysia	2.08	34.58
East Malaysia	1.94	n.a.
Malaysia	2.05	n.a.

Source: Calculations by author based on data from Abdul et al. (1974).
n.a. – not available

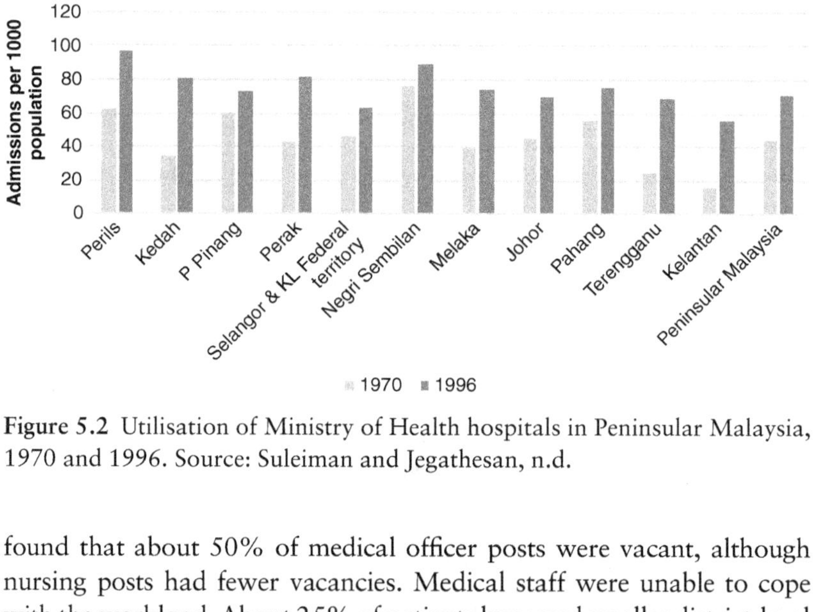

Figure 5.2 Utilisation of Ministry of Health hospitals in Peninsular Malaysia, 1970 and 1996. Source: Suleiman and Jegathesan, n.d.

found that about 50% of medical officer posts were vacant, although nursing posts had fewer vacancies. Medical staff were unable to cope with the workload. About 25% of patients bypassed smaller district-level hospitals to seek care in larger hospitals. The commonest reason reported was the lack of surgical services. Patients were also dissatisfied with ward conditions (Public Health Institute, 1983). Many doctors, frustrated with conditions in the public sector, resigned to become general practitioners in the private sector. This contributed to the continued shortage of doctors in public sector hospitals (see Chapter 8 re. brain drain).

Moreover, it exacerbated the difficulty of improving access in the less-developed states in the country.

5.2.4 STC in the Private Sector Began to Grow

In the meantime, the number of local doctors with specialist qualifications increased steadily, and they served under high pressure in the overcrowded larger hospitals. Recognising the strong demand for more comprehensive STC and exhausted by the high pressure of work, several of them resigned from the public sector during the late 1970s and established four private for-profit hospitals in the largest towns on the West Coast. These hospitals began the trend for the growth in private sector STC in response to demands by the more affluent section of the community for more personalised care and better 'hotel-type' facilities. By 1980, 4.3% of all hospital beds were in private hospitals.

The few established non-governmental organisation (NGO) hospitals that predominantly served the ethnic Chinese population had close links with Chinese traditional practitioners and provided some traditional Chinese medicine (TCM) services.

Supplementary Table 5-a in Appendix II summarises the interaction between different elements in the health system and the larger ecosystem as they influenced the evolution of STC during the first post-independence phase.

5.3 The Second Phase (1980s and 1990s): Drive for Better-Quality Access

5.3.1 Political, Socio-economic and Professional Influences

During the 1980s and 1990s, the population became increasingly urban, and literacy rates and socio-economic status rose, as did the population's expectations of healthcare. Many communicable diseases decreased, while non-communicable diseases (NCDs) increased. A dual thrust in health policy governed the development of STC. The first was the continued struggle to improve equitable access to STC. The second was to respond to the rising expectations of the community and of professional bodies to provide higher-quality care, including care that was:

a. clinically more sophisticated, with more equitable access to surgical interventions, and
b. better quality in terms of
   - effective outcomes,
   - higher client satisfaction, and
   - improved use of resources.

5.3.2 More Sophisticated Clinical Care

Doctors with postgraduate training in specific disciplines had the higher level of competency required to provide comprehensive STC. Specialist training in local universities for doctors began during the 1980s (see Chapter 8) and resulted in the availability of larger numbers of doctors with specialist qualifications and the establishment of a wider range of specialised units in public sector hospitals. This, in turn, triggered the upgrade of laboratory and imaging services and the training of allied health personnel, such as medical laboratory technologists and radiographers, for these services (see Chapter 8). To promote equitable access to specialised medical services, the Ministry of Health (MoH) adopted a regional development approach. State-level and larger district hospitals were categorised into three levels, with Level 1 consisting of five basic medical specialities, Level 2 having six additional specialities and Level 3 consisting of further specialisation within narrow fields of the more general disciplines (such as cardiologists and neurologists within the broader field of internal medicine). Every region in the country had one hospital of Level 3 status and at least one with Level 2 status. The availability of speciality services increased from 12 units per million people in 1970 to 16 units in 1997 (Table 5.2).

With the growing numbers and types of specialist qualifications from various universities and countries, professional bodies and the MoH were concerned about safeguarding the standards of competence to preserve the quality of care. This triggered governance actions in the form of the establishment of procedures for credentialing and certifying specialists (see Chapter 8).

The increasing numbers and types of sophisticated clinical services required better laboratory and imaging services. For example, Table 5.3 illustrates that the upgrading of laboratory services in

Table 5.2 ***Increased availability of specialist care in MoH hospitals, 1970–1997***

	1970	1980	1997
Peninsular Malaysia	121	220	283
Sabah	4	15	31
Sarawak	5	25	38
All	130	260	352
Units[1] per million people	12.1	18.9	16.2

Source: Suleiman and Jegathesan, n.d.

[1] One unit was equivalent to one or more specialists in a specialist unit or department.

Table 5.3 ***Laboratory services increased in sophistication in tandem with the availability of specialist clinicians***

Type of facility	Laboratory service
No specialist doctor	Medical laboratory technologist (MLT)
Specialist doctor but no pathologist	Biochemist OR microbiologist plus MLT
Pathologist	Biochemist AND microbiologist plus MLT
National referral level (IMR)	All plus sub-speciality pathology services
IMR and universities[2]	Very sophisticated tests and research

Sources: Suleiman and Jegathesan, n.d.;

[2] Institute of Medical Research (IMR).

MoH hospitals was linked to the type of specialist services available. The upgraded laboratory services required the appropriate allied health personnel with higher levels of qualifications. Appropriate training programmes and deployment strategies came into place.

The developments required higher investment and maintenance costs. The rising gross domestic product (GDP) facilitated the financing of these investments.

Figure 5.3 provides a summary of the dynamic interactions in the health system as it moved towards providing more sophisticated clinical services.

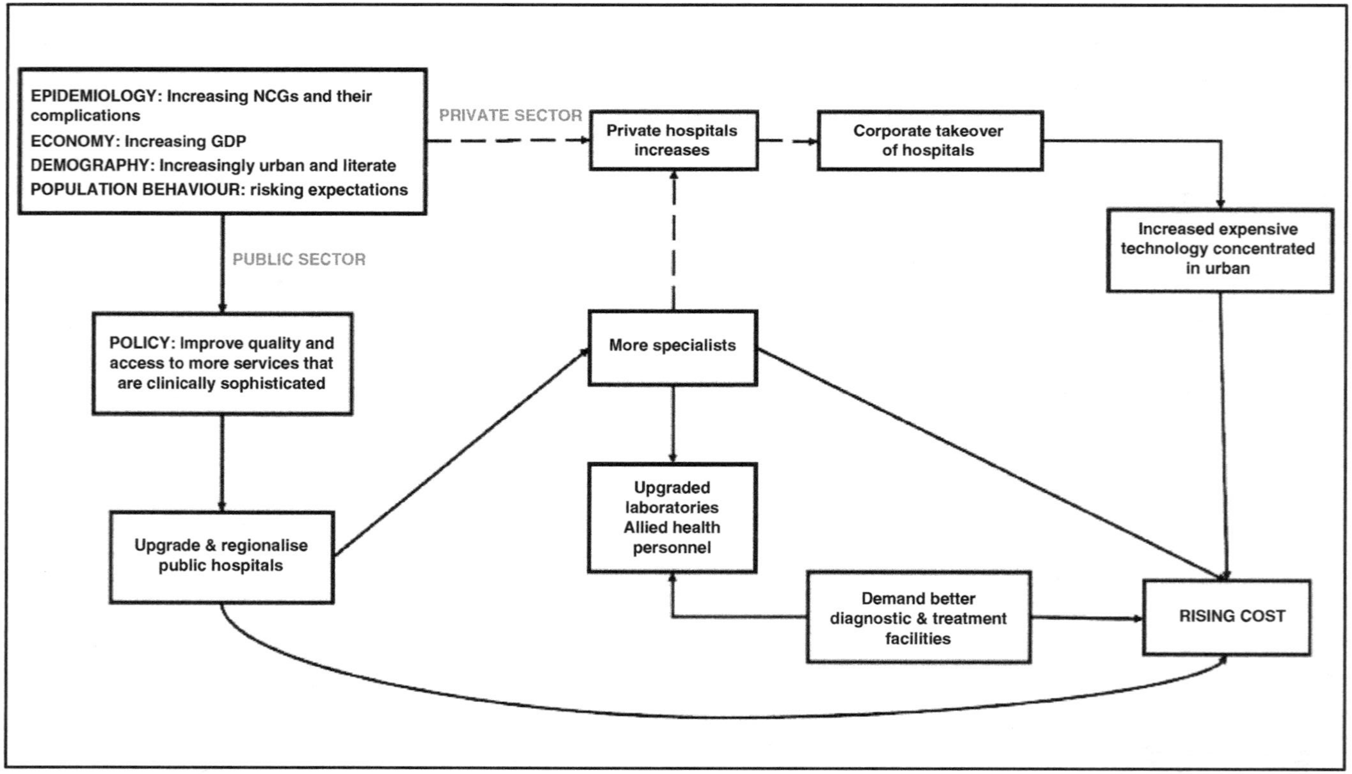

Figure 5.3 Dynamics of providing more sophisticated clinical services.

5.3.3 Private Sector

Meanwhile, there was high demand for STC in the private sector, leading to the rapid expansion of hospitals (Table 5.4). In 1997, 70% of private hospitals were small, with less than 20 beds, and several were in buildings not suited for providing quality care (Suleiman & Jegathesan, n.d.). Concerned about quality standards, the government enacted legislation (Government of Malaysia, 1998) with stringent standards for physical structure and with corporate and clinical governance, including procedures for monitoring quality (see Chapter 12). Enforcement began in 2006.

In parallel, there was high demand for care by the few specialist doctors who had established larger private hospitals since the mid-1970s. Recognising a good business opportunity, corporate entities moved in and bought up the larger hospitals. Corporate ownership led to a change in philosophy. While catering for the demands of the well-to-do who could afford private sector fees, these hospitals now also paid serious attention to profit margins. Their expansion and development plans reflected this change (Suleiman & Jegathesan, n.d.). One evident feature was the trend towards the rapid proliferation of higher-cost technology in the private sector as compared to the public sector (Table 5.5). These hospitals were concentrated in the wealthier regions of the country, thereby challenging the objective of equitable development.

The MoH initiated health technology assessment (HTA) as a means of rationalising the acquisition of newer technology. The output of the

Table 5.4 ***Rapid growth of private hospitals, 1980–1996***

Year	No. of private hospitals	No. of private hospital beds	Private as % of all hospitals	Private as % of all admissions
1980	50	1,171	4.3	n.a.
1985	133	3,559	11.5	12
1990	197	4,675	14.1	14
1996	215	7,417	20.4	17.2

Source: Suleiman and Jegathesan, n.d. (data extracted from Ministry of Health Malaysia annual reports 1981, 1985, 1990 and 1996).
n.a. – not available

Table 5.5 ***Distribution of high-cost imaging technology in MoH and private hospitals, 1997***

	MoH hospitals			Private hospitals		
	CT scan[1]	Mammogram[2]	MRI[3]	CT scan[1]	Mammogram[2]	MRI[3]
Nine West Coast states	11	10	2	42	32	11
Three East Coast states	3	3	0	2	1	0
Sabah and Sarawak	3	2	0	4	3	2

Source: Suleiman and Jegathesan, n.d.

[1] Computed tomography (CT): The MoH had one unit per state except for the capital city, Kuala Lumpur, which had four units. Private hospitals had 17 units in Kuala Lumpur and neighbouring Selangor and 10 units in Penang.

[2] Mammogram: The MoH had one unit per state except Kuala Lumpur, which had three units. Private hospitals had nine units in Kuala Lumpur, four units in Selangor and eight units in Penang.

[3] MRI – magnetic resonance imaging.

HTA unit provided input into the formulation of policies in the public sector and provided the basis for the development of clinical practice guidelines (CPGs), purchasing decisions, drug regulation and health-related advertisements (Roza et al., 2019). However, there is limited information on whether the private sector uses the HTA information for guiding the development of technology.

5.3.4 Quality: Monitoring and Improving Outcomes

In the late 1980s, the government of Malaysia initiated nationwide efforts to improve quality in the public sector. The MoH was one of the agencies that led the way in implementing the national call to action. The National Quality Assurance Programme (QAP) of the MoH spear-headed efforts to instil concern for quality as a culture at all levels of the organisation. It established a system for the explicit measurement of outcomes. This included monitoring performance trends in clinical

Box 5.4 System observations: shifting the healthcare burden to the private sector

The development of the private health sector in Malaysia is an example of how solutions to health system challenges can create long-term, irreversible changes to the system. Rising demand for more sophisticated medical care in the 1960s and 1970s led to a gap in public hospital capacity as limits in financial and human resources caused capacity to lag behind demand. This demand continued to increase in the 1980s and 1990s, so the rise and rapid expansion of private sector hospitals was welcomed by the public sector. While the private sector alleviates the burden of the public sector in some ways, it has become apparent that it draws medical practitioners, especially specialists, away from the public sector (Figure 5.4). The public sector thus has had to invest further resources and change policies to retain medical practitioners to keep up with healthcare demands.

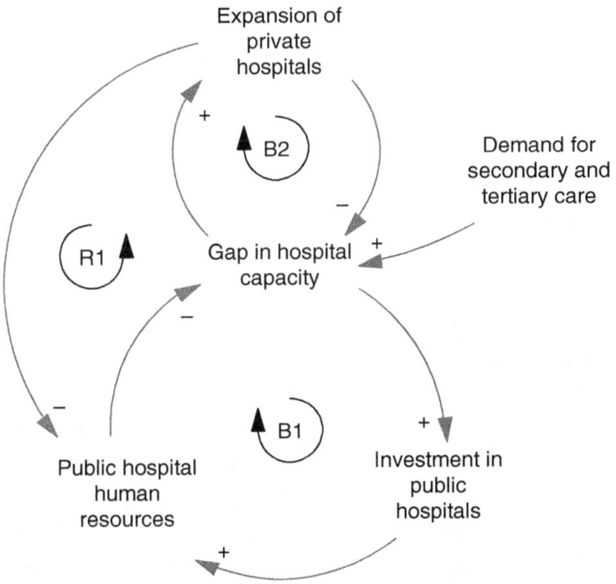

Figure 5.4 Rising demand for medical care outpaced public hospital resources, creating a gap in public sector capacity (B1). The expansion of private sector hospitals (B2 loop) offered a means of bridging this gap with private sector resources. However, private healthcare has drawn on

Caption for Figure 5.4 (cont.)

medical personnel from the public sector, becoming another source of pressure on public sector capacity (R1 loop). This is a well-known system archetype known as 'shifting the burden', in which actions taken to address the outcomes of a problem (a gap in hospital capacity) can exacerbate the underlying causes of that problem (public hospital human resources).

Private sector care has become corporatised and supporting structures such as private insurance and medical tourism have been developed, creating a self-sustaining industry. In addition to health workforce challenges, the resulting fragmentation of healthcare providers and financers has created challenging tensions regarding the locus of responsibility for the provision and payment of healthcare.

care, patient satisfaction and better use of resources (physical, time and human resources). Box 5.5 provides illustrative examples.

The thrust for improving clinical outcomes (Figure 5.5) provided a fillip for strengthening clinical governance measures such as the development and use of Clinical Practice Guidelines (CGPs) and for stronger implementation of existing initiatives such as clinical audits and mortality reviews. It also contributed to improving the quality of data for health information (see Chapter 10), particularly in terms of accuracy of International Classification of Diseases (ICD) coding and timeliness of data, as healthcare providers became aware that this had a critical impact on the accuracy of indicators that measured performance.

The drive for improved outcomes of clinical care led to the establishment of disease registries for selected conditions such as end-stage renal disease (ESRD) and cancer, which are managed largely at the secondary care level. The registries are meant to provide information on disease conditions as well as treatment effectiveness and cost. The National Renal Registry, established in 1993, was a trailblazer, and it monitors trends in the quality, cost and effectiveness of different modalities of care for ESRD (Lim & Lim, 2004). It provided the data for a cost analysis that enabled the move to public–private partnership in the provision of dialysis (Lim et al., 1999).

Box 5.5 Key features of the QAP for secondary and tertiary healthcare services in the public sector

Approach and Methods

- Peer groups in each clinical discipline or hospital management group selected performance indicators.
- The MoH collected data on the indicators, analysed and rank-ordered the performance of individual hospitals, and shared the results with all stakeholders.
- Outliers were encouraged to analyse the factors contributing to their status and were helped to remedy issues.
- Performance trending enabled peer groups to discard or replace indicators periodically to move towards more sensitive and specific monitoring of performance outcomes.

Examples of Results

- Improvement in the management of acute myocardial infarction.
- Decreases in waiting time to see doctors and decreases in rejection rates for X-rays and laboratory specimens.
- Improved client satisfaction with counter services (e.g. pharmacy counters), cleanliness and facilities. For example, a small district hospital (Kuala Krai) in one of the more disadvantaged states won a national award for improving the quality of public services in 1995.

Source: Suleiman and Jegathesan, n.d.

The thrust for better outcomes in patient satisfaction and use of resources (Figure 5.6) stimulated a need for increased managerial competence at all levels of the MoH system (see Chapter 8). It also facilitated the growth of team approaches and the use of health systems research as a management and problem-solving tool. Hospitals won national 'quality awards' for improving client satisfaction and reducing waiting times (Suleiman & Jegathesan, n.d.). Budgeting systems were modified to provide greater authority to hospital managers to manage funds more flexibly to respond to local requirements (see Chapter 9).

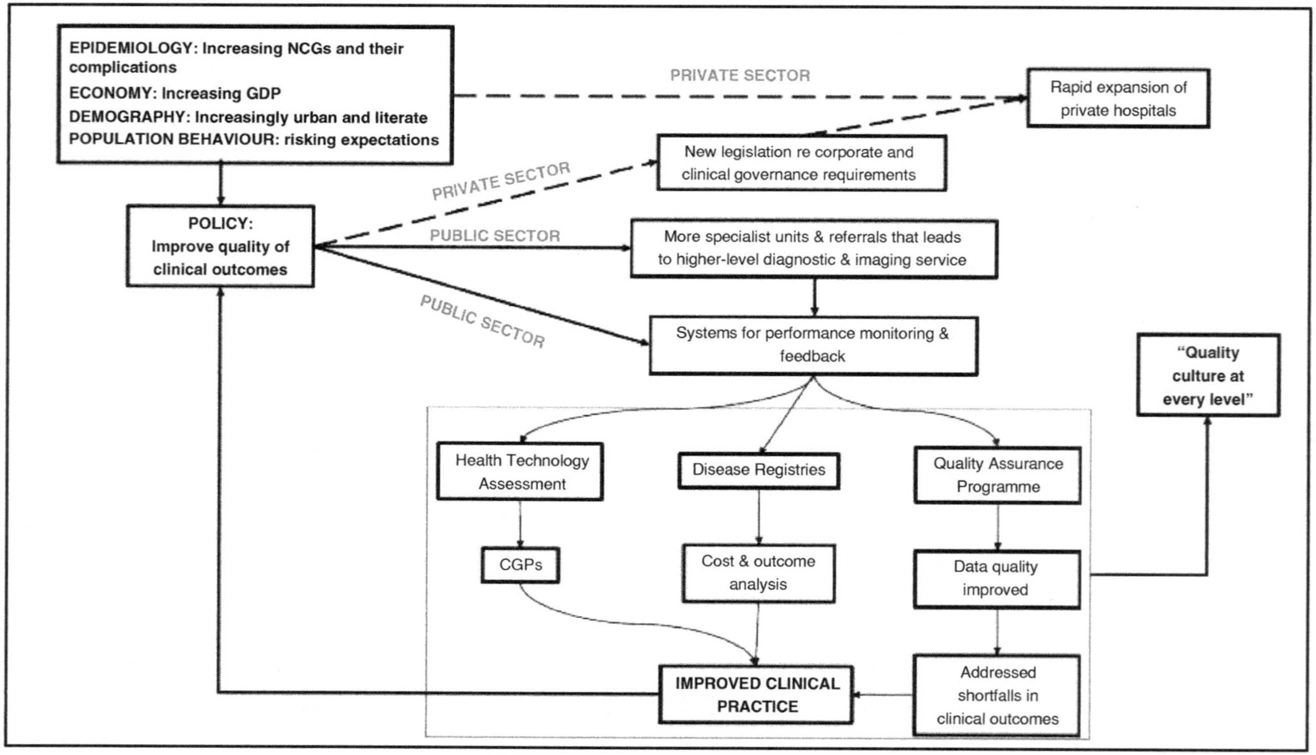

Figure 5.5 Dynamics of improving clinical outcomes and establishing a quality culture at every level.

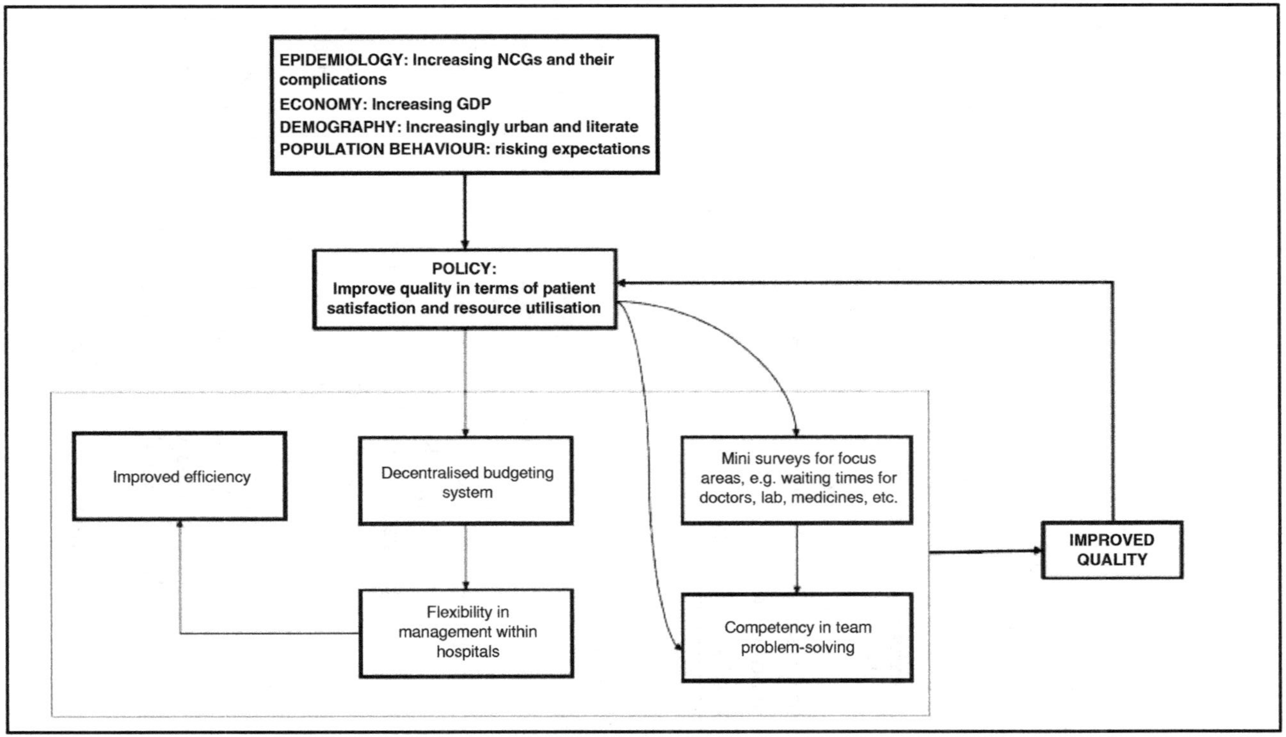

Figure 5.6 Dynamics of improving resource utilisation and client satisfaction.

Box 5.6 Further initiatives strengthened STC support for PHC

Various measures contributed to further strengthening supportive linkages between hospitals and PHC. Examples include:

- In the QAP, the senior specialist for a discipline in each state hospital took responsibility for improving quality in all facilities. For example, the state obstetrician provided oversight to prevent maternal deaths throughout the state and therefore liaised with district hospitals, health centres and rural midwives, resulting in an improvement in the early detection and referral of complications of pregnancy (Pathmanathan et al., 2003).
- Outbreaks of dengue fever resulted in health inspectors visiting hospitals for epidemiological investigations that strengthened communication between STC and PHC. Conversely, health centres and private clinics used clinical management protocols originating from hospital-based specialists to improve the quality of care for dengue patients.

However, as the MoH was part of a larger public sector system, there were constraints. The degree of flexibility that could be decentralised was limited due to financial rules and regulations (see Chapter 9). Similarly, as all MoH staff are part of the federal civil service (see Chapter 8), constraints arose. For example, nurses with training and credentials in one discipline had to move to another discipline to further their careers (Institute of Health Management, 2006).

The thrust for improved resource management extended to strategies for improving the maintenance of building structures and biomedical equipment in public sector hospitals. New posts were created for hospital-based engineers, and maintenance services were outsourced to private contractors, with hospitals retaining oversight of the contractors' performance (see Chapter 7). Performance indicators of quality applied not only to clinical aspects of care but also to support services.

The quality-improvement measures also strengthened support from STC for PHC services (Box 5.6).

Supplementary Table 5-b in Appendix II summarises the interactions in the health system during the 1980s and 1990s (STC development Phase 2).

5.4 The Third Phase (2000–Present): Drive towards Integrated, Seamless, High-Quality Care

By the beginning of the new century, the health sector still fell short of the requirements for equitable access to quality care and faced several threats that arose from the 'successes' of the past. Section 5.4.1 and Case Study 5.1 analyse the interactions between various components of the health system in addressing some of these threats.

The major threats to STC included:

- In the public sector: Rapid increase in specialisation that led to increasing fragmentation at both clinical and managerial levels.
- In the private sector: Increasing conflict between medical care as a profit-oriented business and as a service to improve the welfare of the community.
- Conflicts arising from the changing roles in the public–private split of the health sector.

The health sector reactions to these threats included (but were not restricted to):

- Implementing organisational change to address the fragmentation that arose from increasing trends of specialisation.
- Taking advantage of changes in medical technology and information communication technology (ICT) to improve access and efficiency while reining in escalating costs.
- Attempting to use governance measures (legislation, financing) to address the challenges and governance gaps in dealing with the public–private split in the health sector.

5.4.1 Organisational Change

In the public sector, there was a rapid increase in the types of clinical specialist units in hospitals and the types of programme management units at national and state levels. Communication between organisational units deteriorated. For example, communication between hospitals and health centres, between hospital outpatient departments (OPDs) and wards, between departments of different clinical disciplines and between district- and state-level hospitals became more challenging (Suleiman, 1999). This carried threats to continuity of care for patients, such as people with diabetes, who required long-term care provided by more than one unit or department. There was an increased risk of worse-than-desired health outcomes.

Furthermore, duplications and missed opportunities could contribute to organisational inefficiencies, resulting in rising healthcare costs. The MoH addressed these threats by adopting a policy to 'provide seamless health care by enhancing integration' (Institute for Public Health, 1999). Two structural changes of note occurred. First, OPDs in hospitals were moved to health centres that were better suited to provide seamless preventive, promotive and curative care in ambulatory settings and adopted family and community perspectives in the management of conditions such as NCDs. Chapter 4 discusses this initiative.

The second strategy was the formation of hospital clusters to increase access to specialist care and improve utilisation rates in the smaller hospitals. The smaller hospitals had quite a large proportion of unused beds. During the previous experience in the regionalisation approach to improving access, specialists visited non-specialist hospitals. This proved unsuccessful because the smaller hospitals did not have the facilities or expertise to support specialist care. In the cluster concept, a major hospital that had a wider range of specialities formed a cluster with a few neighbouring smaller hospitals to share financial and human resources and equipment. In addition, there was an initial investment in upgrading surgical facilities in the smaller hospitals. Specialists and their teams from the lead hospital provided specialist services at the smaller hospitals on a visiting basis, negating the need to move patients to the major hospital. There was investment in training to enable staff at the smaller hospitals to provide adequate follow-up care after the team from the major hospital had provided treatment. The pooled budget enabled the sharing of financial and material resources such as drugs, equipment and travel between hospitals. There was shared responsibility for the outcomes of care. Initial assessment indicated that these measures provided relief from overcrowding in the major hospital and increased patient satisfaction and cost–benefit in the management of patients with moderate or

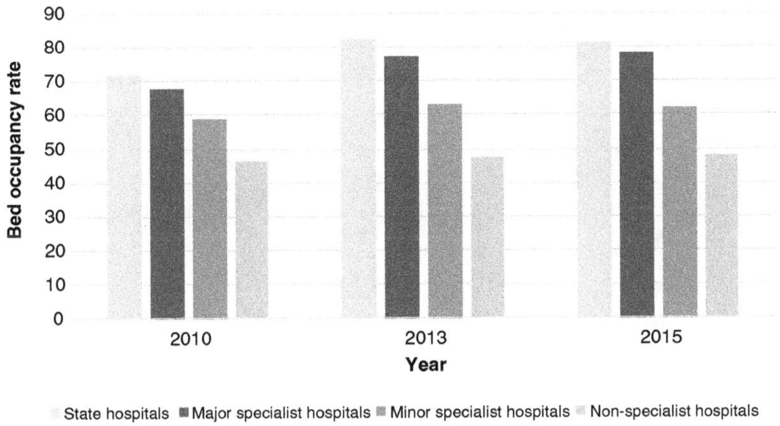

Figure 5.7 Bed occupancy rates in MoH hospitals. Source: Ministry of Health Malaysia, 2016.

serious illness. However, they did not increase utilisation rates in the smaller hospitals. Barriers to sustaining or expanding this initiative included frequent transfer of human resources from the smaller hospitals, thus negating the investment in upgrading capacity, and inadequate recognition of the need for the initial additional investment to prepare smaller hospitals to support specialist services (Institute of Health Management, 2016; 2017). Despite these initiatives, the bed occupancy rates of the non-specialist hospitals remained below 50% (Figure 5.7).

Another aspect was the strengthening of referral systems. Within the MoH system, there were continuing efforts to improve the logistics and communication of referral between primary, secondary and tertiary care levels. This included strengthened governance through the refinement and clarification of procedures, expected standards and technological support, for example, through the telehealth project that enables real-time sharing of patient data between primary and secondary care levels, thereby contributing to quality of continuity of care for patients (Allaudin, 2014). However, other major challenges arose from governance features of the health system. For example, patients have direct access to specialist clinics in both the public and private sectors without going through primary care (Yiengprugsawan et al., 2017). This encourages the bypassing of primary care. In addition, in the private sector, it encourages rivalry between primary and specialist care providers, which in turn raises the risk of failure to refer conditions that require higher levels of competency.

Table 5.6 *Referral experiences reported by doctors in public sector health centres*

	% of doctors stating		
	Usually or always	Occasionally	Seldom or never
Received patient records from previous doctor	36.2	51.6	12.2
Used referral letters	99		
Received feedback from specialists	19	30.8	50.2
Obtained discharge report from hospital	27 (within 4–14 days)	13.7 (delayed > 14 days)	58.4

Source: Sivasampu et al., 2015.

Additionally, evidence suggests that feedback and referral from STC services to primary care in the public sector is weak (Table 5.6). In larger hospitals in both the public and private sectors, rules for referral between different clinical disciplines have not been established.

5.4.2 Advances in Technology

Technological advances affected STC profoundly. Two illustrative examples of the influence of technology on the delivery of STC services are telemedicine and day-care surgery.

Telemedicine. The MoH introduced telemedicine progressively in several districts to increase access and reduce costs by enabling specialists based at larger centres to provide, through teleconsultation, diagnostic and therapeutic advice to doctors in hospitals without specialists or with a smaller range of specialities. Yusof and colleagues (2002) noted that the introduction of telemedicine increased access to STC in the remote, less accessible districts, such as Beluran and Kudat in Sabah, and led to 'enhanced diagnostic options, cost savings and better health outcomes'. By 2016, telemedicine had increased to 45 facilities and 60 stations throughout the country (Ministry of Health Malaysia, 2016). Nurazean and colleagues reviewed the system and noted that the careful selection of sites influenced the usefulness and utilisation of teleconsultation. Factors in selection included sufficient need (i.e. inadequate expertise to address more complex problems), difficulty of physical access between sending and receiving sites, and discipline-specific guidelines (certain types of cases in each discipline are not amenable to distance guidance) (Nurazean et al., n.d.).

Day-care surgery. Medical technology such as advanced anaesthesia and minimally invasive surgical technologies contributed to increasing numbers of day surgeries, for example, cataract surgery, laparoscopy and other endoscopies that require short postoperative monitoring and recovery. The evaluation of day-care cataract surgery has been possible through the National Eye Database, which facilitates the tracking of trends in cataract surgery. It provided evidence that contributed to improvements in techniques and technology, as reflected in practice patterns and outcomes (Table 5.7). An increasing proportion of cataract surgery is being performed as day-care, and visual outcomes have improved, indicating improved quality. The success of the day-care centres for cataract surgery is attributed also to the availability of

Table 5.7 *Cataract surgery profiles, 2002 and 2015*

	2002	2015
Cataract surgeries	12,798	44,534
Day-care (%)	39.3	69
Phacoemulsion (%)	39.7	87.9
Local anaesthesia (%)		93
Intraoperative complications (%)		5
Unaided visual outcome 6/12 or better (%)		55.1
Visual outcome 6/12 or better with spectacles (%)	87	95.1

Source: Goh et al., 2016.

dedicated, well-trained teams of care providers, including highly trained technicians, nurses, specialists and sub-specialists.

Day-care surgery provides an avenue for controlling costs (*Evaluation of Specialist Complex and Ambulatory Care Centre*, 2018). The day-care centre approach has also contributed to integrated care, with specialists from various disciplines managing patients simultaneously. For example, endocrinologists managing problematic diabetic patients have simultaneous input from orthopaedic and vascular surgeons.

5.4.3 Governance Challenges Affecting STC

The fragmentation of clinical services is a challenge and occurs in at least at two dimensions of care. First, several clinical disciplines are compartmentalised into sub-specialties. Sometimes, the care provider in sub-speciality case management focuses on managing a particular condition to the exclusion of co-morbid conditions. At STC level, technological advancement necessitates multidisciplinary knowledge and skills and cross-discipline references in managing patients with multiple complex conditions. Care providers require the appropriate skills and attributes to recognise when cross-referral is needed and facilitate seamless cross-referrals. Currently, in Malaysia, the policies regarding intra- and inter-facility referral in both public and private sector clinical networks are weak.

Furthermore, clinicians at the PHC level who refer patients to STC levels of care have difficulties identifying the person or department in the hospital responsible for co-ordinating and facilitating such referrals. This situation is further complicated because patients have the right to an informed choice

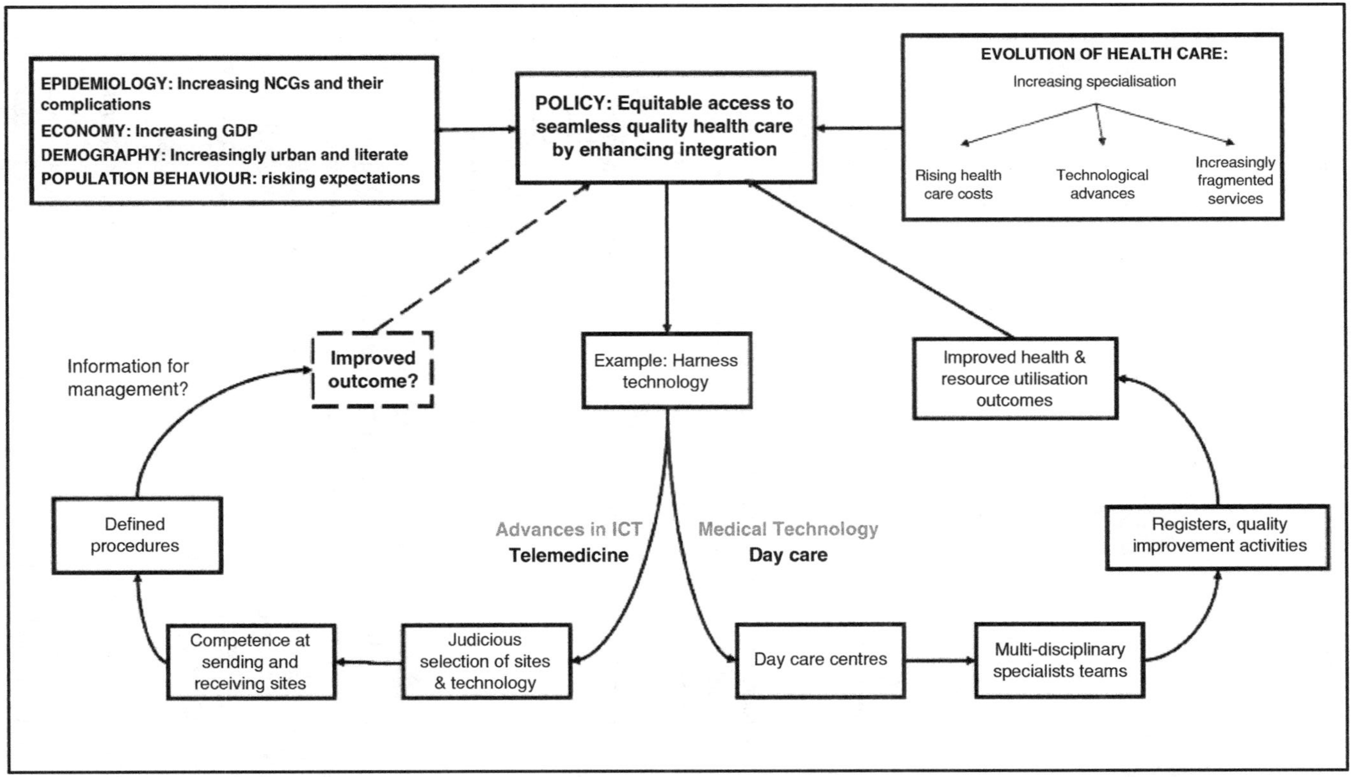

Figure 5.8 Harnessing technology to improve access to seamless, integrated care.

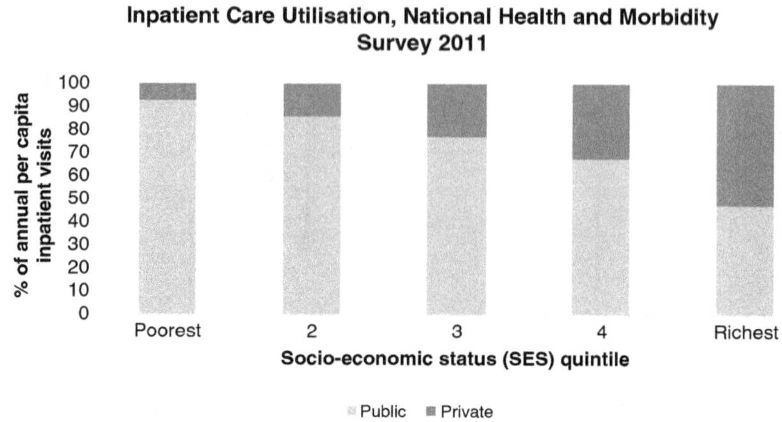

Figure 5.9 Composition of inpatient care utilisation in public and private sector by socio-economic status. Source: Health Policy Research Associates et al., 2013.

of providers that best fit their medical needs and financial resources. Many patients prefer to skip primary care facilities in favour of direct appointments at specialist clinics or hospitals, particularly in the private sector.

Another dimension of the fragmentation of STC is evident in the fragmentation between the public and private sectors, each with different payment and governance mechanisms. During the first 40 years after independence, the fragmentation of the Malaysian healthcare sector into the public and private sectors appears to have assisted the national goal of improving equitable use of healthcare (see Chapters 3 and 9). Although the schism created tensions, particularly in the distribution of the workforce, it also enabled the wealthier segment of the population who could afford it to utilise private hospitals, thereby facilitating the public sector to provide for the lower-income groups (Figure 5.9) (Health Policy Research Associates et al., 2013).

However, during the most recent two decades, fresh challenges have surfaced, arising largely from underlying governance structures and financing mechanisms.

5.4.4 Rising Expenditure and Costs in the Private Sector

STC accounts for a relatively high proportion (55%) of total health expenditure (THE) (Table 5.8). Private sector hospitals are responsible

Table 5.8 ***Expenditure on and utilisation of public and private hospitals, 2012 and 2017***

	2012	2017
THE	42,764	57,361
% public	55.85	51.15
% private	44.1	48.85
All hospitals as % of THE	51	55
Private hospital % of THE	18	24
Public hospital % of THE	33	31
Discharges from private hospitals (millions)	0.9[1]	1.05
Discharges from public hospitals (millions)	2.2[1]	2.49

Source: Ministry of Health Malaysia, 2012; 2018a; 2018b.
[1] 2012 data are reported as admissions, not discharges.

for an increasing proportion of THE, while that of public hospitals remains steady. Yet the proportion of discharges/admissions in public versus private hospitals has not changed during the period 2012–17. It is not clear whether the increased private sector expenditure is due to investment in new hospitals, investment in new expensive technology or higher cost of patient care.

Clients are unhappy with the price of care in private hospitals (Table 5.9).

The rapid increase in high-cost technology experienced in the previous decade continues in the private sector (Table 5.5 and Table 5.10). Are considerations of cost recovery from expensive investments driving costs in private hospitals? In the private sector, there is no overriding guide on technology acquisition. In contrast, reports from health technology assessment guide the acquisition of new technology in the public sector. Furthermore, in contrast to the public sector, no one monitors the outcomes of care and appropriateness of care across the private sector network of hospitals. Therefore, there are no feedback loops to trigger action from the authorities or to modify the behaviour of the providers themselves.

In theory, the public sector could harness the excess capacity of technology in the private sector, and there are examples of small-scale efforts in this direction, such as the purchase of PET (positron emission tomography) and CT (computed tomography) services. Case Study 5.1

Table 5.9 *Client satisfaction with hospital services*

	% good to excellent	
Satisfaction with	Public	Private
Provider behaviour		
Ability to give diagnosis	77	78
Clarity of explanation	77	79
Courtesy and thoughtfulness	78	82
Characteristics of selected system		
Private room/fewer people	44	72
Allowed to choose doctor	45	73
Waiting time to see doctor	38	72
Amount of time spent by doctor	65	75
Treatment charges	80	27
Outcome of service	78	80
Overall impressions	81	72

Source: Institute for Public Health, 2015.

Table 5.10 *Selected medical technology in hospitals, 2011*

	Public	Private
CT scanners[1]	52	91
MRI[2]	30	75
PET[3]	2	6

Source: Sivasampu et al., 2013.
[1] CT – computed tomography
[2] MRI – magnetic resonance imaging
[3] PET – positron emission tomography

on renal dialysis illustrates how imaginative cross-funding between public and private sectors can release private funds for initial investments and facilitate partnership for better utilisation of available private sector healthcare resources. However, this model has not been replicated, suggesting that there are serious barriers, perhaps related to finance and governance.

As there is no social health insurance and individual out-of-pocket payment is the largest source of private sector funding (Table 5.11), no organised entity has the responsibility of influencing rising costs.

Table 5.11 ***Sources of funds in the private sector, Malaysia, 2012 and 2017***

Sources of funds	2012	2017
Private sources of financing (RM million)	19,795	28,023
Out of pocket (%)	78.7	77
Private insurance (%)	14.0	15
MCOs[1] (%)	0.5	4
All corporations (%)		5

Source: Ministry of Health Malaysia, 2018b.
[1] MCOs – managed care organisations

Private insurers are most likely to protect their own pockets by limiting payouts and passing on additional costs to individuals.

Managed care organisations (MCOs) increased their participation in managing private sector funds from 0.5% to 4% of private funds over five years (2012–2017) (Table 5.11). This has raised further issues of gaps in governance, as illustrated by Case Study 4.2 on MCOs.

5.4.4.1 Governance Gaps

Corporate entities whose main driver is profit margins have acquired most of the private hospitals. Ironically, many of the larger corporations are government-linked agencies (Chan, 2015), but they too share the profit motive. Additionally, encouragement of health tourism is now a major government policy (Economic Planning Unit, 2010), thereby accentuating the profit motive in the private sector. Thus, while public sector healthcare retains its vision and goal of the health and wellbeing of the population, including addressing inequitable access, quality, safety and cost containment, the private sector strives for return on investment and competitiveness. There is a conflict in vision about whether healthcare is for social wellbeing or whether it is a business enterprise. Few governance measures are in place to address evident or emerging conflicts.

5.5 Conclusion

In summary, STC evolved in response to demand from the larger ecosystem. Economic growth, population behaviour and epidemiological patterns created political pressures that in turn resulted in an ever-increasing demand for STC.

The evolution of STC has moved from selective secondary care towards increasingly comprehensive STC, moulded by the ability of the health workforce to respond to demands for higher levels of competency and by the availability and capabilities of medical products and technology.

The enabling sub-systems, in turn, have influenced the evolution of the healthcare provider sub-system. These sub-systems comprise finance (sources, recipients and modalities), health information (availability, quality and use) and governance (managerial competence, governance structures and legislative tools) that either enable or constrain the evolution of the provider sub-system.

The outcomes of the healthcare system, in turn, have influenced the larger ecosystem, thereby creating a perpetual cycle (Figure 5.10).

5.6 Key Messages from Malaysia's Experience

5.6.1 *What Went Well?*

- STC ability to respond to people's desire for more sophisticated care and professionals' desire to provide the best care available effectively and efficiently. Key factors are:
  - Human resource production and use (see also Chapter 8).
  - Systematic quality improvement strategies.
  - Use of technology assessment for production of practice guidelines.
- Investment in strengthening management, and decentralised decision-making.

5.6.2 *What Did Not Go So Well?*

- Smaller hospitals built in response to public demand for access remain underutilised because of system inability to provide the human and material resources expected by the public.
- Rapid growth of private sector STC affects social efficiency of STC and PHC.
- In private sector STC: Unresolved conflict between the interests of shareholders (of companies owning hospitals) and those of stakeholders (users, providers, public sector STC).

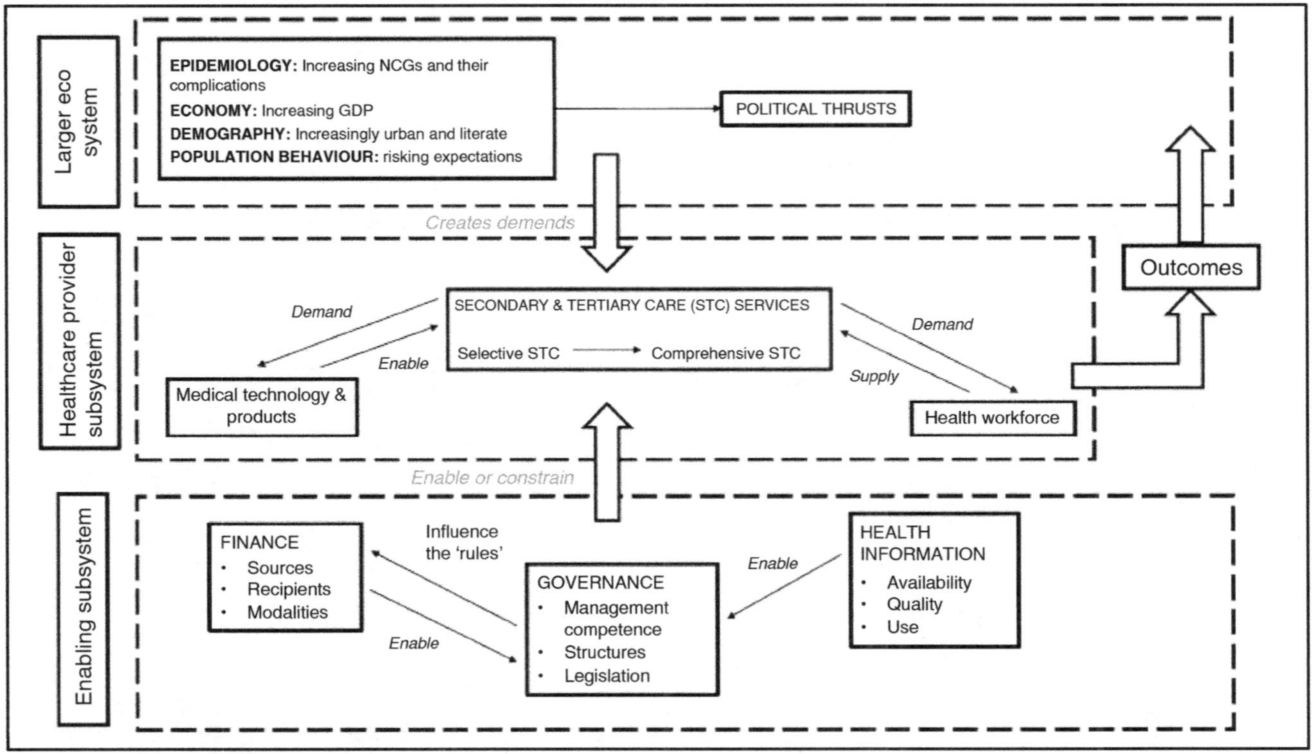

Figure 5.10 Interactions between the larger ecosystem and the healthcare provider sub-system with its enabling or constraining sub-systems.

5.6.3 Trends and Challenges

- The rapid growth of technology will require adaptive responses from STC and its support systems (e.g. day-care surgery).
- Increasing medical tourism will have an impact on the health system and the societal view of healthcare.

References

Abdul, W., Gurmukh, S. and Matinez, E. (1974). *Regionalisation of Patient Care Services in Malaysia*. Kuala Lumpur: Percetakan Semanjung Malaysia.

Allaudin, F. S. (2014). *National eHEALTH: Moving towards Efficient Healthcare*. Putrajaya: Ministry of Health Malaysia.

Chan, C. (2015). State and healthcare in Malaysia: provider, regulator, investor. In Chan, C. K., *The Third World Resurgence*. Third World Network, pp. 34–7. www.twn.my/title2/resurgence/2015/296-297/cover06.htm

Economic Planning Unit. (2010). *Tenth Malaysia Plan 2011–2015*. Putrajaya: Economic Planning Unit.

Evaluation of Specialist Complex and Ambulatory Care Centre. (2018). Kuala Lumpur: Hospital Kuala Lumpur.

Goh, P. P., Aziz Salowi, M., Adnan, T. and Sa'at, N. (eds.). (2016). *The 9th Report of the National Eye Database 2015*. Kuala Lumpur: Clinical Research Centre Network.

Government of Malaysia. (1998). *Private Healthcare Facilities and Services Act 1998 (Act 586)*. Kuala Lumpur: Percetakan Nasional Malaysia Bhd.

Health Policy Research Associates (HPRA), Institute for Health Systems Research (IHSR) and Institute for Health Policy (IHP). (2013). *Malaysia Health Care Demand Analysis: Inequalities in Healthcare Demand and Simulation of Trends and Impact of Potential Changes in Healthcare Spending*. Putrajaya: Institute for Health Systems Research, Ministry of Health Malaysia.

Institute for Public Health. (1983). *Study of Hospital Utilization in Peninsular Malaysia*. Putrajaya: Ministry of Health Malaysia.

Institute for Public Health. (1999). Executive summary. In *Proceedings of the Directors Conference: Challenges in Optimization of Health Services through Enhancing Integration*. Putrajaya: Ministry of Health Malaysia, p. 13.

Institute for Public Health. (2015). *National Health and Morbidity Survey*. Setia Alam: Institute for Public Health.

Institute of Health Management. (2006). *Health Workforce Development Strategies in the Public Sector*. Setia Alam: Institute of Health Management.

Institute of Health Management. (2016). *Cost Effectiveness Analysis of Cluster Hospital Pilot Projects in Transforming the Healthcare Service in Malaysia*. Putrajaya: Ministry of Health Malaysia.

Institute of Health Management. (2017). *Compilation of Reports of the Hospital Cluster Implementation*, 2nd ed. Putrajaya: Ministry of Health Malaysia.

International Bank for Reconstruction and Development. (1955). *The Economic Development of Malaya*. Washington, DC: International Bank for Reconstruction and Development.

Ismail, A. M. (1975). *Our Health Services in the Seventies*. Kuala Lumpur: Ministry of Health Malaysia.

Lim, T. and Lim, Y. (2004). *11th Report of the Malaysian Dialysis and Transplant Registry 2003*. Kuala Lumpur: National Renal Registry.

Lim, T. O., Lim, Y. N., Wong, H. S., Ahmad, G., Singam, T. S., Morad, Z. et al. (1999). Cost effectiveness evaluation of the Ministry of Health Malaysia Dialysis Programme. *Medical Journal of Malaysia*, 54(4), 442–52.

Mahler, H. (1980). *Address to the XXII Biennial World Congress of the International College of Surgeons: Surgery and Health for All*. Mexico City: World Health Organization.

Md. Yusof, F. A., Goh, A., Lim, T. O., Ahmad, G. and Morad, Z. (2007). *Cost Utility Analysis of the Ministry of Health Dialysis Programme*. iHEA 2007 6th World Congress: Explorations in Health Economics paper. Online paper. https://ssrn.com/abstract=993376

Ministry of Health Malaysia. (2012). *Health Facts (2012)*. Putrajaya: Ministry of Health Malaysia.

Ministry of Health Malaysia. (2016). *Annual Report*. Putrajaya: Ministry of Health Malaysia.

Ministry of Health Malaysia. (2018a). *Health Facts (2018)*. Putrajaya: Ministry of Health Malaysia.

Ministry of Health Malaysia. (2018b). *Malaysia National Health Account: National Health Expenditure Report 1997–2017*. Putrajaya: Ministry of Health Malaysia.

Nurazean, M., Win, K. T., Singh, H. S. S. and Masrom, M. (n.d.). *Teleconsultation Service Utilization Key Issues in the Context of Malaysia: An Organizational Perspective*. Online report. https://people.utm.my/nurazean/files/2017/10/Nurazean_ICCRIS_2019.pdf

Pathmanathan, I., Liljestrand, J., Martins, J. M., Rajapaksa, L. C., Lissner, C., de Silva, A. et al. (2003). *Investing in Maternal Health: Learning from Malaysia and Sri Lanka*. Washington, DC: World Bank.

Prime Minister's Department. (1961). *Second Malaya Plan 1961–65*. Kuala Lumpur: Government of Malaysia.

Prime Minister's Department. (1966). *First Malaysia Plan 1966–1970*. Kuala Lumpur: Government of Malaysia.

Roza, S., Junainah, S., Izzuna, M. M. G., Ku Nurhasni, K. A. R., Mohd Yusof, M. A., Noormah, M. D. et al. (2019). Health technology assessment in Malaysia: past, present and future. *International Journal of Technology Assessment in Health Care*, 35(9), 446–51.

Sivasampu, S., Arunah, C., Kamilah, D., Fatihah, M., Goh, P. P. and Hisham, A. N. (eds.). (2013). *National Healthcare Establishment and Workforce Statistics (Hospital) 2011*. Kuala Lumpur: Clinical Research Centre, Ministry of Health Malaysia.

Sivasampu, S., Lim, T. O. and Hisham, A. N. (eds.). (2011). *National Healthcare Establishment and Workforce Statistics (Hospital) 2008–2009*. Kuala Lumpur: Clinical Research Centre, Ministry of Health Malaysia.

Sivasampu, S., Mohamad Noh, K. and Chin, M. C. (2015). *Quality and Costs of Primary Care (QUALICORP) Malaysia: Phase 1 – Public Clinics*. Putrajaya: Ministry of Health and Harvard T. H. Chan School of Public Health, Harvard University.

Suleiman, A. B. (1999). Keynote address. In *The Directors Conference: Challenges in Optimization of Health Services through Enhancing Integration. Proceeding of the Conference*. Putrajaya: Institute for Public Health and Ministry of Health Malaysia, pp. 27–34.

Suleiman, A. B. and Jegathesan, M. (eds.). (n.d.). *Health in Malaysia: Achievements and Challenges*. Putrajaya: Ministry of Health Malaysia.

Tahrani, P. K., Sivasampu, S., Goh, P. P., Faizah, A. and Hisham, A. N. (eds.). (2012). *National Healthcare Establishment and Workforce Statistics (Hospital) 2010*. Kuala Lumpur: Clinical Research Centre, Ministry of Health Malaysia.

Tate, D. J. M., Khoo, K. K. and Gabriel, S. (2005). *History of Medicine in Malaysia: The Foundation Years*. Kuala Lumpur: Academy of Medicine of Malaysia.

Tung Shin Hospital. (n.d.). *Annual Report (Various Years)*. Kuala Lumpur: Tung Shin Hospital.

World Health Organization. (1978). *Primary Health Care: Report of the International Conference on Primary Health Care, Alma-Ata*. Geneva: World Health Organization.

Yiengprugsawan, V., Healy, J., Kendig, H., Neelamegam, M., Karunapema, P. and Kasemsup, V. (2017). Reorienting health services to people with chronic health conditions: diabetes and stroke services in Malaysia, Sri Lanka and Thailand. *Health Systems & Reform*, 3(3), 171–81.

Yusof, K., Neoh, K. H., Hashim, M. A. and Ibrahim I. (2002). The role of teleconsultation in moving the healthcare system forward. *Asia-Pacific Journal of Public Health*, 14(1), 29–34.

Appendix I

Systems Thinking Analysis of STC

David T. Tan and Indra Pathmanathan

In the 1960s and 1970s, demand for more sophisticated medical care increased. Unable to obtain such care in clinics and smaller hospitals, patients bypassed those in favour of major hospitals, which became overcrowded. Public hospital capacity lagged behind demand, creating a gap that reduced the quality of care. The government attempted to upgrade hospitals and increase the number of specialists to reduce the gap (B1 loop) but was limited by the availability of funding (Figure 5-a).

Despite continued government investment, a gap remained between the demand for healthcare and public sector capacity to provide it. Figure 5-b demonstrates how, in the 1970s and 1980s, rising societal affluence increased the demand for sophisticated healthcare while also growing the population segment that could afford to pay for private care. This created private sector

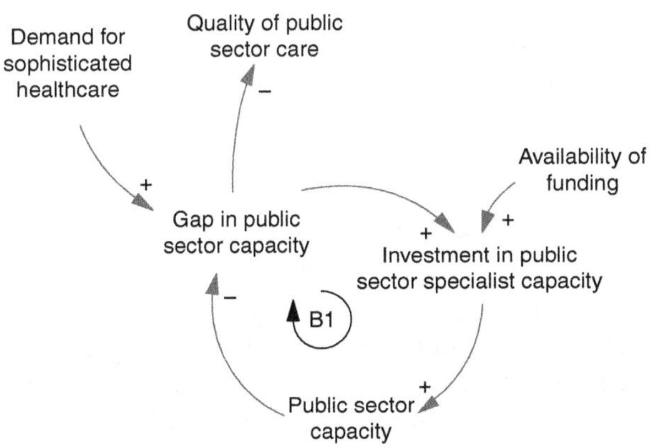

Figure 5-a The rising demand for more sophisticated STC stressed the capacity of the public sector, thereby requiring greater investment.

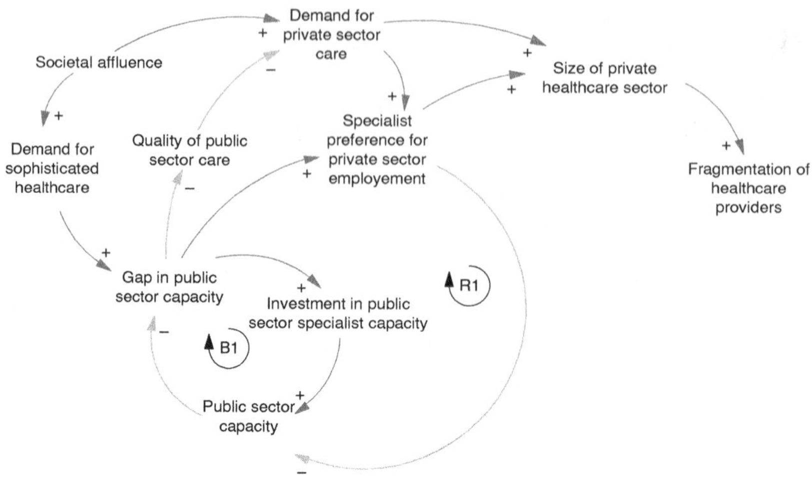

Figure 5-b In the 1970s and 1980s, rising societal affluence further increased the demand for sophisticated healthcare, resulting in the growth of the private sector STC, drained specialists from the public sector to the private sector and counteracted efforts to increase public sector capacity.

opportunities that were welcomed by public sector specialists facing high patient loads and inadequate support. However, the movement of these specialists out of the public sector further undermined public sector capacity, as illustrated by the reinforcing loop R1. Meanwhile, the growth of the private sector created a fragmentation of healthcare providers both between the public and private sectors and within the private sector.

Figure 5-c illustrates that the public sector used new strategies to address capacity shortfalls. The public sector further invested in increasing clinical specialists (B1 loop) and emphasised health management and quality improvement (B2 loop), including information for performance monitoring and managerial strategies for quality improvement. While outcomes improved, unintended effects surfaced from the growing numbers and types of specialisation. Clinical treatment expertise and service delivery modalities in the public and private sectors became increasingly compartmentalised, with the development of silos in caregiving (R2 loop).

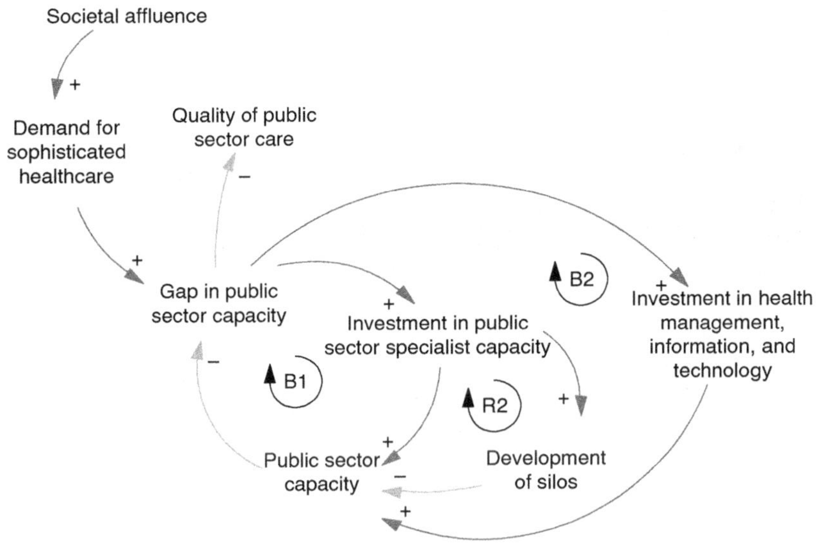

Figure 5-c Increased investment resulted in increased availability of specialist services but was associated with the unanticipated effect of increased compartmentalisation of care.

Figure 5-d demonstrates that in the 2000s onward, the public sector responded to the development of silos by investing in organisational structure (B3 loop) to bridge silos. This includes the creation of hospital clusters to share specialists and other resources, integrating hospital OPDs with PHC facilities, and creating new modalities of treatment such as telemedicine and day-care centres to improve access and integration.

Despite continual improvements to the public healthcare system, demand for private sector care has remained strong. Private sector care has become corporatised and supporting structures such as private insurance and medical tourism have developed, creating a self-sustaining industry and supplier-driven demand (R3 loop). While the private sector alleviates the burden of the public sector in some ways, it continues to draw medical practitioners, especially specialists, away from the public sector and creates challenging tensions regarding the locus of responsibility for the provision and payment of healthcare.

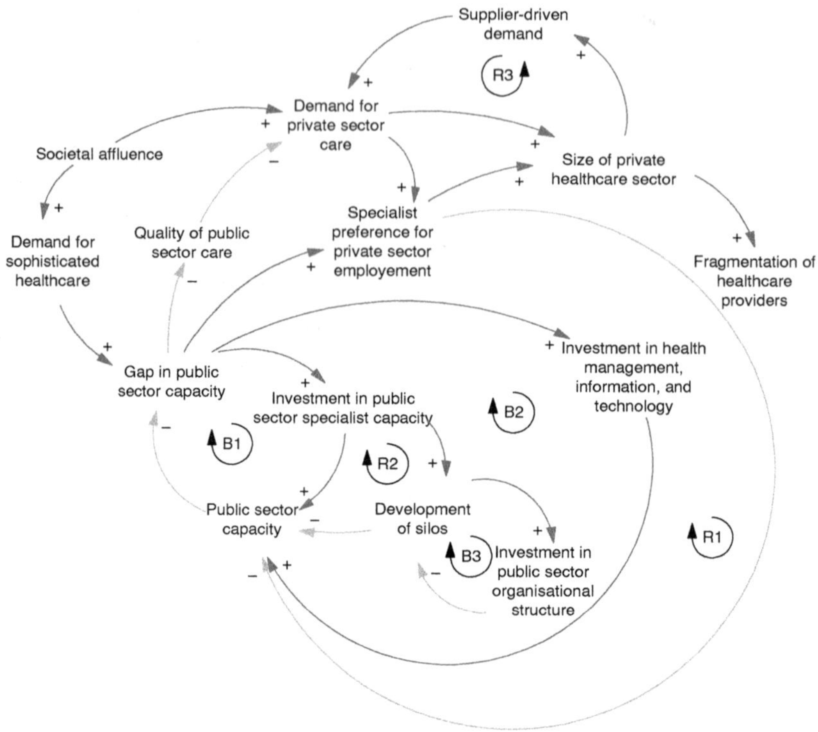

Figure 5-d Investment in public sector organisational structure improved the capacity to deal with compartmentalisation.

Appendix II
Supplementary Tables

Supplementary Table 5-a ***Interaction of forces that shaped the evolution of STC during the 1960s and 1970s***

Larger ecosystem	(A) Influence of the larger ecosystem on STC	(B) Influence of STC on the larger ecosystem OR other components of health system
Population behaviour and demographic profile	**During the 1960s and early 1970s** Largely rural population (74%) Low literacy (58%) Low health literacy *Resulted in:* Need and demand for access to hospital care by the rural population **By the mid-1970s** Rising demand for more complex secondary care, evidenced in the bypassing of district hospitals to seek care in larger hospitals able to provide better investigations and surgical services	**During the period** Probably increased awareness of hospital services (no data) **By the end of the period** Improved availability of hospitals in rural areas (no data on access or utilisation at that time)
Morbidity and mortality profile	High rates of maternal and infant mortality, vaccine-preventable diseases, malaria, TB, water- and soil-borne diseases, malnutrition *Resulted in:* Need for hospital care for treatment of more severe illness (TB, malaria, complications of childbirth)	**By the end of the period** Deaths from serious illness and pregnancy-related causes declined

Supplementary Table 5-a (*cont.*)

Larger ecosystem	(A) Influence of the larger ecosystem on STC	(B) Influence of STC on the larger ecosystem OR other components of health system
Economy and macro policies	Steady increase in GDP Rapid integrated rural development, including rural agriculture land development schemes (roads/bridges, schools, clinics, women's mobilisation for income generation, basic literacy, nutrition and health) *Resulted in:* Improved transportation to hospitals Expanding network of hospitals	Increased political awareness of the popularity of provision of healthcare services
Education sector	Rapid expansion of primary and secondary schools Rising education level of school leavers *Resulted in:* Better-qualified candidates for the health workforce Probably increasing health literacy and empowerment of women, particularly for use of health services (no Malaysian data)	
Components of the health system		
Health services (STC)	**Public sector** 1. Inherited dilapidated hospitals, mostly in urban areas in state capitals – some were refurbished during this period. 2. New district-level hospitals were constructed.	

3. District hospitals had staff and basic investigation facilities capable of managing major communicable diseases (malaria, TB, leprosy) and childbirth to reduce maternal deaths. Few had surgical facilities.
4. Ambulances provided free transport for patients from health centres and district hospitals to larger hospitals.
5. State-level hospitals provided more sophisticated imaging, laboratory and surgical services and specialists for basic specialties.
6. There were strong linkages (referrals, case finding, leadership support) with rural maternal and child health (MCH) services and TB and malaria programmes.

Private sector

7. A few not-for-profit missionary hospitals had specialist services.
8. Several small nursing homes catered mainly for childbirth.
9. In the late 1970s, a few specialists resigned from the public sector and set up the first few doctor-owned private for-profit hospitals.

	Influence of other components of the health system on STC	Influence of STC on other components of the health system
Other modalities of service delivery	*Public sector:* Rural MCH services and TB control programme formed close bidirectional links with hospitals, especially for maternal health, which helped to popularise safe childbirth, and for TB treatment. *Private sector (NGOs):* Private hospitals had links with TCM providers.	

Supplementary Table 5-a (*cont.*)

	Influence of other components of the health system on STC	Influence of STC on other components of the health system
Health workforce	Shortage of doctors and specialists dictated the types of services available at each type of hospital. Introduction of compulsory year of post-registration service in the public sector for all doctors to provide staff for more rural facilities. Nurses, midwives and medical assistants were the backbone of district-level hospitals.	Demand for expanded health workforce to provide services in the expanding network of hospitals. Demand for health workforce willing and able to work in less developed states (e.g. East Coast states of Peninsular Malaysia). 'Task shifting' – the MoH granted authority to nurses and medical assistants to perform some tasks of doctors in remote locations where doctors were unavailable (e.g. anaesthesia, trauma care, some complications of childbirth).
Governance and financing of health sector	**Financing** *Public sector:* Provision of highly subsidised medical care funded by the government was almost free at point of delivery. *Private sector:* Payment was on a fee-for-service basis, being mostly out-of-pocket expenditure for patients and their families. **Governance** Laws and regulations under the MoH regulated the practice of the medical, nursing, midwifery, dental and pharmacy professions. The Boards also had oversight of recognition of qualifications.	

Health information	Very little information was available on hospital utilisation (only volume of admissions, childbirth, deaths and attendance at clinics). *Resulted in:* Inadequate data for management of hospital services.	*As a result:* At federal level, the MoH began the process of strengthening hospital information systems and monitoring the quality of information.
Medical products	Standardised essential drug lists were implemented for different categories of public sector hospitals based on types of services available. This facilitated the implementation of clinical management protocols. Central procurement at federal level and improved supply logistics. *Resulted in:* Better availability (volume, continuous supply) of medical products in hospitals.	

Supplementary Table 5-b *STC services: interaction of forces that shaped the evolution during the 1980s and 1990s*

Larger ecosystem	(A) Influence on STC	(B) Influence of STC on the larger ecosystem
Population behaviour and demographic profile	Increased rural–urban migration By 1991, 51% of the population was urban Rapid rise in female literacy By 1997: 49% of primary school enrolment was female *Resulted in:* Rising literacy rate (72%) Improving health literacy Increased demand for allopathic medical care	Improved access to basic STC services Increased demand for more sophisticated clinical care (investigation facilities, surgical services, specialist services) *Outcome by the end of the period:* Reduced disparities in access to care between geographic regions, especially between the West and East Coast states of Peninsular Malaysia
Morbidity and mortality profile	Decline in major communicable diseases (CDs) Remaining burden from re-emerging (dengue, TB) and new CDs (HIV/AIDS) Rise in NCDs (cardiovascular, metabolic, neoplastic) and accidents	Recognition of need for more sophisticated clinical care by policy-makers and politicians across the country *Outcome by the end of the period:* Improved quality of care in the public sector in terms of clinical outcomes, patient satisfaction and resource utilisation
Economy and macro policies	Budget constraints Macro policy directed towards: • Private sector as engine of growth • Improving efficiency to counter budget constraints • Nationwide quality-improvement initiatives in the public sector	Rise in private sector expenditure on health care (see Chapter 9)

	• Addressing imbalance between regions • Poverty-reduction programmes *Resulted in initiatives to:* • Improve quality (clinical outcomes, patient satisfaction, resource utilisation) • Outsource some hospital support services • Begin the growth of private sector hospital and specialist services	
Education sector	Better-qualified school levers were now demanding tertiary education. Tertiary education was expanded, including local production of doctors and various allied health professionals (see Chapter 8). This contributed to changing the profile of the health workforce in hospitals.	Increased the demand for medical education by increasing the visibility and prestige of doctors and specialists (see Chapter 8)
	Influence of other components of the health system on STC	**Influence of STC on other components of the health system**
Other modalities of healthcare delivery	Notification of CDs (dengue) improved through collaboration between the disease control programme and STC services. Support from STC to the PHC level was strengthened through the QAP, whereby senior specialists in state-level hospitals had to take responsibility for quality in their discipline in district hospitals and health centres (e.g. maternal health, paediatrics, surgery).	

Supplementary Table 5-b (*cont.*)

Larger ecosystem	(A) Influence on STC	(B) Influence of STC on the larger ecosystem
Health workforce (see Chapter 8 for details)	More doctors became available. There was brain drain of doctors and nurses from the public to the private sector. The competence and remuneration of nurses and hospital assistants (medical assistants) was upgraded. More specialised categories of allied health personnel were recruited or trained to support the growing number of specialist services. Management skills in public sector hospitals were upgraded.	Increased demand for doctors, dentists, pharmacists and nurses *Resulting in:* • Increased local production • Increased financial support for foreign training of local candidates (doctors and dentists) • Establishment of local training programmes for a wider range of allied health personnel
Governance	**Public sector** • 'Regionalisation' of hospitals to improve geographic distribution of specialist services • Improved financial literacy of hospital managers • Improved community participation (hospital boards) **Private sector** • Fee schedules agreed on for private sector doctors and specialists	Increased recognition of safety and quality issues in smaller private sector providers of inpatient care Increasing influence of clinical specialists in health policy and programme management Improved linkages with some public sector health programmes (disease control, e.g. dengue notification, clinical management protocol)

Healthcare financing	Progressive decentralisation of financial authority and responsibility to state-level hospitals (modified budgeting system)	In 1985: • % national budget allocated to health: 4.3% • % GNP for health: 1.68% • Public sector funded 75% of THE • 13% of MoH budget spent on development Demand for increasing share of the government budget for the health sector because of higher-cost personnel and high-cost technology
Health information	Better quality and timeliness of hospital data facilitated Better allocation of resources (human, materials) Improved monitoring of performance (utilisation, clinical quality, patient satisfaction) Strengthened capacity for and production of health technology assessment contributed to rational acquisition of technology and products in the MoH network	Monitoring of quality of care in hospitals strengthened the quality of data generated in hospitals, e.g. causes of death, ICD coding Strengthened capacity for clinical trials and management research in hospitals Improved communication with patients (health promotion, patient education)

System Analysis Case Study 5.1: Expanded Access to Dialysis Services through Public Funding of Private Delivery

Indra Pathmanathan, Milton Lum, Anuar Zaini and David T. Tan

This study applies systems thinking methodology to a paper by Teck-Onn Lim, Adrian Goh, Yam-Ngo Lim, Zaki Morad bin Mohamad Zaher and Abu Bakar Suleiman entitled 'How Public and Private Reforms Dramatically Improved Access to Dialysis Therapy in Malaysia', published in *Health Affairs* in December 2010.

The major precursors of end stage renal disease (ESRD) are uncontrolled hypertension and diabetes. The prevalence of hypertension in Malaysia increased from 29.9% in 1995 to 30.3% in 2015, and one in two patients were undiagnosed. The prevalence of diabetes mellitus increased from 8.3% in 1996 to 17.5% in 2015, and three out of five patients were undiagnosed (Institute for Public Health and Ministry of Health Malaysia, 2008; 2015). In 2015, a staggering 61% of ESRD was reported to be caused by diabetes mellitus (National Renal Registry, 2018).

ESRD is treated through renal replacement therapy (RRT). The types of RRT are haemodialysis, and peritoneal dialysis with or without renal transplantation.[3] ESRD requires long-term dialysis, which comes at a high cost.

The first patient with ESRD to be given long-term dialysis was in the private sector in 1966. Until the 1980s, dialysis treatment was available only in Kuala Lumpur, but during the 1970s, the seeds for future development in the public sector were sown by a team of nephrologists and urologists who established service modalities using team approaches with allied health personnel, and haemodialysis equipment with a very limited budget. Facilities were gradually expanded to larger towns, mostly in MoH hospitals. Access was very limited. Constraints to the expansion of access were lack of budget for establishing the infrastructure, and the very small number of qualified staff. Many patients were considered ineligible for treatment in the public sector and were forced to resort to the private sector, but several could not afford the cost. The National Kidney Foundation (NKF) and other non-governmental organisations (NGOs) tried to alleviate the situation by raising funds and were able to supplement the public sector service to a small extent. Figure 5-A illustrates the increasing gap between demand and supply. Theoretically, the

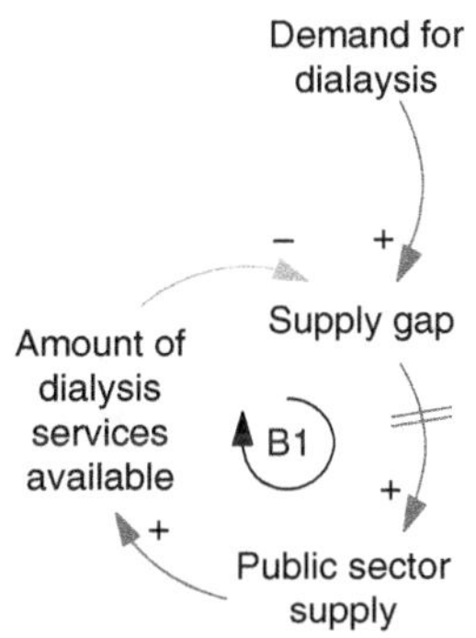

Figure 5-A The gap between demand and supply. A simple balancing (B1) loop caused the rapidly increasing demand for dialysis in the 1990s to outpace the ability of the Malaysian public health sector to respond. Factors in the wider system kept the supply rate low and the supply gap large.

supply gap should have induced the private sector to step in and meet the demand (Loop B2). However, patients' ability to pay for services was a strong limiting factor. Consequently, private sector involvement was limited to a few charitable organisations and private clinics that catered to those who could afford to pay. Figure 5-B demonstrates that the persistent supply gap kept the price of private dialysis services high (R1a). Furthermore, the relatively low number of dialysis services prevented economies of scale from lowering the cost, as equipment and consumables suppliers had to keep prices high to remain profitable in the absence of large-scale demand (R1b).

Lim and colleagues (2010) noted that rapid economic growth from 1990 to 2005 was accompanied by an eightfold increase in dialysis rates to reach levels comparable with that of developed countries (Supplementary Table 5-A). They noted that 'In spite of the resource constraints that all developing countries face, popular demand in Malaysia, combined with effective stewardship of public funds, resulted in a mix of public and private financing and provision of dialysis services.'

This remarkable transformation was triggered by the government's large-scale purchase of dialysis services from the private sector.

In the Malaysian scenario, there was a total dichotomy between the public and private sectors. For the first time, the government departed from its standard policy of monopolising healthcare provision and

Supplementary Table 5-A *Haemodialysis in Malaysia: prevalence, 1990–2015*

Increased funding	1980	1990	1995	2000	2005	2010	2015
Dialysis prevalence per million population	4	46	108	285	512	830	1,238
Total number of patients on dialysis at year end	59	836	2,230	6,693	13,385	23,740	37,729
% patients on dialysis by sector							
Public		88	65	42	37	33	31
Private		7	15	26	30	41	48
NGO		5	20	32	32	26	21

Sources: National Renal Registry, 2003; 2008; 2018.

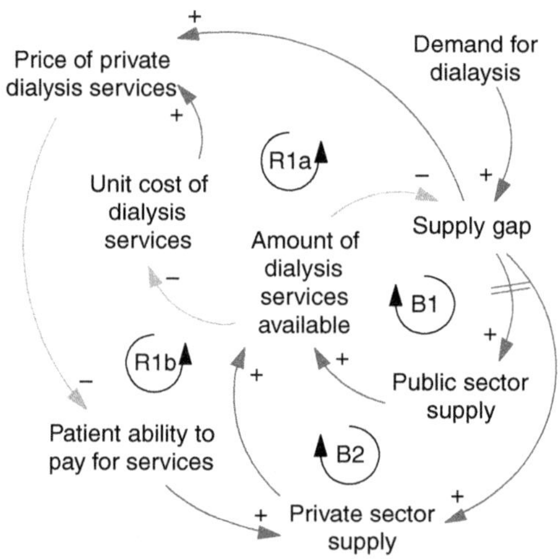

Figure 5-B A view of the wider system affecting dialysis demand and supply. The balancing loop in Figure 5-A interacts with a second balancing (B2) loop. The two reinforcing loops (R1a, R1b) show some of the factors that kept private sector involvement low.

purchased clinical services from the private sector. This was done by subsidising payment for private dialysis and setting a reimbursement rate. In Figure 5-C, the B2 loop represents the delivery of dialysis

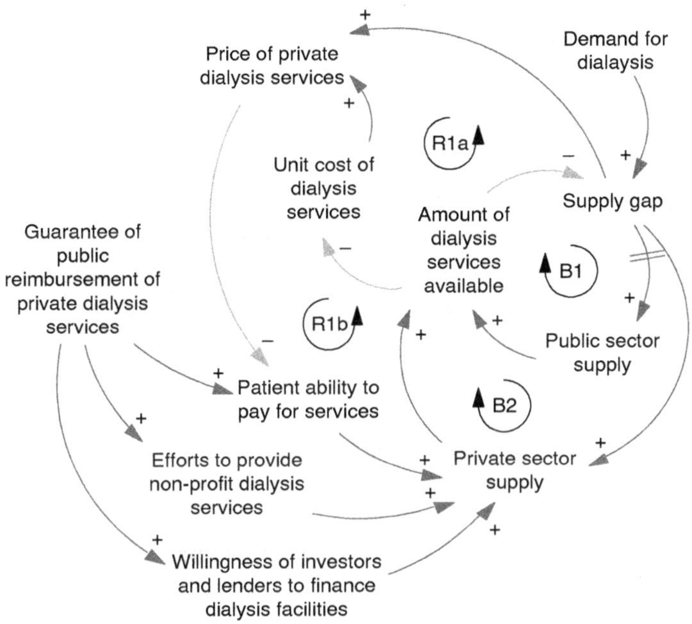

Figure 5-C Changing the behaviour of the system through new policy. To increase supply, the Malaysian government subsidised private provision and fixed payment rates for dialysis services.

treatment by the private sector and the R1 loop indicates how the cost per treatment was reduced. Patients' ability to pay for services increased. This initiative also unlocked private investment and charitable contributions that provided capital for setting up and operating many new dialysis centres.

Government funding was disbursed through multiple channels (Box 5-A). Reimbursement rates were set after an initial costing study followed by extensive consultations with the private sector and negotiations with suppliers based on arguments of economies of scale. The reimbursement rate was fixed, with no mechanism for revision, and does not account for inflation. Service providers were allowed to charge patients above the government reimbursement rate, and patients had to pay the difference out of pocket. The government also ensured a level playing field for all qualified providers who could offer services to patients eligible for public subsidies. Eligible patients had a choice of

Box 5-A Key features in the rapid expansion of dialysis

- Financing: Increased funding, expanded access, improved efficiency
  - Increased funding
  - Public financing of private sector services through:
    - Matching grants for NGOs
    - Subsidised payment based on pre-determined fixed rate
    - Payment through multiple channels (MoH, Social Security Organisation (SOCSO), Baitulmal, Public Services Division (PSD))
    - Level playing field in terms of eligibility of private providers to participate
  - Efficiency gains: Total spending increased 15-fold, but the number of patients increased 16-fold (13.4% more patients treated because of efficiency gain)
- Governance – legislative: Removed barriers but improved oversight
  - Lifting of restrictions on importation and marketing of equipment
  - Exemption from import duties
  - Mandatory reporting (Private Health Care Facilities Act)
- Information
  - Established National Renal Registry – has very good coverage
  - Monitors quality, efficiency and equity in utilisation
  - Analyses data regularly and provides feedback for decision-making
- Health workforce
  - Innovation in task shifting, training private sector in public facilities

providers, who therefore had to compete with each other; that is, the money followed the patient. The private sector responded by investing in physical capacity and human resources.

The result was a spectacular expansion of private dialysis services. Competition led to an increase in efficiency. This was reflected in the reduction in the price per treatment (Supplementary Table 5-B). However, the government continued to bear the major financing of dialysis (Table 5-C).

The rapid expansion of dialysis facilities could have been expected to create a demand for workforce that exceeded supply (B3 loop), and

Supplementary Table 5-B *Dialysis: price pre-treatment*

	1990 RM	1995 RM	2000 RM	2005 RM
Private sector	302	254	194	165
Public sector	163	182	201	219

Source: Lim et al., 2010.

Supplementary Table 5-C *Dialysis: financing by sector*

	1990	1995	2000	2005	2010	2015
Public	64.4%	56.1%	45.6%	67.3%	65.8%	67.1%
Private	33.1%	36.3%	40.0%	20.7%	21.6%	19.7%
NGO	2.5%	7.5%	14.4%	11.9%	12.6%	13.2%

Sources: National Renal Registry, 2008; 2018.

training new personnel would have required time (B4 loop) (Figure 5-D). These bottlenecks were anticipated, and policies to supply the necessary workforce were enacted and successfully carried out (Box 5-A). Legislation reduced import restrictions and costs, and it established mandatory reporting that enabled oversight of quality and efficiency.

The reforms were driven by a small group of public sector nephrologists who provided strong leadership and commitment in building consensus among key stakeholders on policy details. They also overcame resistance to reforms by various stakeholders.

Lim and colleagues (2010) noted that, contrary to expectations, the rapid increase in dialysis in the private sector had 'no adverse trends in several measures of quality including patient mortality, quality of life, dialysis adequacy . . .' Their analysis also implied that the private sector was catering for the more affluent, while the public sector services were directed towards patients with low socio-economic status.

The development of the dialysis service system has successfully increased access to dialysis treatment through the provision of financing and workforce development. This system, however, increases government exposure to dialysis costs, and this cannot be easily changed without major disruption to the service delivery system that has been built upon government reimbursement. The total ESRD expenditure increased from 2.95% of the public sector THE in 2010

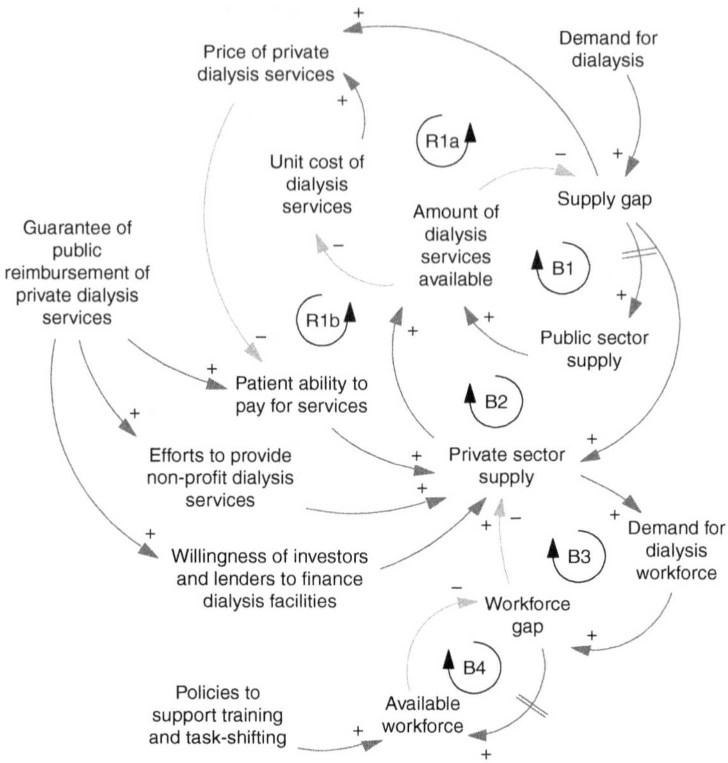

Figure 5-D Effect of the rapid expansion of services on the workforce (B3 and B4).

to 4.2% in 2016, with only 6% of total ESRD expenditure on renal transplantation and the remaining 94% on dialysis (Ismail et al., 2019). Thus cost control must come by reducing the causes of renal failure and the consequent demand for dialysis.

Systems Lessons

Systems analysis illustrates how successful interventions require consideration of and planning for the dynamic interactions between various components of the health system, such as modalities of financing and service delivery, medical products, human resources, and information systems as well as the larger ecosystem, such as taxation policies. Mapping out the key components enables policies that align incentives to enable action.

References

Institute for Public Health and Ministry of Health Malaysia. (2008). *National Health and Morbidity Survey 2006*. Putrajaya: Ministry of Health Malaysia.

Institute for Public Health and Ministry of Health Malaysia. (2015). *National Health and Morbidity Survey 2015*. Putrajaya: Ministry of Health Malaysia.

Ismail, H., Abdul Manaf, M. R., Abdul Gafor, A. H., Mohamed Zaher, Z. M. and Nur Ibrahim, A. I. (2019). Economic burden of end-stage renal disease to the Malaysian healthcare system. *Kidney International Reports*, 4(9), 1261–70.

Lim, T. O., Goh, A., Lim, Y. N., Mohamad Zaher, Z. M. and Suleiman, A. B. (2010). How public and private reforms dramatically improved access to dialysis therapy in Malaysia. *Health Affairs*, 29(12), 2214–22. DOI: http:// 10.1377/hlthaff.2009.0135

National Renal Registry. (2003). *Eleventh Report of the Malaysia Dialysis and Transplant Registry 2003*. Kuala Lumpur: National Renal Registry, Malaysia.

National Renal Registry. (2008). *Fifteenth Report of the Malaysian Dialysis and Transplant Registry 2007*. Kuala Lumpur: National Renal Registry, Malaysia.

National Renal Registry. (2018). *Twenty-Fourth Report of the Malaysian Dialysis and Transplant Registry 2016*. Kuala Lumpur: National Renal Registry, Malaysia.

Notes

1. Essential, emergency and comprehensive obstetric care as defined by the United Nations Population Fund (UNFPA, www.unfpa.org).
2. West Coast states: Perlis, Kedah, Penang, Perak, Selangor, Negri Sembilan, Melaka and Johor. East Coast states: Kelantan, Terengganu and Pahang. East Malaysia: Sarawak and Sabah.
3. In Malaysia, dialysis is the most frequent mode of therapy. In 2015, there were 33,965 haemodialysis and 3,764 peritoneal dialysis patients. Transplant rates in Malaysia have remained low, with rates of 6 and 3 per million population in 2006 and 2015, respectively (Dialysis and Transplant Registry Reports, Clinical Research Centre, www.crc.gov.my/ report-registry).

6 Health Service Delivery

Disease Prevention and Control

SHIANG CHENG LIM

6.1 Introduction

Disease prevention and control programmes aim to reduce disease incidence, prevalence, and morbidity or mortality (Dowdle, 1998). Within the first thirty years since independence in 1957, Malaysia successfully eradicated or drastically reduced the occurrence of several serious communicable diseases (CDs) (Figure 6.1). During the next thirty years, Malaysia had some success as well as limited or no progress in dealing with non-communicable diseases (NCDs), re-emerging CDs (such as dengue) and other new and emerging CDs (such as influenza H1N1). This chapter analyses the development and evolution of disease control in Malaysia over the sixty years since independence (1957–2017). It explores and analyses the influences and interactions of various components of the health system and beyond the healthcare system in controlling diseases. The chapter does not attempt to address all the threads of disease control efforts in Malaysia. Instead, specific examples of disease control programmes illustrate key features that contributed to the success or limited progress of control efforts.

Disease control programmes in low- and middle-income countries commonly use vertical or campaign-style programmes. Horizontal programmes, on the other hand, rely on a system of health services. Atun, Bennett and Duran (2008) discuss the advantages of vertical programmes (rapid response; quick, economical and efficient solutions; better accountability within limited resources and timeframe) and constraints (donor- and value-driven (responsive to disease, lacking in people-centred care); expensive to sustain; creating subsequent redundancies, inefficiency and fragmentation in the health system). They note that some vertical programmes are standalone, completely separate and parallel to mainstream health services, and continue to remain in that mode. Others are designed as time-limited programmes that are

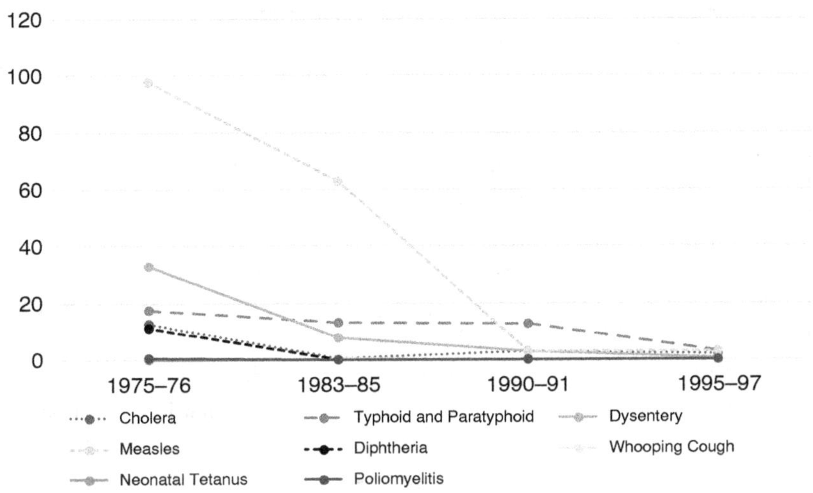

Figure 6.1 Incidence rate of communicable diseases per 100,000 population, Malaysia, 1975–1997.
Sources: Ministry of Health, 1983; Suleiman and Jegathesan, n.d.

then integrated with extant health services; yet others have varying degrees of integration from inception.

This chapter describes Malaysia's developmental experience in disease control and explores how the characteristics of prevalent diseases and the health system have combined to influence the design of disease control programmes and their subsequent integration into the mainstream health service.

6.2 The First Phase (1957 until the Mid-1980s): Control of Communicable Diseases

By the time it gained independence, Malaysia had already controlled several major epidemic contagious diseases (smallpox, cholera, plague). The main CDs of concern were vaccine-preventable diseases (neonatal tetanus, diphtheria, pertussis (whooping cough)), which took a heavy toll of infant lives; vector-borne and water borne diseases (malaria, dysentery, typhoid and paratyphoid, and endemic cholera), which affected the productivity and lives of the work-aged population groups; and tuberculosis (TB), which caused illness and premature death in both adults and children (Box 6.1).

Box 6.1 The major communicable diseases of concern in Malaysia (1960s to mid-1980s)

- **Malaria and TB** were the fifth and sixth leading causes of hospital admissions and deaths, respectively (Supplementary Table 6.a) (Ismail & Martinez, 1974; Suleiman & Jegathesan, n.d.).
- **TB:** An estimated 25% of all hospital beds were occupied by TB patients, most lt in advanced stages of the disease, and 75% of children had been infected by age 15 (MAPTB, 2012).
- **Malaria:** A 1965–66 survey showed 168,500 malaria cases reported from static and mobile clinics in Peninsular Malaysia, an annual 40,000 cases in Sarawak and 250,000 cases in Sabah (Suleiman & Jegathesan, n.d.).
- **Dysentery, typhoid and cholera** were endemic.
- **Yaws** was reported at 140.85 per 100,000 population in 1958 (Lo, 1985).
- **Filariasis** was present in 20,000 of 600,000 people clinically examined between 1960 and 1984 (Suleiman & Jegathesan, n.d.).
- **Leprosy:** An estimated 11,900 to 15,000 cases in Peninsular Malaysia in 1969 (Kamaludin, 1990).
- **Tetanus, diphtheria, pertussis, poliomyelitis and measles** contributed to high infant and child mortality rates (Figure 6.1 and Supplementary Table 6.b).

See Supplementary Tables 6.a, 6.b and 6.c for further information.

As elaborated in Chapters 3, 4 and 5, during the 1960s until the mid-1980s, healthcare for the predominantly rural population increased gradually, with expanding rural health centres and district hospitals and gradually increasing availability of nurses, midwives, hospital assistants (later known as assistant medical officers) and sanitation staff. Training and competence in public health and programme management was limited and concentrated mainly at the national and state levels. Monitoring systems were rudimentary. The high incidence and prevalence of the common CDs was a heavy burden for the nascent health services. The rationale for adopting vertical approaches for controlling selected CDs was to provide additional resources targeted at rapidly reducing specific disease burdens to enable the young health service to assume responsibility without being overcome by these diseases to the detriment of other functions.

A distinctive feature of Malaysian development was that disease control programme funding was from domestic sources and channelled through the budget allocated to the Ministry of Health (MoH). Malaysia generally does not receive significant bilateral aid for health (World Health Organization, 2017). Foreign aid was mainly in terms of consultant expertise for designing programmes and training staff, management and treatment protocols, and designing monitoring and surveillance systems. Therefore, the new programmes aligned as closely as possible to national health development strategies. There was no need to provide accountability to external donors. On the other hand, there were strong incentives to avoid unnecessary domestic financial burdens by using existing facilities and staff and avoiding human resource issues arising from redundant staff.

The factors that influenced the design of prevention and control programmes included:

- the access of affected population groups to, and coverage provided by, the rural health service and public sector hospitals
- the availability and technical skills of the staff in those facilities
- the management capacity of the health services
- the clinical nature of the diseases in question, which partly influenced how and when those who were affected made contact with health services
- the epidemiological characteristics of the diseases in question, for example, the mode of transmission, the types of vectors and their habits, and the habits and lifestyles of human population groups
- the availability of effective and affordable technology or medical products to address the diseases

The initiatives for preventing and controlling CDs during this period could be categorised in three groups:

1. No dedicated 'programme', for example, waterborne diseases, such as endemic cholera, typhoid and paratyphoid.
2. National programmes (or campaigns) with dedicated organisational entities for planning, training, monitoring and evaluation

but service delivery through the mainstream health services. Examples are the vaccine-preventable diseases of childhood and TB.
3. National- or state-level programmes with dedicated management structures as well as service delivery mechanisms. Examples include vector-borne diseases such as malaria and filariasis.

Table 6.1 illustrates the key features that differentiated the various degrees of verticality in the spectrum of vertical programme designs.

Dedicated vertical programmes were suited for diseases that required the delivery of medical care (immunisation, diagnostic, medication) to specific target population groups or measures aimed at disrupting the lifecycle of specific vectors. In contrast, waterborne diseases required environmental control approaches coupled with surveillance and outbreak control. Therefore, instead of a dedicated disease-specific vertical national programme, preventing waterborne disease was the responsibility of environmental health services (see Chapter 7), while surveillance and control of disease outbreaks was the purview of mainstream health services for CD epidemiology and control.

6.2.1 Socio-economic Development Influenced the Development of Disease Control Programmes

The overall improvement of the country's socio-economic and living conditions (see Chapter 3) facilitated the successes in controlling CDs. The gross domestic product (GDP) per capita increased substantially, with an annual growth of 7.7% between 1970 and the mid-1980s, improving standards of living for the majority of the population, making them less vulnerable to infectious diseases (Tan et al., 1987; UN Country Team, 2005). Significant improvements in roads and transportation made healthcare more accessible.

In addition to economic growth and infrastructure development, social development also progressed. The percentage of women (aged 15–19 years) who attended secondary school increased from 15% in 1960 to 75% in 1980, while the percentage of living quarters with piped water and flush toilets rose from 48% and 18% in 1970 to 68% and 60%, respectively, in 1980 (Tan et al., 1987). The increase in women's education levels as well as improved environmental health contributed to the decline of infant mortality caused by CDs; in

Table 6.1 ***Examples illustrating key features in the spectrum of Malaysian vertical disease control approaches that subsequently merged with mainstream health services (see Supplementary Table 6.c for programme details)***

	Examples of vertical disease control programmes		
	Vaccine-preventable diseases of childhood	Tuberculosis	Malaria
Pressures that led to the adoption of national programmes	Professional and political awareness of the value of vaccines, influence of the WHO and availability of affordable vaccines	Strong advocacy by civil society (MAPTB) leading to political awareness and commitment	International pressure to move from control measures (based on species sanitation in cities and rubber estates) to nationwide eradication to avoid becoming a pool of infection dangerous to neighbouring countries
Key organisational features of vertical national programmes at inception: • Dedicated programme[1] • Mainstream[2] • Legislation governing notification of diseases and vector control applied to all the relevant CDs	*Dedicated programme:*[1] • Procurement and distribution of vaccines *Mainstream*[2] *health services (rural health services (RHS) and hospitals):* • Delivery of immunisation • Programme monitoring • Notification of disease and control of outbreaks	*Dedicated programme:*[1] • Planning, monitoring and evaluation • Training and treatment protocols • Supervision of implementation • Community education and mobilisation	*Dedicated programme:*[1] • Planning, monitoring and evaluation • Training and management protocols • Service delivery – vector control, case finding and treatment

Table 6.1 (*cont.*)

	Examples of vertical disease control programmes		
	Vaccine-preventable diseases of childhood	Tuberculosis	Malaria
	• Pre-condition of immunisation as eligibility for school entry	• Supplementary periodic mass screening campaigns *Mainstream[2] health services (RHS and hospitals):* Delivery of treatment Notification of cases Contract tracing Provision of financial aid for travel and work absenteeism	*Mainstream[2] health services (RHS and hospitals):* Passive case detection, i.e. detection of malaria in patients who attended clinic services for any illness Use of laboratory facilities Notification of cases and laboratory screening
Duration and criteria for merging vertical programmes into mainstream health services	*Duration:* ongoing *Criteria:* eradication (polio) or sustained elimination of vaccine-preventable diseases *Strategies:* Other vaccines were added when they became available and affordable. Vaccine distribution and cold-chain management merged	*Duration:* 15 years of dedicated funding Dedicated management structure was dismantled in gradual stages and completed after 30 years (1995). *Criteria:* High vaccine coverage (95%), reduced incidence of new cases (<60 per	*Duration:* Began as a malaria eradication programme but converted to malaria control after 10 years (in East Malaysia) and 15 years (in Peninsular Malaysia) 'due to operational, administrative and technical problems' (Mak et al., 1992).

	into maternal and child health (MCH) programme.	100,000 population) and good cure rate (>85%). *Strategies:* Monitoring and surveillance systems and dedicated staff were absorbed into the public sector health services and some were re-trained for other programmes.	*Criteria:* Reduce morbidity (<2 per 1,000 population) and mortality (<0.5%) and prevent spread to non- endemic areas. *Strategies:* Over the next 5-year period, vector control activities merged into national programmes for vector-borne diseases. Surveillance, health education and control of outbreaks merged into the gamut of other CD control activities within the public sector health services.

[1] Separate funding and staffing with vertical authority and accountability structure.
[2] Involved the use of existing organisational and service delivery structures, staff and accountability mechanisms.

particular, vaccine-preventable diseases and food-borne and water borne diseases (DaVanzo & Habicht, 1986).

6.2.2 *Programmatic Features that Influenced Outcomes*

6.2.2.1 Collaborative and Co-ordinated Activities at Various Levels of Service Delivery

The national disease control programmes carried out promotion, prevention and early detection activities (education, vaccination and case detection) mostly at the primary care level. In the rural health units, disease control activities complemented maternal and child health and outpatient care, sanitation and environmental health services, and dental care. District and general hospitals served as training, treatment and referral centres. For example, hospitals supported rural health units by providing training for bacillus Calmette-Guerin (BCG) vaccination and served as referral points for case finding and contact tracing for TB control programmes (Suleiman & Jegathesan, n.d.). The dedicated management teams of the national disease control programmes played a critical role in aligning and co-ordinating disease control funding, strategies, processes, activities and services across different actors, sectors, levels and facilities. For example, TB managerial teams were formed at state level to provide continuous supervision, consultation and support and to ensure seamless co-ordination at all levels of care with available resources (Ismail & Martinez, 1974; Suleiman & Jegathesan, n.d.).

The rapid expansion of rural health facilities and services between the 1960s and 1970s and its linkages to district and general hospitals contributed to the reduction of morbidity and mortality from CDs. However, most of the disease control programmes included a unilateral (one-way) referral system from clinics to primary/district hospitals or national referral hospitals, and this system soon became established as the norm in the health services. The lack of a counter-referral system was workable when the country dealt with CD control that mainly required acute care and response. However, it would later create difficulties in the management of patients with diseases that required long-term care, such as NCDs and HIV.

6.2.2.2 Human Resources

Similar to the public sector health services, the disease control programmes relied on allied health personnel, including nurses, medical assistants, medical laboratory technologists and junior laboratory technicians rather than doctors. As discussed in Chapters 4, 5 and 8, this strategy enabled Malaysia to reach wider populations, especially those in rural areas, while there was a shortage of medical professionals. The allied health personnel received technical information and skills training and acted as front-line staff. For example, junior laboratory technicians trained by the Institute for Medical Research (IMR) did most of the sputum examination for TB (Cheong, 2010). Allied health staff from rural health clinics assisted in case detection for malaria screening (Jaafar et al., 2007). Not only did the front-line staff provide medical care, they also raised community awareness regarding early detection and treatment.

Staff employed by or deployed to the national disease control programmes were mostly from the same categories as those in the health services, and qualifications and employment conditions were the same. By the time the vertical programmes merged into the mainstream health services, economic and health service growth created the need for more of these personnel as well as the capacity to absorb them. Thus, career paths and absorption were not problematic, and the issue of redundancy was avoided.

6.2.2.3 Surveillance Systems

Each disease control programme developed a tailored surveillance system. For example, a central TB registry established in 1973 under the National TB Control Centre monitored TB cases. Chest clinics in hospitals in each state collected and compiled data for submission to the national level. The malaria eradication programme had a case registry system and entomological surveillance activities. Similarly, leprosy had a surveillance system.

Meanwhile, a standard epidemiological surveillance system had been developed for the Epidemiology Unit since 1971 (Suleiman & Jegathesan, n.d.). The separate surveillance systems were integrated into the standard epidemiologic surveillance system of the MoH during late 1980s and early 1990s when the vertical programmes merged into the mainstream. Although Malaysia has not evaluated the impact of the separate surveillance systems, it is possible to conjecture about both their advantages and their constraints. The dedicated surveillance and monitoring systems of the disease control programmes were probably of better quality because of special efforts in training, tighter supervision and less staff mobility. However, they would have created duplication and an additional burden on the reporting staff, particularly at the front line. However, the skills and experience gained through the better-quality surveillance in the vertical programmes probably carried over to the mainstream health services when the programmes merged.

6.2.2.4 Community Education and Mobilisation

The disease control programmes used the same strategies of community mobilisation and education as used successfully in primary healthcare (PHC), using local community organisations, particularly in rural areas (see Chapter 4). Also, the MoH programmes partnered with major non-governmental organisations (NGOs), which earlier had advocated for national disease control efforts, mobilised funding from civil society and developed care models. Examples are the Malaysian Leprosy Relief Association (MaLRA) and the Malaysian Association for the Prevention of Tuberculosis (MAPTB). Evidence of the success of such efforts is, for example, the fact that over 80% of registered TB cases in 1975–79 were self-referred by symptom-motivated patients (Cheong, 2010). Not only did such partnerships address ignorance, scepticism and cultural prejudices, they also established practical measures for facilitating and supporting individuals and families to benefit from the disease control efforts. Examples include the provision of a TB allowance to compensate for travel and sickness absenteeism, and the provision of living allowances as well as housing and income-generation opportunities in sheltered communities for cured leprosy patients who carried the stigma that isolated them from their own communities (Suleiman & Jegathesan, n.d.).

However, there were failures. For example, resistance by the population in Sabah to spraying with DDT (dichlorodiphenyltrichloroethane) under the malaria control programme in the 1980s is attributed to the lack of engagement with the communities and failure to understand local needs and concerns (Rahman, 1982; Mak et al., 1992; Ministry of Health et al., 2015).

6.2.2.5 Introduction and Availability of Vaccines and Effective Medicines/Medical Products

The introduction of new technology, vaccines and medicine contributed to the prevention, early detection and control of CDs. The incidence of childhood TB declined sharply in the 1970s after the introduction of the BCG vaccination programme (Cheong, 2010). Effective treatment such as single-dose penicillin with 2% aluminium monostearate (PAM) for yaws (Lo, 1985), multiple drug therapy (MDT) for leprosy and a shorter duration of TB treatment (from two years to six months) led to reductions in morbidity (i.e. deformity among leprosy patients) and mortality rates (Lo, 1985; Jayalakshmi, 1994; Cheong, 2010). The IMR played a significant role in introducing new vaccines and diagnostic tests in the early days (Box 6.2).

6.2.2.6 Outcomes

The BCG vaccination programme realised its initial objective of providing at least 75% coverage of the susceptible population within a short period (Ismail & Martinez, 1974). The mass survey and treatment campaign with PAM under the yaws control activities also reduced the reported cases from 9,462 in 1958 to 335 in 1968 (Lo, 1985).

The incidence of most CDs declined dramatically (Figure 6.1). The incidence of TB declined from 151.5 per 100,000 population in 1961 to 56.8 per 100,000 population in 1985 (Suleiman & Jegathesan, n.d.); malaria cases reduced significantly from 150,000 to below 50,000 in the late 1970s, but the goal of disease

Box 6.2 The role of the IMR in vaccine production and diagnostic services

- The production of vaccines for cholera, typhoid, plague, smallpox and rabies was started by the IMR in the 1940s (Ramanathan et al., 1976). The IMR initiated field trials and developed them as a standard protocol before any new vaccines were released to the public. In 1986, a trial on measles vaccines was conducted by the MoH and supported by the IMR before it was included as part of the national immunisation programme (UN Country Team, 2005).
- The IMR acted as a central reference laboratory for the whole country for more specialised diagnostic and public health laboratory tests for diseases such as yaws, typhoid and cholera (Ramanathan et al., 1976).

eradication had yet to succeed fully (Mak et al., 1992). Yaws and filariasis were no longer a concern; the country had successfully eliminated leprosy in 1994 and achieved polio-free status in 2000 (Suleiman & Jegathesan, n.d.). With the increase of childhood immunisation coverage (Table 6.2), the infant and child mortality rates had also declined significantly in 1990 (Table 6.3).

Table 6.2 *Percentage coverage of immunisation in Malaysia, 1970–2017*

% of childhood immunisation coverage	1970	1980	1990	2000	2010	2016/17
BCG for infants	46.6	88.2	97	99.3	99	98.55
DPT (diphtheria, pertussis, tetanus) for infants (3rd dose)	15.0	67.0	89.9	98.7	101.14	99.34
Polio for infants (3rd dose)	15.0	72.0	89.6	93.4	94.13	99.34
Measles/MMR (measles, mumps, rubella) for infants	10.0	20.0	87.1	93.9	96.1	88.8

Sources: Suleiman & Jegathesan, n.d.; Ministry of Health, 2010; 2018b.

Table 6.3 *Infant and child mortality rates, 1957–2017*

	1957	**1970**	**1983**	**1990**	**2000**	**2010**	**2016/17**
Infant mortality rate (per 1,000 live births)	68.9	39.4	20.2	13.1	6	6.7	7.3
Neonatal mortality rate (per 1,000 live births)	29.6	21.4	12.3	8.5	3.1	4.3	4.2
Toddler mortality rate (per 1,000 population aged 1–4 years)	8	4.2	1.7	0.9	0.5	0.4	0.4
Under-5 mortality rate (per 1,000 live births)	110.4	55.9	26.6	16.8	7.9	8.5	8.6

Sources: Jayalakshmi, 1994; Department of Statistics, 2009; 2011a; Ministry of Health et al., 2015.

Box 6.3 System observations: understanding feedback loops through communicable diseases

The role of feedback loops in CDs is well known among epidemiologists. They use stock-and-flow models, such as the susceptible-infectious-recovered (SIR) model, to predict and curb the spread of disease. Successful control of CDs relies on disrupting biological transmission feedback loops via vaccination, quarantine, culling of vectors, etc. The wide acceptance of such models in the health profession provides a useful entry point to many important system dynamics concepts.

The two programmes that failed to live up to their initial promise were those for TB and malaria. Although greatly reduced during the 1990s, TB incidence remained a problem. There were two contributing factors: first, the large concentration of foreign workers from neighbouring countries were a continual pool of infection. Local surveillance and control systems were ill-prepared to detect and manage them (Suleiman & Jegathesan, n.d.). Second, the HIV/AIDS epidemic brought with it an associated increase in TB due to impaired immune systems (Suleiman & Jegathesan, n.d.). The treatment modalities available at that time and programme strategies were inadequate for addressing this threat. For malaria, although incidence declined significantly, pockets of transmission and endemic levels persisted. There were several contributing factors, including people movement that was difficult to monitor, insecticide resistance, drug resistance and changes in vectors.

6.3 The Next 30 Years: The Era of the Integrated/Horizontal Approach to Disease Control (Mid-1980s to the Present)

6.3.1 The Changing Disease Profile

6.3.1.1 The Rise of Non-communicable Diseases

After the late 1980s, socio-economic development, urban migration, changes in work and lifestyles, and demographic transition to fewer children and more people of working age resulted in an evolving disease profile (see Chapter 3). NCDs such as cardiovascular disease, diabetes

Table 6.4 *Prevalence of selected NCD risk factors in Malaysia for adults aged ≥18 years, 1996–2015*

NCD risk factor	1996 (%)	2006 (%)	2011 (%)	2015 (%)
Diabetes mellitus	8.3[1]	11.6	15.2	17.5
Hypertension	29.9[1]	32.2	32.7	30.3
Hypercholesterolemia	–	28.2	43.9	47.7
Overweight	16.6	29.1	29.4	30.0
Obesity	4.4	14.0	15.1	17.7
Physical inactivity	–	43.7	35.2	33.5
Smoking[2]	24.8[3]	21.5[4]	23.1[4]	22.8[4]
Alcohol (current drinker)	–	7.4	11.6	7.7

1 Data for population aged ≥30 years.
2 Data for population aged 15 years and above.
3 NHMS II definition: respondent who reported to be smoking at the time of the survey.
4 Centers for Diseases Control and Prevention (CDC) definition: respondent who reported to have smoked ≥100 cigarettes in their lifetime and smoked daily or some days in the past 1 month.

Sources: Institute for Public Health, 1996; 2008; 2011; 2015; Department of Statistics, 2011b; Ministry of Health Malaysia & Harvard T. H. Chan School of Public Health, 2016.

mellitus and cancer emerged as major contributors to the disease burdens (Supplementary Table 6.a). There was also a shocking rise in the prevalence of NCD risk factors over the years, as shown in the National Health and Morbidity Surveys (NHMS) (Table 6.4). In 2016, NCDs accounted for 74% of all deaths (World Health Organization, 2018), while NCD-related morbidities and disabilities had increased by 80% between 1990 and 2013 (Ministry of Health Malaysia & Harvard T. H. Chan School of Public Health, 2016).

6.3.1.2 Emerging and Re-emerging Infectious Diseases

Since the 1990s, Malaysia has experienced emerging diseases, including HIV infection, dengue, Nipah virus and severe acute respiratory syndrome (SARS), and re-emerging diseases, including resurgent TB and measles, while malaria persisted in endemic areas, perpetually threatening to spread to other areas. (Table 6.5).

The first case of HIV was detected in 1986, and by 2017, there were a cumulative 115,263 HIV cases (Ministry of Health, 2018a). Initially

Table 6.5 *Incidence rate of emerging and re-emerging communicable diseases (per 100,000 population)*

	1990	1995	2000	2005	2010	2017
HIV	4.30	20.30	26.97	23.42	12.89	10.33
Dengue fever	9.54	10.68	58.93	60.71	148.73	257.6
Dengue haemorrhagic fever	1.29	1.87		3.82	14.23	1.25
Tuberculosis	61.2	56.93	63.29	61.20	68.25	80.78
Measles	3.17	3.16	2.83	5.39	0.26	5.28

Sources: Suleiman and Jegathesan, n.d.; Ministry of Health 2005; 2010; 2018b.

confined largely to injecting drug users (IDUs), sexual transmission thereof became more prevalent in recent years and has proved a challenge to control measures. First recognised as a public health issue in 1973, dengue incidence has increased tremendously, from 969 cases in 1973 to more than 100,000 cases, with 200 deaths per year, since 2014 (Ministry of Health, 2016).

The factors contributing to the emergence of new diseases or the resurgence of longer-standing diseases are complex and include population movements and lifestyle changes, globalisation and the movement of goods, adaptive mutations in pathogens and vectors, and environmental changes that facilitate or support changes. Table 6.6 shows the illustrative key features of emerging diseases in Malaysia.

The Nipah virus outbreak in 1998–1999, SARS in 2002–2003 and the H1N1 pandemic influenza in 2009 not only posed an increased healthcare burden but also caused social disruptions and economic loss. Up to 40% of cases, or 105 people, with acute encephalitis (out of 265 cases) died during the Nipah virus outbreak (Looi & Chua, 2007), while H1N1 caused 77 deaths (out of 12,307 reported cases) in 2009, the majority of whom were children (Sam, 2015).

Meanwhile, re-emerging diseases such as TB and measles continue to be a public health challenge. TB cases per 100,000 population declined over 30 years from 350 cases to about 60–68 cases but increased to about 84 cases in the subsequent 30-year period (Ministry of Health, 2016). Similarly, despite a strong childhood immunisation programme, measles increased during the 30 years after 1990, from an incidence of 3.1–5.18 per 100,000 population, and one-third of the cases during the

Table 6.6 *Illustrative examples of the rapid emergence of and varied challenges posed by emerging diseases in Malaysia*

Year	Virus	Location	Relevant features illustrating the complexity of the disease
1997 2000 & 2003, re-emergence	Enterovirus 71 Known to be circulating widely in the region. Danger of mutation into a more virulent variety.	Sibu	• Hand, foot and mouth disease (HFMD). Transmission: faecal–oral route. Mostly asymptomatic but could cause severe illness with deaths. • In 2000 and 2003, novel variants emerged in Peninsular Malaysia.
1998 Re-emerged 2006	Chikungunya virus Factors potentially responsible for spread include migrant labour and climate changes favouring vector mutation.	Port Klang and Kuala Lumpur Perak (50 km from earlier site)	• Vector-borne disease. Sporadic outbreaks, febrile illness with polyarthritis similar to dengue and thereby masking early recognition. • Re-emergence coincided with wider epidemic in Indian Ocean countries. More serious and higher rate of illness symptoms.
1998	Nipah virus Believed to be 'spill over' from wild fruit bats to commercially reared pigs, and subsequently to humans.	Ipoh, Seremban	• Previously existing as infection in pigs, the virus adapted to infect humans, causing fever, encephalitis and a high mortality rate of about 40%. Genotyping and epidemiological studies in Malaysia and several neighbouring countries resulted in better understanding of natural reservoirs of the virus family and raised the international alert on potential danger in the future.

1986	HIV type 1	Kuala Lumpur	• First case in Malaysia.
2003, new variant appeared in Malaysia	HIV type 1 CRF33_01B		• The new variant is widespread in all risk groups. New variants pose a challenge for diagnosis and the development of antivirals and vaccine candidates.
2004 2006 2007	Avian influenza H5N1	Kelantan, Kuala Lumpur, Perak, Penang	• Highly pathogenic virus originating in poultry. Adaptation to infect humans, causing fever; deaths reported in other countries. Outbreaks detected in poultry in Malaysia. Linked to fighting cocks smuggled from neighbouring countries. Rapid and effective control measures prevented the spread to humans.

Source: Adapted from Tee et al. (2009).

recent 2-year period involved children who had never been vaccinated (Ministry of Health, 2016).

6.3.2 *Drivers of Change in the Responses to the Disease Profile*

6.3.2.1 Health Information Systems

Improved information systems provided information that spurred policy-makers and leaders in the health sector to review and revise national strategies for disease control (see Chapter 10). For example, surveillance systems provided information on emerging and re-emerging CDs. The NHMS provided evidence of the rapid increase and high levels of risk factors and disease prevalence for NCDs, while NCD disease registers provided information on disease trends and disease burdens, early detection and effective control. In some cases, the information also energised social activists to advocate for revised approaches, for example, for HIV/AIDS.

6.3.2.2 International Movements

International movements such as the United Nations' millennium development goals (MDGs), sustainable development goals (SDGs) and the WHO Framework Convention on Tobacco Control (FCTC, ratified on 16 September 2005) served to focus attention and provide impetus for stronger efforts. For example, in 2005, the Cabinet Committee on AIDS agreed to pilot test a harm reduction programme for HIV prevention among IDUs despite it being incompatible with the country's zero-tolerance policy on drugs (see Case Study 6.1). In 2018, the Cabinet Committee decided not to reintroduce 'kiddie pack' cigarettes (packs of ten) despite the possibility of increasing tax revenue (Bernama, 2018).

International concerns about cross-border transmission of emerging diseases contributed to stronger collaboration and co-ordination between Malaysia, regional and international agencies such as the ASEAN[1] and the WHO[2], and bilateral co-ordination with neighbours (e.g. the Thailand-Malaysia Border Health Goodwill Committee, the Health Task Force of the Asia-Pacific Economic Cooperation (APEC) group) (Barraclough & Phua, 2007).

6.3.2.3 Leadership, Governance and Competing Priorities

The examples of cross-sectoral collaboration for NCDs quoted above also provide evidence of the government's commitment and the influence of leaders from the health sector and of the MoH in shaping policy that transcended several sectors. However, balancing the competing priorities in health with other opportunities for economic growth and development remains a challenge for Malaysia, especially in NCD prevention. Several factors and entities outside of health have considerable influence. For example, food, beverages and tobacco are deemed promising industries for driving growth in the manufacturing sector in the Eleventh Malaysia Plan (2016–20). However, they might not contribute to the promotion of a healthy lifestyle for reducing CDs and NCDs (Economic Planning Unit, 2015). Population health outcomes require multi-actors and sectors to work together to address social, economic and environmental risk factors. There is top-level commitment in the form of a Cabinet-level committee comprised of ministers from various sectors and chaired by the deputy prime minister and several task forces for establishing priorities and developing strategies (Box 6.4).

However, progress in translating the top-level commitment into genuine collaborations across ministries and agencies is slow, especially at implementation level. The MoH faces a continuing challenge to advocate for and create an enabling environment and an integrated approach for implementing multi-sectoral strategic plans. Such plans require the acceptance of roles, responsibilities and incentives for each agency to contribute to disease control efforts as well as for monitoring and evaluation mechanisms to track performance and accountability.

6.3.2.4 Programme Management and Service Delivery

Disease control programmes require considerable structural and functional change to address the changing epidemiologic picture. The previous national control programmes for CDs had tightly knit management structures at MoH level, together with a high level of authority. Hitherto, leadership for managing NCDs had primarily been the purview of various clinical disciplines, such as cardiology, nephrology or oncology. The introduction of a more holistic perspective to NCD control required a more collaborative management structure that allowed inputs from various disciplines and shifted the focus from patient care to population outcomes. This required shared leadership between public health, clinical and laboratory specialist disciplines. Inevitably, the authority structure and interrelationships changed. Also, disciplines that had previously worked within a small

Box 6.4 National committee/task force/strategic plan/policy

Communicable diseases

National committee/task force

- HIV and AIDS
  - o 1985: National AIDS Task Force
  - o 1992
    - Inter-Ministerial Committee on AIDS
    - National Coordinating Committee on AIDS
    - National Technical Committee on AIDS
  - o 2000: Cabinet Committee on AIDS
- Dengue
  - o 2014: National Committee on Dengue

Laws and regulations

- Prevention and Control of Infectious Diseases Act 1988

National Strategic Plan (NSP)

- National Plan of Action on AIDS, 1988, 1998
- NSP on HIV and AIDS, 2006–10 and 2011–15
- NSP for Ending AIDS, 2016–30
- NSP for Leprosy, 2016–20
- NSP for Tuberculosis Control, 2011–15 and 2016–20

Non-communicable diseases

National committee/task force

- NCDs
  - o 2010: Cabinet Committee for a Health Promoting Environment
- Tobacco Control
  - o National Coordinating Mechanism for Tobacco Control

Laws and regulations

- Control of Tobacco Products Regulation 2004 and Control of Tobacco Product (Amendment) Regulations 2008, 2009, 2010 and 2011 under the Food Act 1983

National Strategic Plan (NSP)

- NSP for Non-Communicable Disease, 2010–14 and 2016–25
- NSP for Tobacco Control, 2015–20
- National Cancer Control Blueprint, 2008–15
- NSP for Cancer Control Programme, 2016–20
- National Action Plan for Healthy Kidneys, 2018–25
- Salt Reduction Strategy to Prevent and Control of NCD for Malaysia, 2015–20
- Policy Options to Combat Obesity in Malaysia, 2016–25
- NSP for Active Living 2016–25
- Malaysia Alcohol Control Action Plan 2013–20

circle of related disciplines had to gain competence in collaborating at multi-sector level and aim at population-wide behaviour change, working with communities and using mainstream and social media.

The Epidemiology Unit, previously established under the Health Division of the MoH in 1971, had focused on CDs. It was re-organised in 1992 (Suleiman & Jegathesan, n.d.) to expand its scope to include NCDs, disease surveillance, HIV/AIDS, vector-borne diseases, occupational and environment health and tobacco control, and public health laboratories. Its responsibilities include policies, planning and strategic management, building integrated and collaborative efforts with other agencies including healthcare providers in the private sector, and providing a platform within the MoH to co-ordinate inputs from the various clinical disciplines as well as with the research institutions[3] that provide laboratory expertise or programme evaluation and investigative skills.

As discussed in Chapters 4 and 5, since the early 1990s, the service delivery system was re-organised and upgraded with the appropriate technology and staff, particularly at the primary care level, to strengthen comprehensive management of CDs and NCDs. Box 6.5 provides examples of the initiatives. Public sector clinics have standardised clinical management protocols to guide service providers, but the process of placing fully trained multi-disciplinary teams is a slow, ongoing process and far from complete (see Chapter 4). For example, healthcare providers' insufficient interpersonal and communication skills contributed to gaps in managing diabetic patients (Lim et al., 2018). Chan (2015) highlighted the need for trained diabetic nurse educators to empower patients for self-care. Additionally, efforts at addressing NCD management are hampered by inadequate referral systems, lack of continuity of care between primary, secondary and tertiary care, and inadequate involvement of private general practitioners in the co-ordinated management of NCDs (see Chapters 4 and 5).

NCD monitoring evolved from early ad hoc initiatives from various clinical disciplines that established patient registries[4] to monitor their disease speciality. This resulted in over 31 separate disease registries by 2012, most of which had resource constraints. There were over 70 databases with no linkages to each other, and data standards varied (Clinical Research Centre, 2012). Efforts to centralise the registries and standardise the quality of data face several challenges, including the lack of resources (workforce, funding and information communication

Box 6.5 Examples of integration of disease prevention and control activities (prevention, early detection, management and treatment) in PHC clinics

- 1995: Breast self-examination (BSE) and annual breast examination by trained health workers
- 1996: Decentralisation and transfer of general outpatient services in hospitals to PHC clinics
- 1998: HIV screening and management services such as prevention of mother-to-child transmission (PMTCT) programme
- 2000 onwards: Integration of diabetes screening and management, methadone services for IDUs, management of other NCDs

technology (ICT) infrastructure), a governing body and data sharing between registries. The more successful registries are those that deal with single diseases or interventional entities and that require data input from fewer sources. Examples are the renal and cataract registries that contribute to continuous improvement in quality of care.

Recognising the high cost of managing and treating NCDs, the MoH adopted a key strategy of encouraging healthier lifestyles that would reduce NCD risk factors in the community. A series of national healthy lifestyle programmes targeted at the general population (Suleiman & Jegathesan, n.d.) disseminated key messages through a variety of channels. Also, specially designed community mobilisation efforts were implemented to empower communities to foster behaviour change with the involvement of multiple agencies such as the Ministry of Education and the Ministry of Information. Despite these efforts, diabetes, obesity and overweight increased dramatically, and smoking rates remained unchanged (Table 6.4). Malaysia has yet to find effective means of addressing these challenges.

The health system had to respond to emerging and re-emerging CDs with better tools for rapid diagnosis, rapid and effective analysis of epidemiological data and rapid response capability to control outbreaks – this required sophisticated technology at multiple levels: field, laboratory, clinical and digital information. The effort required financial resources and higher levels of competency in human resources. The continuing burden of dengue, malaria and TB required multi-agency collaboration.

Box 6.6 Key milestones in the evolution of responses to emerging communicable diseases

1999: Inter-ministry committee for the control of zoonotic diseases
2002: Epidemic intelligence programme
2006: National influenza pandemic preparedness plan
2007: Crisis preparedness and response centre
2008: Risk communication plan

Source: Sulaiman, 2011.

Earlier years had seen the development of surveillance and systems to respond to CD outbreaks. The new challenges, illustrated in Table 6.6, resulted in further evolution, and the key milestones in Box 6.6 demonstrate the range of stakeholders and activities involved.

New procedures required the district health office to act as a gatekeeper to collect data routinely from a wider range of stakeholders, including health facilities in the public and private sectors, such as laboratories, clinics and hospitals (clinical-based surveillance); the Department of Veterinary Services and FOMEMA (Foreign Workers' Medical Examination); and communities (Ministry of Health, 2004).

Monitoring systems established by the earlier national control programmes for CDs such as TB had been merged into the mainstream by 1995, whereby district health offices were the nodal points for integrating data from hospitals and clinics. Nevertheless, at the national level, separate programme entities maintained some elements of their original structure. For example, the chest clinics maintained their own TB registry, and most of the district health offices had limited access to such data, leading to a lower priority for TB control (Ministry of Health, 2002). The situation only improved in 2002 when the National TB Information System (TBIS) gave the district health office full responsibility for co-ordinating and monitoring the information. Nonetheless, contact tracing for CDs such as TB and HIV remains a concern, particularly among the key populations, that is, migrant and rural populations, including the indigenous populations (Suleiman & Jegathesan, n.d.).

Box 6.7 System observations: considering feedback loops in behavioural change

The health system has frequently struggled when it has had to change human behaviour for successful disease control. Health promotion often follows a knowledge gap theory, assuming that providing the right information will yield the right behaviour, but with very limited results. Positive feedback from unhealthy behaviour – for example, the satisfaction from eating unhealthy foods – is often immediate, whereas negative feedback – for example, cardiovascular disease – is distant, vague and uncertain. More immediate feedback that promotes healthy behaviour and discourages unhealthy behaviour, such as social approval, may provide useful tools for individual behavioural change. On a larger scale, we need to consider what types of feedback loops will create health-promoting environments.

6.4 Conclusion

Malaysia has successfully reduced the burden of several CDs through time-limited dedicated programmes aimed at specific diseases. These programmes largely avoided the well-known disadvantages of vertical programme approaches. There are several contributing factors: programme designs recognised and relied on the existing and developing healthcare delivery system. Thus, at the front line, service delivery was in the hands of the PHC providers.[5] This avoided unnecessary duplication and inefficiencies and subsequent potential redundancy and wastage of human resources and physical facilities. On the other hand, the dedicated vertical approach enabled the development of competencies in programme management, supervision, monitoring and evaluation that later transferred to the public health sector. Conceivably, reliance on domestic and not foreign funding ensured that programme design was accountable to domestic authorities and therefore aligned to national health and development priorities and strategies. (Other chapters elaborate on these priorities and strategies.)

Emerging and re-emerging infectious diseases pose continuing challenges, some of which have been easier to address. The underlying factors are the adaptive behaviour of pathogens, changes in the habits and immune levels of communities that expose them to virulent pathogens, and changes in the environment that facilitate change in either pathogens or humans. There is insufficient knowledge on how the emergence of a new disease can be prevented. Therefore, health systems rely on rapid recognition and effective control of outbreaks. Quick to recognise that Malaysia has the climatic and geographic features that place it at risk of emerging diseases, particularly those arising from zoonotic pools of infection (Ministry of Health, 2002; 2004), the country rapidly developed the capacity for early recognition and containment of outbreaks (Lim, 1999). There has been less success in dealing with re-emerging diseases caused by human behaviour such as migration and drug use or by the adaptive behaviour of pathogens and vectors compounded by human behaviour, such as antibiotic-resistant microbes and dengue.

Malaysia has had less success in the field of NCDs. The reasons for this are unclear. The range of diseases is much broader and their causative and contributory factors more varied. For some, such as several neoplastic diseases, medical knowledge about their prevention and management is limited. For others, such as cardiovascular and metabolic diseases, the contributory factors require a change in human behaviour, which is complex and dependent on a wide variety of influences. The health sector has yet to devise effective means of addressing many of those influences.

6.5 Key Messages from Malaysia's Experience

6.5.1 What Went Well?

- The design of disease-specific control programmes, as far as possible, used existing healthcare delivery systems. They also developed specific competencies in programme management, supervision, monitoring and evaluation, which later transferred to the public health delivery system.
- The health system rapidly developed the capacity for prompt recognition and effective control of outbreaks of new diseases, as knowledge on prevention was insufficient.

6.5.2 *What Didn't Go So Well?*

- The health system has had less success in dealing with NCDs and CDs caused by:
  - Human behaviour such as migration and drug use.
  - The adaptive behaviour of pathogens and vectors compounded by human behaviour, such as antibiotic-resistant microbes and dengue.

6.5.3 *Trends and Challenges*

The increasing prevalence of diseases whose root causes lie outside the traditional jurisdiction of the health system will require innovative leadership and new approaches.

References

Atun, R., Bennett, S. and Duran, A. (2008). *Policy Brief: When Do Vertical (Stand-Alone) Programmes Have a Place in Health Systems?* Copenhagen: WHO Regional Office for Europe.

Barraclough, S. and Phua, K.-L. (2007). Health imperatives in foreign policy: the case of Malaysia. *Bulletin of the World Health Organization*, 85, 225–9.

Bernama. (2018). *Malaysia Says No to Kiddie Pack Cigarettes.* Kuala Lumpur: Edge Markets.

Chan, S. P. (2015). Diabetes care model in Malaysia. *Journal of the ASEAN Federation of Endocrine Societies*, 30, 100.

Cheong, P. S. (2010). *Tuberculosis Control Programme in Malaysia 1961–1980. History of Medicine in Malaysia: Vol II – the Development of Medical and Health Services.* Kuala Lumpur: Academy of Sciences of Malaysia.

Clinical Research Centre (CRC). (2012). *Situational Analysis of Patient Registries in Malaysia.* Kuala Lumpur: Clinical Research Centre, Ministry of Health, Malaysia.

DaVanzo, J. and Habicht, J. P. (1986). Infant mortality decline in Malaysia, 1946–1975: the roles of changes in variables and changes in the structure of relationships. *Demography*, 23, 143–60.

Department of Statistics. (2009). *Vital Statistics Time Series Malaysia, 2000–2009.* Kuala Lumpur: Department of Statistics, Malaysia.

Department of Statistics. (2011a). *Vital Statistics: Time Series, Malaysia, 1963–1998.* Kuala Lumpur: Department of Statistics, Malaysia.

Department of Statistics. (2011b). *Vital Statistics Malaysia, 2010*. Kuala Lumpur: Department of Statistics, Malaysia.

Department of Statistics. (2018). *Vital Statistics Malaysia, 2018*. Kuala Lumpur: Department of Statistics, Malaysia.

Dowdle, W. R. (1998). The principles of disease elimination and eradication. *Bulletin of the World Health Organization*, 76, 22–5.

Economic Planning Unit (EPU). (2015). *Eleventh Malaysia Plan, 2016–2020*. Putrajaya: Economic Planning Unit, Malaysia.

Institute for Public Health (IPH). (1996). *Second National Health and Morbidity Study (NHMS 2)*. Kuala Lumpur: Ministry of Health Malaysia.

Institute for Public Health (IPH). (2008). *The Third National Health and Morbidity Survey 2006 (NHMS III)*. Kuala Lumpur: Ministry of Health Malaysia.

Institute for Public Health (IPH). (2011). *National Health and Morbidity Survey 2011 (NHMS 2011)*. Kuala Lumpur: Ministry of Health Malaysia.

Institute for Public Health (IPH). (2015). *National Health and Morbidity Survey 2015–VOLUME II: Non-communicable Diseases, Risk Factors and Other Health Problems*. Kuala Lumpur: Ministry of Health Malaysia.

Ismail, H. A. M. and Martinez, E. J. (1974). *Our Health Services in the Seventies*. Kuala Lumpur: Ministry of Health Malaysia.

Jaafar, S. H., Suhaili, M. R. H., Mohd Noh, K. and Lee, F. S. (2007). *Primary Health Care: Key to Intersectoral Action for Health and Equity*. Geneva: World Health Organization.

Jayalakshmi, P. (1994). Leprosy in Malaysia. *Malaysian Journal of Pathology*, 16, 7–9.

Kamaludin, F. (1990). Leprosy control programme in Malaysia. *Nihon Rai Gakkai Zasshi*, 59, 169–82.

Lim, S. C., Aagaard-Hansen, J., Mustapha, F. I. and Bjerre-Christensen, U. (2018). Malaysian diabetes patients' perceptions, attitudes and practices in relation to self-care and encounters with primary health care providers. *Malaysian Journal of Medical Research*, 2, 1–10.

Lim, V. K. E. (1999). Emerging and re-emerging infections. *Medical Journal of Malaysia*, 54(2), 287–92.

Lo, E. K. (1985). Yaws in Malaysia. *Reviews of Infectious Diseases*, 7(Supplement 2), S251–3.

Looi, L.-M. and Chua, K.-B. (2007). Lessons from the Nipah virus outbreak in Malaysia. *Malaysian Journal of Pathology*, 29, 63–7.

Mak, J. W., Jegathesan, M., Lim, P. K., Hakim, S. L., Rain, A. N., Ambu, S. and Chong, H. K. (1992). Epidemiology and control of malaria in Malaysia. *Southeast Asian Journal of Tropical Medicine and Public Health*, 23, 572–7.

MAPTB. (2012). *Tuberculosis in Malaya – the Early Days, Kuala Lumpur: Malaysian Association for the Prevention of Tuberculosis.* Online paper. www.maptb.org.my/info/history.htm

Ministry of Health. (1983). *Health Indicators 1983.* Kuala Lumpur: Ministry of Health Malaysia.

Ministry of Health. (1990). *Health Indicators 1990.* Kuala Lumpur: Ministry of Health Malaysia.

Ministry of Health. (1997). *Health Indicators 1997.* Kuala Lumpur: Ministry of Health Malaysia.

Ministry of Health. (2002). *National Tuberculosis Information System: TBIS Manual.* Kuala Lumpur: Ministry of Health Malaysia.

Ministry of Health. (2004). *Standard Operating Procedure for Potential Infectious Disease.* Putrajaya: Ministry of Health Malaysia.

Ministry of Health. (2005). *Health Indicators 2005.* Putrajaya: Ministry of Health Malaysia.

Ministry of Health. (2010). *Health Indicators 2010.* Putrajaya: Ministry of Health, Malaysia.

Ministry of Health. (2016). *Annual Report.* Putrajaya: Ministry of Health Malaysia.

Ministry of Health. (2018a). *Country Progress Report on HIV/AIDS 2018: Malaysia.* Putrajaya: Ministry of Health Malaysia.

Ministry of Health. (2018b). *Health Indicators 2018.* Putrajaya: Ministry of Health Malaysia.

Ministry of Health Malaysia and Harvard T. H. Chan School of Public Health. (2016). *Malaysian Health Systems Research Volume 1: Contextual Analysis of the Malaysian Health System March 2016.* Putrajaya: Ministry of Health Malaysia.

Ministry of Health, World Health Organization and University of California. (2015). *Eliminating Malaria: Case-study 8 | Progress towards Elimination in Malaysia.* Geneva: World Health Organization.

Rahman, K. M. (1982). Epidemiology of malaria in Malaysia. *Reviews of Infectious Diseases*, 4, 985–91.

Ramanathan, K., Cheah, W. C. and Dondero, T. J. (1976). *75 Years of Medical Research in Malaysia: 1901–1976.* Kuala Lumpur: Institute for Medical Research.

Sam, I. C. (2015). The burden of human influenza in Malaysia. *Medical Journal of Malaysia*, 70, 127–30.

Sulaiman, L. H. (2011). *Emerging and Re-emerging Diseases.* Paper presented at the Asia Pacific Conference on Public Health, 2011.

Suleiman, A. B. and Jegathesan, M. (eds.). (n.d.). *Health in Malaysia: Achievements and Challenges.* Kuala Lumpur: Ministry of Health, Malaysia.

Tan, P. C., Kwok, K. K., Tan, B. A., Nagaraj, S., Tey, N. P. and Zulkifli, S. N. (1987). Socio-economic development and mortality patterns and trends in Malaysia. *Asia-Pacific Population Journal*, 2, 3–20.

Tee, K. K., Takebe, Y. and Kamarulzaman, A. (2009). Emerging and re-emerging viruses in Malaysia, 1997–2007. *International Journal of Infectious Diseases*, 13(3), 307–18.

UN Country Team. (2005). *Malaysia: Achieving the Millennium Development Goals: Successes and Challenges*. Kuala Lumpur: United Nations Development Programme.

World Health Organization. (2017). *Malaysia: WHO Country Cooperation Strategy 2016–2020*. Geneva: World Health Organization.

World Health Organization, 2018. *Noncommunicable Diseases (NCD) Country Profiles – Malaysia*. Geneva: World Health Organization.

Appendix III
Supplementary Tables

Supplementary Table 6.a ***Ten principal causes of admissions and deaths, 1960, 1974 and 1996***

	1960, rank (%)		1974, rank (%)		1996, rank (%)
Causes	Admissions	Deaths	Admissions	Deaths	Deaths
Accidents	1 (10.14)	7 (5.63)	1 (13.48)	3 (10.53)	3 (9.44)
Skin diseases	2 (4.11)	–	6 (2.58)	–	–
Gastroenteritis/digestive system diseases	3 (3.90)	3 (8.93)	3 (3.71)	8 (2.87)	7 (4.60)
Complications of pregnancy	4 (3.72)	10 (2.64)	2 (4.97)	–	–
Tuberculosis	5 (2.88)	5 (7.36)	–	7 (4.40)	–
Malaria	6 (2.65)	–	–	–	–
Mental illness	7 (2.42)	–	4 (3.10)	–	–
Bronchitis	8 (2.34)	–	10 (1.95)	–	–
Pyrexia of unknown origin	9 (2.21)	–	8 (2.16)	–	–
Heart diseases	10 (1.77)	2 (9.94)	5 (2.59)	2 (15.02)	1 (15.61)
Disease of early infancy	–	1 (15.2)	7 (2.29)	1 (18.99)	6 (7.82)
Cardiovascular/cerebrovascular diseases	–	8 (3.17)	9 (2.08)	4 (7.32)	4 (9.27)
Pneumonia	–	4 (8.48)	–	6 (6.50)	8 (4.17)
Neoplasms	–	6 (6.03)	–	5 (6.71)	5 (8.92)
Deficiency diseases	9 (2.81)	–	–	10 (1.43)	–
Liver diseases	–	–	–	9 (2.32)	–
Septicaemia	–	–	–	–	2 (10.12)

Sources: Ismail and Martinez, 1974; Suleiman & Jegathesan, n.d.

Supplementary Table 6.b *Infant and child mortality rates, 1957–2017*

	1957	1970	1983	1990	2000	2010	2016/2017
Infant mortality rate (per 1,000 live births)	68.9	39.4	20.2	13.1	6	6.7	7.3
Neonatal mortality rate (per 1,000 live births)	29.6	21.4	12.3	8.5	3.1	4.3	4.2
Toddler mortality rate (per 1,000 population aged 1–4 years)	8	4.2	1.7	0.9	0.5	0.4	0.4
Under-5 mortality rate (per 1,000 live births)	110.4	55.9	26.6	16.8	7.9	8.5	8.6

Sources: Department of Statistics, 2009; 2011a; 2011b; 2018.

Supplementary Table 6.c *National disease control programmes*

Disease control programme	Key strategies			Supporting strategies			Outcomes
	Prevention	Screening/ detection	Treatment and management	Human resource and capacity building	Surveillance system	Community participation	
Yaws Elimination Campaign, 1954 – with assistance from WHO and UNICEF (UN Children's Fund)		Mass survey campaign, with annual re-surveys. When the incidence rates declined, modified school surveys were deployed every 6 months. If infectious cases were found, the entire area would be studied.	Mass treatment using procaine penicillin for open cases, latent cases and contact.	Yaws elimination unit was set up.			Incidence rate declined from 140.85 per 100,000 population in 1958 to <2 in 1974. Yaws control activities were integrated into the general health services in 1974. All health workers were trained to recognise yaws cases.
Filariasis Control Programme, 1960		Case detection: House and population censuses and nocturnal mass blood survey. Whenever a nocturnal survey was not feasible, the diethylcarbamazine (DEC) stimulation technique was used during follow-up of cases or in school surveys.	Mass treatment in the locality using DEC: Individual case follow-up was carried out after 3–5 months while the locality was resurveyed after about 2–3 years.	Peninsular Malaysia: Control team (medical assistant, public health auxiliary, junior laboratory technician, driver and vehicle). Sabah and Sarawak: Ad hoc team to conduct surveys and treatment in specific areas.			1988–90: There appeared to be a decreasing trend in the number of filariasis cases detected country-wide. 1983: incorporated into the Vector-Borne Disease Control Programme.

Supplementary Table 6.c *National disease control programmes* (continued)

Disease control programme	Key strategies			Supporting strategies			Outcomes
	Prevention	Screening/ detection	Treatment and management	Human resource and capacity building	Surveillance system	Community participation	
National TB Control Programme, 1961 – monitored and co-ordinated by the Division of TB and National TB Control Centre	National health education campaigns: To increase public awareness of TB signs and symptoms and early diagnosis. BCG vaccination programme: Between 1961 and 1974, at least 75% of the susceptible population had been vaccinated (total BCG vaccinations performed: 4,965,982).	Case finding programme: Early case detection among symptomatic and high-risk groups (at least 66%) in the community using mass miniature radiography (MMR), X-ray, bacteriological and sputum examination and referred for appropriate treatment.	Treatment programme: 20-month standard treatment regimen (streptomycin with isoniazid or isoniazid with para-aminosalicylic acid or thiacetazone) for patients to render them non-infective (at least 95%). The National TB Control Centre served as the national referral hospital for patients with complicated TB.	Countrywide training programme conducted by the National TB Centre, supported by hospitals, for different categories of personnel (doctors, nurses, hospital assistants, health inspectors, medical students and lab technicians). Formation of State TB Control/Managerial Teams in 1973 to supervise and monitor the treatment programme and contact tracing.	1973: The TB registry was established.	Working with MAPTB to provide socio-economic aid and increase community participation to reduce defaulter rates for treatment.	TB is no longer the major cause of death. The National TB Control Programme was integrated with public health and general medical services in 1995.

Supplementary Table 6.c ***National disease control programmes*** **(continued)**

Disease control programme	Key strategies			Supporting strategies			Outcomes
	Prevention	Screening/ detection	Treatment and management	Human resource and capacity building	Surveillance system	Community participation	
Malaria Eradication Programme, 1967–82: Part of the Global Malaria Eradication Programme	Vector control: Residual insecticide spraying using DDT (started with DDT wettable powder and replaced by DDT emulsion) - Abate 500 E was applied in drains and canals - Automatic siphons, tidal gates and sluice gates were constructed to manage water movement. Health education for the community.	Active case detection in high-risk areas. Passive case detection in patients seeking medical and health services. Mass blood screenings every 6 months in areas with increase of cases, influx of foreign workers, interior Orang Asli settlements and where there were cases in non-endemic areas.	Presumptive treatment (Darachlor (chloroquine/pyrimethamine)) was given to suspected cases, especially those from malarious areas before blood examination. Radical and follow-up treatment (sulfadoxine/pyrimethamine, chloroquine and primaquine) was given for all reported cases.	Vertical organisational structure: - Director and deputy director - Administration bureau - Spraying bureau - Health education and training bureau - Epidemiology bureau - Entomology bureau - Malariologist - District chief and multi-purpose/special team Specially trained personnel deployed to map and spray all houses and structures, perform census counts, perform mass blood surveys and general surveillance activities.	Case registries Entomological surveillance activities to study vector habits.		Substantial decline in reported cases in West Malaysia and Sarawak, from 150,000 at the start of the programme to <50,000 a year in the late 1970s. Did not succeed in eliminating malaria, re-orientated strategy to malaria control. 1985: Incorporated into the Vector-Borne Disease Control Programme.

Supplementary Table 6.c *National disease control programmes* (continued)

	Key strategies			Supporting strategies			
Disease control programme	Prevention	Screening/ detection	Treatment and management	Human resource and capacity building	Surveillance system	Community participation	Outcomes
			Introduction of multiple drug therapy (MDT) and decentralisation of treatment: patients were hospitalised only during the intensive phase of treatment, and follow-up treatment was available at 23 skin clinics throughout the country.				
National Leprosy Control Programme Peninsular Malaysia (1969), Sarawak (1974), Sabah (1985)		Early case finding by staff of the 'skin clinics'.	Institutional treatment only for infectious cases and non-infectious cases with severe reactions from drug cases requiring reconstructive surgery.		A Central Registry of cases was established at the National Control Centre: it registered 50% or 8,710 estimated cases in 1969.	Worked with MaLRA to reduce stigma and facilitate social integration of patients.	1994: achieved WHO elimination status of <1 per 10,000 population.

Supplementary Table 6.c *National disease control programmes* (continued)

Disease control programme	Key strategies			Supporting strategies			Outcomes
	Prevention	Screening/ detection	Treatment and management	Human resource and capacity building	Surveillance system	Community participation	
National Immunisation Programme – Expanded Immunisation Programme was adopted as part of the National Immunisation Programme in the late 1980s. • Smallpox (early 1950s) • DPT (1958) • BCG (1961) • Poliomyelitis (1972) • Measles (1984) • Rubella (1988) • Hepatitis B (1989)	Immunisation campaigns jointly organised with NGOs. Dissemination of health education messages through mass media. Delivered through the rural health units or the MCH clinics in urban areas as part of MCH services.	Focus on low-coverage groups: • Estate population • Indigenous people • Religious subgroups • Urban poor • Defaulter tracing • Missed opportunities	Strengthening of the cold chain: • Provision of suitable refrigerators, ice packs and vaccine carriers • Training on the management, maintenance and monitoring of the cold chain		Development of a mapping system and improved monitoring system at district and local levels.		Almost 90% childhood immunisation coverage for BCG, DPT, polio and MMR in 1990 Decline of the infant and children mortality rate.

System Analysis Case Study 6.1: Adoption of Harm Reduction Strategies for Preventing HIV among Injecting Drug Users

Shiang Cheng Lim and David T. Tan

The HIV Epidemic and Drug Abuse in Malaysia

HIV was first reported in Malaysia in 1986. Following this, infection rates rose sharply over two decades, culminating in the peak incidence of approximately 7,000 new cases per year in 2002 (Ministry of Health Malaysia, 2016b), of which 70–80% were injecting drug users (IDUs), followed by female sex workers (FSWs), transgender people (TG) and men who have sex with men (MSM) (Malaysian AIDS Council & Malaysian AIDS Foundation, 2012). Injecting drugs was associated with drug abuse. Malaysia had declared drugs the 'Nation's Number One Enemy' since 1970 and had aimed to create a drug-free nation by 2015.

Malaysia's efforts to combat drug use and trafficking took a criminalisation approach, including: (1) mandatory death penalty for drug trafficking, (2) preventative education for young people and school children, and (3) compulsory detention and rehabilitation programmes for drug users. Treatment and rehabilitation centres adopted the total abstinence method, that is, 'cold turkey' detoxification, focusing mainly on vocational, spiritual, psychosocial and military-style physical training with little or no medical intervention to assist drug users in quitting their drug habits (Kamarudin, 2007). The rising number of cases led to increased criminal enforcement, education and rehabilitative efforts under the criminalisation approach (Figure 6-A). This was expected to reduce

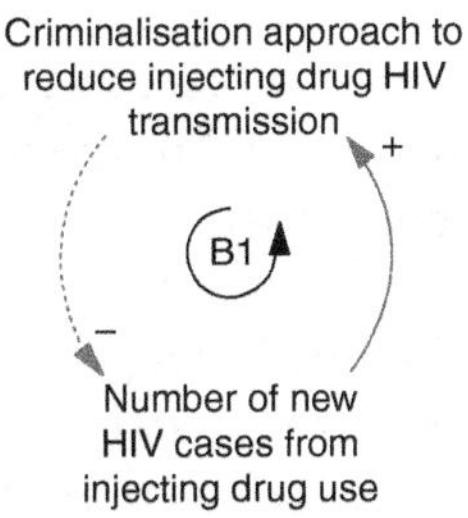

Figure 6-A A criminalisation approach emphasising criminal enforcement, education and rehabilitative efforts failed to reduce the number of new HIV cases from injecting drugs use.

HIV spread to acceptable levels, creating a balancing loop (B1). Unfortunately, this strategy did not yield the desired outcomes.

Indeed, although Malaysia's efforts in the war on drugs were expected to prevent and curb drug use, the number of drug users instead continued to grow. The criminalisation of drug use also led to riskier injecting behaviours among IDUs because many of them feared being caught in possession of any injecting equipment (Reid et al., 2007). This increased the sharing of needles and consequent transmission of HIV. In the early 2000s, the HIV prevalence rate among IDUs was 10–27% (UNAIDS, 2001). The ineffectiveness of the criminalisation approach (Figure 6-A, dotted line, B1) created an urgent demand for alternative solutions, such as harm reduction.

Barriers to the Adoption of Harm Reduction Strategies

Harm reduction principles (see Box 6-A) were gaining traction globally. However, there were several barriers to the introduction of such an approach in Malaysia. Social stigmatisation and criminalisation of drug users were major obstacles to the feasibility of carrying out needle exchange and drug replacement therapy – reinforcing existing practices instead. With a predominantly Muslim population, strong religious and cultural views on drugs and stigmatisation of users were major barriers to public acceptability of harm reduction (Kamarulzaman & Saifuddeen, 2010).

Jurisdiction over the prevention of drug use and HIV was split between enforcement under the Ministry of Home Affairs (MOHA) and healthcare under the MoH. In practice, the enforcement paradigm took priority. Medical practitioners were obligated to report persons with drug dependency who sought medical treatment so that they could be detained and rehabilitated under the Drug Dependants (Treatment and Rehabilitation) Act 1983. Consequently, most IDUs did not seek HIV testing or early diagnosis and would only discover their status at treatment and rehabilitation centres due to compulsory testing or when forced to undergo testing due to suspected HIV-related symptoms (Positive Malaysian Treatment Access and Advocacy Group, 2012).

Additionally, negative societal attitudes towards IDUs were also prevalent within the healthcare workforce (World Health Organization, Regional Office for the Western Pacific & Ministry of Health, Malaysia, 2011). IDUs did not trust healthcare providers –

Box 6-A Harm reduction principles and strategies

Harm reduction focuses on preventing and reducing drug-related harm rather than preventing drug use. It is modelled around humanistic values that uphold human dignity and rights (Hunt et al., 2003). Focused on public health rather than criminal justice, harm reduction goals include reducing injecting drug use and the sharing of injecting equipment, reducing drug abuse, and increasing abstinence from all drug use.

Examples of Harm Reduction Strategies

1. **Needle and syringe exchange programme (NSEP):** Emphasises the use of sterile equipment and the return of used needles and syringes to prevent sharing, which proliferates HIV transmission.
2. **Methadone maintenance treatment (MMT):** Offers an oral, long-acting opioid substitute for reducing the use of illicit parenteral substances and for improving the person's social health status (e.g. enabling them to take on full-time employment).
3. **Condom distribution:** A structural intervention usually complemented with other education strategies aimed at reducing the risk of sexual exposure to HIV.

Early success of harm reduction strategies came from the Netherlands, where success was noted in the reduction of acute hepatitis B incidence and stabilisation of HIV prevalence (Buning, 1991).

particularly with regard to maintaining confidentiality of their HIV status. Most preferred to turn to peers, including former IDUs, as they were more supportive (Positive Malaysian Treatment Access and Advocacy Group, 2012). These attitudes made it very difficult for government health services to be an effective conduit for harm reduction approaches. Some civil society organisations already engaged with the IDU community were better positioned and equipped to do so. Examples included handing over activities from the MoH to civil society, modifying national-level policies that criminalised drug users and addressing stigmatisation of IDUs by multiple stakeholders, including religious leaders and healthcare providers (Figure 6-B).

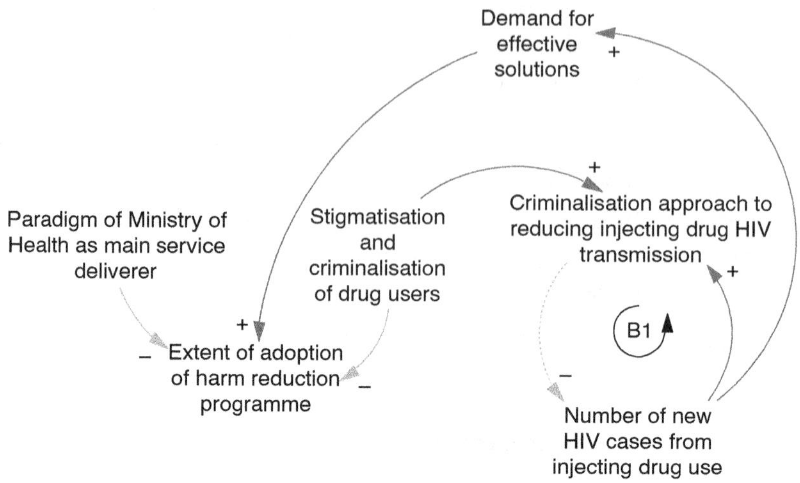

Figure 6-B Stigmatisation and the paradigm of regarding the MoH as the main provider of outreach and services were barriers to a harm reduction programme.

Window of Opportunity and Leadership Resulting in Pilot Programmes

Two key events created a window of opportunity for government leadership to change existing policies (Figure 6-C). First, the Millennium Development Goals (MDGs) mid-term review in 2005 reported that Malaysia was not on track to achieve MDG No. 6 of halting the spread of HIV/AIDS by 2015. This triggered concerns at the highest political levels. At around the same time, local advocacy efforts led by prominent Malaysian individuals hit a high-water mark (see Box 6-B). Together, these events created institutional and public acceptability for the piloting of the methadone maintenance treatment (MMT) programme and needle and syringe exchange programme (NSEP) in October 2005 and February 2006, respectively. Government leadership and strategic partnerships with non-governmental organisations (NGOs) played key roles in the implementation of these harm reduction initiatives. The paradigm that required the MoH to be the main service deliverer changed.

Methadone is a controlled substance and its use requires medical supervision. While the MoH had the authority to implement MMT, it required strong partnerships with NGOs who were able to reach out and win the trust of the IDU community. Implementation of the NSEP

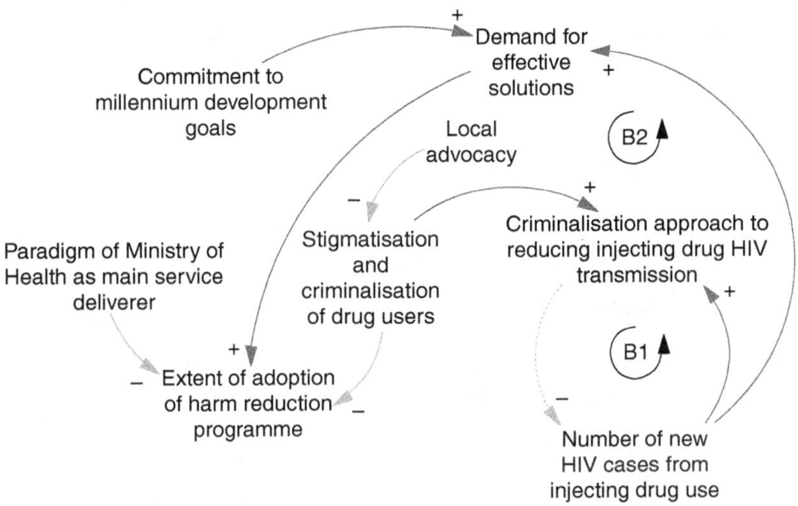

Figure 6-C Commitment to MDG goals and local advocacy were critical enabling factors that overcame barriers to the adoption of the harm reduction approach.

by the government agencies was seen as contradictory to existing drug policies, and there was a fear of inciting resistance from the conservative parties. Civil society organisations, therefore, became an attractive platform. The government provided financial backing to the Malaysian AIDS Council (MAC) (Box 6-B) and allocated RM 4 million annually for their NSEP outreach activities (Malaysian AIDS Council & Malaysian AIDS Foundation, 2007). In turn, the MAC provided a rich resource pool of community healthcare and peer outreach workers with a pre-existing and long-standing rapport with the IDU community. This partnership marked a significant milestone in changing the paradigm for service delivery.

The pilots proved effective. There was a significant reduction in IDUs sharing used equipment as well as a reduction of IDUs using the services of street or port doctors (people who inject drugs for IDUs) across the three NSEP pilot sites (Ibrahim, 2007). Within the MMT pilot project, there were high compliance and retention rates and improved employment rates and performance among the clients who came for MMT programmes (Reid et al., 2007); (Babu, 2009).

Box 6-B Key involvement by the MAC in the government's adoption of harm reduction strategies

The MAC was established in 1992 and serves as the umbrella organisation for partner organisations to advocate, support and co-ordinate all HIV-related activities.

Advocacy

Harm reduction initiatives in Malaysia were propelled by the MAC, which was led by the following influential figures:

- Datin Paduka Marina Mahathir (daughter of the prime minister, Mahathir Mohamad (1981–2003 and 2018–20), president of MAC between 1994 and 2005).
- Dato' Prof Dr Adeeba Kamarulzaman (related to Malaysian royalty and graduated with a medical degree from Australia, MAC board member since early 2000) (Narayanan et al., 2011).
    - Led the Harm Reduction Working Group (HRWG) and used evidence-based research to advocate for harm reduction by focusing on drug use and HIV/AIDS as a public health problem – the pilot project for MMT and NSEP was approved by the Cabinet Committee on Drug Use in 2005 based on the HRWG proposal (Reid et al., 2007).
    - Generated bottom-up support among the religious agencies and scholars in the community by conducting workshops and engaging in theological exchanges (Narayanan et al., 2011).

Implementation

With continuous allocated funding from the Malaysian MoH since 2003 and being the principal recipient of the Global Fund later on (Tanguay, 2011), the MAC and its partner organisations would be the primary implementers of harm reduction initiatives, which include (Malaysian AIDS Council & Malaysian AIDS Foundation, 2015; Ministry of Health Malaysia, 2015; Ministry of Health Malaysia, 2016b):

- Community-based peer outreach programmes
- Drop-in centres
- Shelter care
- HIV treatment and adherence support programme (TAPS)

Sustaining and Replicating Success

The conditions for action described above will not necessarily sustain the acceptability of harm reduction indefinitely. However, the successes achieved in reducing HIV risk and prevalence among IDUs have created acceptance and ownership of the harm reduction programme within the MoH and provided justification to other stakeholders and actors for the continuation and scaling up of the programme, which creates a reinforcing loop (Figure 6-D, R1). Harm reduction has been recognised as the right HIV prevention strategy by the MoH, which has taken ownership of the programme and its successes (Ministry of Health Malaysia, 2013; Institute for Public Health, 2016).

Despite persistent mixed attitudes towards drug users, the success provided justification to other stakeholders and actors for the continuation and scaling up of the programme. Top-level politicians have thrown their weight behind harm reduction policies and programmes. To increase the buy-in from religious groups, the deputy prime minister justified the programme to religious authorities on the grounds that drastic action is needed in emergencies that could lead to death,

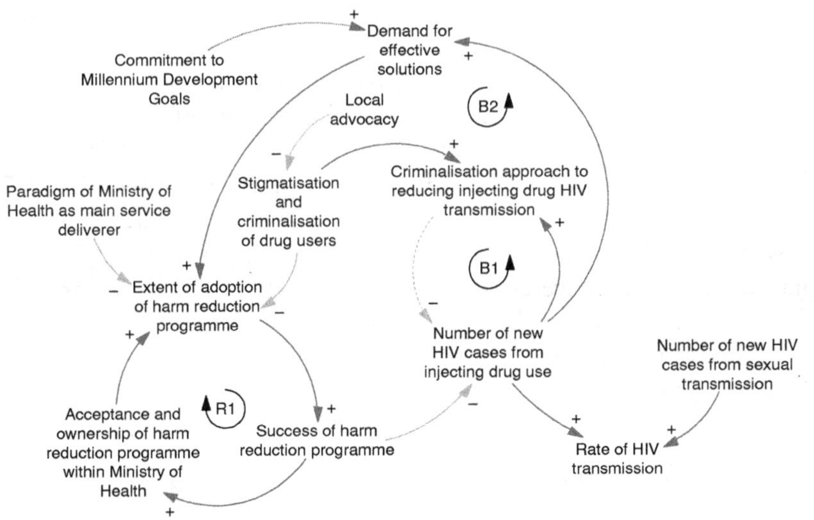

Figure 6-D Success of the pilots created favourable conditions for institutional changes that persisted even after key enabling factors for the adoption of the harm reduction approach (MDGs and local advocacy) receded.

which is permissible under the rule of *darūra* (the rule of necessity) in Islamic law (Narayanan et al., 2011). These political commitments were translated into organisational re-structuring as well as financial support for the harm reduction programme. A National Harm Reduction Task Force, comprising representatives from health and drug control authorities, the police, prison and religious authorities, academics and NGOs was set up in 2005. It provided opportunities for different government agencies to work across and increase the partnership with NGOs (Kamarulzaman, 2009). There was increased funding from the government to finance human resource costs, facility overheads, methadone procurement for MMT services in public facilities and the delivery of NSEP services by NGOs, and the government remained the single largest funding source even as the programme scaled up (Naning et al., 2014). This financial commitment is an indication of the acceptance and ownership of the harm reduction programme within the MoH.

Service delivery through NGOs has proven to be very important, with 70% of needle exchange services delivered through such organisations. The drug replacement therapy wing of the intervention had to be delivered through government (or private) clinics due to methadone being a controlled substance, and penetration has been much lower.

The number of new HIV infections fell from its peak in 2002 to an average of 3,400 cases per year in 2010 and has since plateaued (Ministry of Health Malaysia, 2018). The risk of HIV transmission among IDUs fell from 70–80% to about 10% in 2017, and HIV prevalence among IDUs also decreased from 22.1% in 2009 to 13.4% in 2017 (Ministry of Health Malaysia, 2018). A cost analysis study reported savings of RM 47.1 million in direct healthcare costs and 12,653 HIV infections averted since 2006 (Naning et al., 2014). These remarkable successes have ensured the sustainability of the harm reduction programme even after the initial conditions that enabled it (i.e. the MDGs and the highwater mark of local advocacy) had passed.

New Problems Emerge

The harm reduction programme has achieved and sustained substantial results in reducing HIV transmission among IDUs. These gains have been maximised, however, and further progress in reducing HIV transmission requires new strategies. Sexual transmission is now the leading

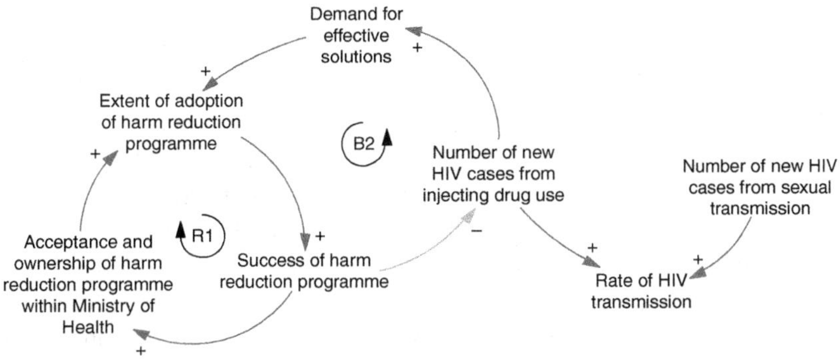

Figure 6-E While harm reduction strategies have reduced HIV in IDUs, the gains are being threatened by the increasing incidence of sexual transmission of HIV.

cause of HIV infection. Evidence shows that the number of new cases has remained persistent and may even be increasing, threatening to reverse gains against the spread of HIV (Figure 6-E).

The MoH acknowledges this challenge. *'The MDGs were vital for the Malaysian government's decision to adopt harm reduction initiatives in the year 2006, however current and ongoing efforts are built upon previous successes and are streamlined towards meeting SDG goals such as Fast Tracking to Zero and Ending AIDS'* (Ministry of Health Malaysia, 2015).

Conclusion and Lessons Learnt

This experience provides lessons on how to test potentially effective strategies for improved health outcomes when the stigmatisation and criminalisation of culturally 'deviant' behaviours are major obstacles. International commitments such as the MDGs, together with evidence-based research, proper data collection and accountability, can help government leadership undertake the necessary interventions even if they may be locally unpopular. Civil society groups may be vital in the delivery of services, particularly services targeted towards marginalised populations. And early success, as seen from the pilot programmes, will probably be necessary in order to sustain interventions in the face of societal suspicion.

The existing harm reduction strategies targeted at IDUs may have reached their limits for reducing the spread of HIV in the Malaysian context, particularly as sexual transmission has overtaken injecting drug use as the major mode of HIV transmission since 2011 (Malaysian AIDS Council & Malaysian AIDS Foundation, 2012). To progress further and meet the new targets of '90-90-90' (90% diagnosed, 90% on treatment, 90% virally suppressed) and to end AIDS by 2030, the MoH will require new strategies that can address sexual transmission effectively. The adoption of such strategies will probably encounter similar barriers related to the stigmatisation and criminalisation of culturally 'deviant' behaviours, so the previous experience holds valuable lessons. At this time, however, the evidence base for interventions to curb the sexual transmission of HIV is low, whereas a high likelihood of substantial success will be needed for key actors to take the political risks of pushing through such an intervention.

Systems Lessons

Systems analysis illustrates that conditions that enable a change in practice are often transient, especially when there is doubt about and hostility to the new practice. For such changes to be sustainable, feedback loops that reinforce the new practice have to be built. Good narrative-building that captures and communicates successes in ways that fit organisational paradigms are valuable for this.

References

Babu, R. (25 April 2009). *Malaysia: Helping the Addicts with Methadone.* Online blog post. www.ssig.gov.my/blog/2009/04/25/malaysia-helping-the-addicts-with-methadone

Buning, E. C. (1991). Effects of Amsterdam needle and syringe exchange. *International Journal of the Addictions*, 26(12), 1303–11.

Hunt, N., Ashton, M., Lenton, S., Mitcheson, L., Nelles, B. and Stimson, G. (2003). *A Review of the Evidence-Base for Harm Reduction Approaches to Drug Use*. London: Forward Thinking on Drugs.

Ibrahim, F. H. (2007). Needle syringe exchange program in Malaysia. *Jurnal Anti Dadah Malaysia*, 29–58.

Institute for Public Health. (2016). *Malaysian Methadone Treatment Outcome Study (MyTOS): Review of Methadone Maintenance Therapy in Malaysia (2005–2014)*. Kuala Lumpur: Ministry of Health Malaysia.

Kamarudin, A. R. (2007). Misuse of drugs in Malaysia: past and present. *Jurnal Anti Dadah Malaysia*, 1–24.

Kamarulzaman, A. (2009). Impact of HIV prevention programs on drug users in Malaysia. *JAIDS: Journal of Acquired Immune Deficiency Syndromes*, 52, S17–19. DOI: https://doi.org/10.1097/QAI.0b013e3181bbc9af

Kamarulzaman, A. (2016). *Islam and Harm Reduction*. Paper presented at the Faculty of Medicine, University of Malaya. Kuala Lumpur: Faculty of Medicine, University of Malaya.

Kamarulzaman, A. and Saifuddeen, S. M. (2010). Islam and harm reduction. *International Journal of Drug Policy*, 21(2), 115–18. DOI: https://doi.org/10.1016/j.drugpo.2009.11.003

Malaysian AIDS Council and Malaysian AIDS Foundation. (2007). *Annual Report 2007*. Kuala Lumpur: Malaysian AIDS Council and Malaysian AIDS Foundation.

Malaysian AIDS Council and Malaysian AIDS Foundation. (2012). *Annual Report 2011: Getting to Zero*. Kuala Lumpur: Malaysian AIDS Council and Malaysian AIDS Foundation.

Malaysian AIDS Council and Malaysian AIDS Foundation. (2015). *Annual Report 2014*. Kuala Lumpur: Malaysian AIDS Council and Malaysian AIDS Foundation.

Ministry of Health Malaysia. (2006a). *Malaysian Needle and Syringe Exchange Program Pilot Project: Standard Operating Procedures for NSEP Pilot Sites (Guidelines for NGOs)*. Putrajaya: Ministry of Health Malaysia.

Ministry of Health Malaysia. (2006b). *National Strategic Plan on HIV/AIDS: Malaysia 2006–2010*. Putrajaya: Ministry of Health Malaysia.

Ministry of Health Malaysia. (2011). *National Strategic Plan on HIV and AIDS 2011–2015*. Putrajaya: Ministry of Health Malaysia.

Ministry of Health Malaysia. (2013). *Mid-term Review: The National Strategic Plan on HIV/AIDS, 2011–2015*. Putrajaya: Ministry of Health Malaysia.

Ministry of Health Malaysia. (2015). *The National Strategic Plan for Ending AIDS 2016–2030*. Putrajaya: Ministry of Health Malaysia.

Ministry of Health Malaysia. (May 2016a). *Polisi dan Prosedur Operasi Piawai Program Rawatan Methadone*. Putrajaya: HIV/STI Sector, Disease Control Division, Ministry of Health Malaysia.

Ministry of Health Malaysia, Disease Control Division. (2016b). *Global AIDS Response Progress Report 2016: Malaysia*. Online report. www.moh.gov.my/images/gallery/Report/Malaysia%20GARPR%202016_Final.pdf

Ministry of Health Malaysia. (2018). *Country Progress Report on HIV/AIDS 2018: Malaysia*. Putrajaya: Ministry of Health Malaysia.

Ministry of Health Malaysia and Royal Malaysia Police. (2006). *The National Needle and Syringe Exchange Programme: Guidelines for Police*. Putrajaya: Ministry of Health Malaysia.

Naning, H., Kerr, C., Kamarulzaman, A., Dahlui, M., Ng, C.-W. and Wilson, D. P. (2014). *Return on Investment and Cost-Effectiveness of Harm Reduction Programmes in Malaysia (No. 88083)*. Washington, DC: World Bank.

Narayanan, S., Vicknasingam, B. and Robson, N. B. M. H. (2011). The transition to harm reduction: understanding the role of non-governmental organisations in Malaysia. *International Journal of Drug Policy*, 22(4), 311–17. DOI: https://doi.org/10.1016/j.drugpo.2011.01.002

Positive Malaysian Treatment Access and Advocacy Group (MTAAG+). (2012). *PLHIV Stigma Index*. Petaling Jaya: MTAAG.

Reid, G., Kamarulzaman, A. and Sran, S. K. (2007). Malaysia and harm reduction: the challenges and responses. *International Journal of Drug Policy*, 18(2), 136–40. DOI: https://doi.org/10.1016/j.drugpo.2006.12.015

Tanguay, P. (2011). *Policy Responses to Drug Issues in Malaysia*. International Drug Policy Consortium. DOI: http://dx.doi.org/10.2139/ssrn.1908799

UNAIDS. (2001). *The Asian Harm Reduction Network: Supporting Responses to HIV and Injecting Drug Use in Asia*. Geneva: UNAIDS.

World Health Organization, Regional Office for the Western Pacific and Ministry of Health, Malaysia. (2011). *Good Practices in Asia: Effective Paradigm Shifts towards an Improved National Response to Drugs and HIV/AIDS: Scale-Up of Harm Reduction in Malaysia*. Online report. www.wpro.who.int/publications/docs/GoodPracticesinAsia_WEB_270411.pdf

Notes

1. Association of South East Asian Nations.
2. World Health Organization.
3. Examples are the IMR, the Institute of Health Management and the Institute of Health System Research.
4. Patient registries collect uniform data on demographics, diagnostics, treatment and outcomes for patients.
5. The exception was malaria, which required special categories of workers for the limited initial phase of the programme.

7 Health Service Delivery

Environmental Health Services

MUKUNDAN SUGUNAN PILLAY AND DEBBIE SIRU

7.1 Introduction

The protection and management of the natural and built environment and monitoring its relation to and impact on health are important components of any country's health system. The ever-expanding global population and increasing urbanization place a strain on the environment and create new risks and exposures that exacerbate health problems. The first line of defence in disease prevention is controlling the physical, chemical and biological agents in the environment that have the potential to affect populations. Thus, every aspect of the environment that impacts on health falls within the scope of environmental health services (EHS). Clean water, safe disposal of solid waste and wastewater, vector and rodent control, air pollution control, food quality control and climate change are just some examples. In this chapter, we focus on providing a broad overview of the evolution of EHS in Malaysia as part of the overall health system.

7.2 Overview of EHS and Its Evolution in Malaysia

In the 1960s, after independence, 70% of the population was poor and resided in rural areas (see Chapter 3). Limited water accessibility and communicable diseases were major problems, which were addressed by the Rural Environmental Sanitation Programme (RESP), an integral component of the Rural Health Services (Suleiman & Jegathesan, n.d.). Highly effective community mobilization by allied environmental health officers and technical expertise from engineers trained in public health are credited as two success factors of the RESP, which achieved high levels of coverage and drastic reduction of the disease burden from waterborne diseases.

With increasing economic development, more than 70% of the population moved to urban areas, life expectancy increased, and there was a decline in infant mortality rates and incidence of communicable diseases (see Chapter 3) (Ministry of Health Malaysia, 1988–2017). However, population growth, increasing urbanization and industrialization introduced other environmental hazards, creating the need to address a wider range of environmental health issues such as sewerage, water quality, solid and hazardous waste, and radiation protection.

EHS in Malaysia began in an organized and structured manner with the establishment of the Environmental Health Engineering Programme in the Ministry of Health (MoH), pioneered by engineers seconded from the Public Works Department (PWD) in the 1970s. This pool of engineers, often assisted by sanitary engineers from the World Health Organization (WHO), went on to strengthen the EHS as an integral part of the MoH's public health programme.

As the Constitution of Malaysia apportions responsibility for health to the federal government, and water supply and urban sanitation to state and local governments, the responsibility for managing EHS was split among different government agencies (see Chapter 12).

To provide leadership and the relevant authority, some public health engineers were seconded from the MoH to some of these departments. Thus EHS in Malaysia grew primarily because of the leadership and governance role the MoH took. EHS established an organizational structure and staffed it with trained personnel while at the same time empowering the organizational units with the required funding. The initial batch of public health engineers provided the leadership on the ground to support the health inspectorate and health officers. Human resources training and development were crucial to achieving success. Environmental health was introduced into postgraduate public health programmes. Engineers who had training in public health helped to upgrade the training of health inspectors and health overseers. The upgraded three-year course for health inspectors (see Chapter 8) included aspects of newer technologies in wastewater treatment, water treatment and waste disposal. Also, environmental health was included in the training of microbiologists and biochemists. Expertise was shared with other ministries and departments. The WHO contributed by establishing the Centre for the Promotion of Environmental Planning and Applied Studies (PEPAS), which conducted valuable research and training programmes that in turn led to policy and programme formulation such as the National Solid Waste Management Strategy (WHO Western Pacific Region, 1977). Introducing health impact assessment (HIA) to other agencies for development projects was a concerted effort using many existing channels available at the state and federal government levels (Hashim & Hashim, 2009).

7.2.1 *Examples of Malaysia's EHS Programmes*

Some of the main environmental health programmes that were developed successfully are described in this section.

7.2.1.1 Rural Environmental Sanitation Programme (RESP)

Concerns about the quality of water supply and sanitation led to an environmental survey of Peninsular Malaysia in 1968. It revealed that only 3.6% of the population had piped water, while 85.3% used water from unprotected wells and 11.1% from untreated surface water (Pillay et al., n.d.). As a result, an environmental sanitation pilot project was carried out. The pilot project indicated that a national environmental health programme needed to have four basic elements to succeed: community participation, health education, appropriate technology and training. The initial efforts of EHS were directed to rural areas of the country that lacked safe water supply and sanitation and were plagued by waterborne diseases (Suleiman & Jegathesan, n.d.). The national programme was successful in increasing coverage of the rural population of safe water supply to 68.6% and sanitary latrines to 72.5% in 1987 (Ministry of Health Malaysia, 1989). This coverage reached 93.5% for safe water supply and 98.2% for sanitary latrines in 2000 (Ministry of Health Malaysia, 2002). The MoH had contributed to 22.2% of the water supply for rural communities. The MoH provided a high percentage of water supply in states such as Sarawak (62.3%), Sabah (43.5%), Kelantan (32.5%) and Terengganu (30.4%) (Pillay et al., n.d.).

This programme was not only a paradigm shift, with the MoH taking on a function that was traditionally that of state governments and the PWD, it also became an important programme under the MoH public health programmes. It complemented the other programmes, such as communicable disease control, vector hygiene, food quality control and others, and was implemented in all states (Ministry of Health Malaysia, 1988). The Environmental Health Engineering Unit

Box 7.1 System observations: cross-boundary problems

One of the challenges in the application of systems thinking is that the actual system surrounding a particular problem often does not correspond to disciplinary or organizational structures. Therefore, solutions to these problems are often partial, with partial results. Indeed, while the 'social and environmental determinants of health' is a well-known concept, it largely remains on the periphery of health systems. A whole-system approach towards environmental health requires interfacing with non-health sectors as well as re-thinking the responsibilities and functions of the health system. The expansion of the MoH to create an engineering department and take on the task of rural water and sanitation is an excellent example of such cross-boundary work. Future advances in tackling non-communicable diseases are likely to require such re-thinking of what health services look like.

grew and was later expanded with the recruitment of more public health engineers and health inspectors. The unit provided the needed policies, technical guidance and training, and it also monitored budget allocations. Initially, public health engineers were stationed in critical states such as Kedah, Perak, Pahang, Terengganu and Kelantan, but they are now present in every state nationwide. Health inspectors were trained in appropriate technologies for rural water supply and sanitation. RESP, later called the BAKAS (*Bekalan Air dan Kebersihan Alam Sekeliling*) or Water Supply and Environmental Sanitation Programme, clearly demonstrated the close interaction between the different levels of government. The federal government provided the funds and technical advisory services while the state governments provided the needed managerial support through the district levels right up to the village action committees (Suleiman & Jegathesan, n.d.). This was a key success factor, as was the people's involvement through community participation (see Case Study 7.1 for more details).

7.2.1.2 National Drinking Water Quality Surveillance Programme (NDWQSP)

Having succeeded in the BAKAS programme, the MoH engineering unit was entrusted with monitoring the quality of urban water supplies.

This decision was made following a survey in 1983 that attributed the outbreak of diseases to poorly operated water supply systems. This programme, known as the National Drinking Water Quality Surveillance Programme (NDWQSP), had the objective of improving the standard of health by ensuring the safety and acceptability of public water supply systems (Suleiman & Jegathesan, n.d.). The components of the programme included monitoring, sanitary surveys, data processing and evaluation, remedial action and institutional examination such as evaluating the capacity of the water supply agency to perform its functions. Under the programme, all public water supplies were monitored, and samples were sent to the Department of Chemistry (DOC) for bacteriological and chemical analysis (Pillay & Sinha, n.d.). The relevant water authority was required to take immediate action if there were any violations of the standards set by the MoH. A quality assurance programme (QAP) was formulated in 1993 to strengthen the effectiveness of the programme (Suleiman & Jegathesan, n.d.). By 2001, the percentage of water samples that met the national standards of bacteriological quality, residual chlorine and turbidity was 98%, 96% and 96%, respectively (Pillay & Sinha, n.d.).

Significant co-operation was established between the state governments, water authorities and relevant agencies such as the DOC, the Department of Environment (DOE) and the federal Drainage and Irrigation Department as well as local authorities. The reports generated under this programme were presented at state- and federal-level meetings and critically examined by many agencies. The training of water operators and health inspectorate staff and public health engineers, coupled with inter-departmental co-operation, were key success factors of this programme. Due to the limited capacity of the DOC, the MoH also developed its water testing capabilities (Ministry of Health Malaysia, 1988) by purchasing field test kits and training the health inspectorate staff and public health engineers on their use.

The leadership and promotional role of the MoH was important in the absence of legislation. The Safe Drinking Water Act was drafted in the 1980s but never came into force for numerous reasons. However, since then, the National Water Services Commission (SPAN) has been formed to address some of the constitutional problems, such as division of responsibility and authority between federal and state government, and the Water Services Industry Act 655 was formulated and enforced in 2008 (National Water Services Commission, 2019).

7.2.1.3 Urban Sanitation

The role played by public health engineers at the state level was recognized as crucial, and over time they played a key role in advising state governments of the sad state of urban sanitation. Together with the Economic Planning Unit (EPU) of the Prime Minister's Department, the MoH engineering unit initiated Master Plan Studies on sewerage and drainage in many towns (Economic Planning Unit, 1981). Such studies identified a grave concern: bucket latrines were widely used in urban centres. Eliminating bucket latrines became a priority, together with studies on suitable sewerage systems for larger towns.

Other than bucket latrines, individual septic tanks were the predominant disposal system. Substantial funds were needed to convert centralized sewerage systems and this would, therefore, take a long time. The MoH adopted an incremental strategy by promoting the use of centralized sewerage systems as opposed to individual septic tanks (Ujang, 2006). All new development projects were directed to follow the guidelines developed by the MoH and to instal centralized sewerage systems with treatment plants such as oxidation ponds. There was no legislation at that time; this was purely based on the MoH's insistence and promotion through its expanded numbers of well-trained public health engineers (Ujang, 2006).

Similar efforts were made in solid waste management. All urban centres had poor waste management systems. Open burning was rampant. Crude landfills were the norm. With support from the WHO, the MoH initiated national forums to develop strategic plans for waste management. Through the environmental health engineering programme, the MoH also provided support to the Prime Minister's Department and the Ministry of Housing and Local Government (MHLG) in matters related to sewerage, urban waste management, urban drainage and urban environmental management (Ujang, 2006; Ministry of Housing and Local Government, Malaysia, 2005).

In 1980, a special technical unit with engineers seconded from the MoH was formed to serve as the technical arm of the Local Government Department of the MHLG. This unit provided technical advisory services to all local authorities and state governments. Numerous studies were undertaken, and guidelines were developed. A major achievement was the total elimination of the bucket latrine system. Policies for urban sewerage systems became entrenched in local development plans, and efforts moved towards the formulation of laws on sewerage and waste management (Ujang, 2006). This then progressed to the privatization of both the national sewerage service and the municipal waste management services. The enactment of these laws and privatization were unprecedented moves by the federal government to take over services traditionally performed by state and local governments. It paid off handsomely, as this led to the systematic development of these two services throughout the country (Japan International Cooperation Agency (JICA), Malaysia Office, 1999).

The privatization of sewerage services was undertaken through the enactment of the Sewerage Services Act, which allowed the federal government to take over the responsibility for sewerage services, which was a traditional function of local authorities. A national sewerage company called Indah Water Konsortium (IWK) was established (Japan Sanitation Consortium, 2011). IWK took over all sewerage assets from local authorities and moved to upgrade and maintain these systems to acceptable standards by ensuring all domestic wastewater was adequately treated before discharging to surface water (Sewerage Services Department, Ministry of Housing and Local Government, 2001). Another significant move was the creation of the Sewerage Services Department (SSD) to regulate sewerage services, and this was staffed with engineers seconded from the MoH (Ujang, 2006).

7.2.1.4 Clinical Waste Management

Recognizing the hazardous nature of clinical waste generated in healthcare settings, the Engineering Division of the MoH undertook a national survey that highlighted the poor conditions in the handling, storage, transportation and disposal of clinical waste. The division went on to issue guidelines for the management of clinical and related waste in hospitals and healthcare establishments, followed by training for selected hospital personnel (Ministry of Health Malaysia, 1991). The gaps identified in the system were addressed by outsourcing clinical waste management to hospital support services. The rapid progress under this strategy was self-evident and is further outlined in Case Study 7.2 at the end of this chapter.

7.2.1.5 Air Pollution

Air pollution in Malaysia is generally at a low level except for sporadic incidents of haze during certain periods of the year. Maintaining good air quality sustainably throughout the year will drastically reduce the burden on the healthcare system. For this purpose, Malaysia built inter-departmental co-operation, involving agencies such as the DOE, the MoH, the Ministry of Transport, the Ministry of Natural Resources and Environment, the Meteorology Department and the Ministry of Foreign Affairs. The private sector was also mobilized by outsourcing air quality monitoring to a private company, Alam Sekitar Malaysian Sdn Bhd (ASMA), which has fifty-two monitoring stations throughout the country (Sahani et al., 2016).

As mentioned earlier, public health engineers were seconded from the MoH to the DOE, and they contributed to the formulation of the Environmental Quality Act 1974 (EQA) and its subsidiary regulations, which included among others the Clean Air Regulations. The MoH was a member when the Environmental Quality Council was launched in 1973, and its membership was subsequently formalized in the EQA. The council is responsible for advising the Minister of the then Ministry of Science, Technology and the Environment, now known as the Ministry of Natural Resources and Environment, regarding environmental matters, and this includes, among other things, air pollution (The Commissioner of Law Revision Malaysia, 2006).

The MoH also contributed the development of guidelines on indoor air quality (IAQ), which is under the purview of the Department of Occupational Safety and Health (DOSH), and continues to play a critical role in providing health advisory notices via news media, their website and so on. The MoH has also developed several guidelines on IAQ for healthcare settings and is training a pool of engineers to be certified by DOSH as indoor air quality assessors. To kickstart its IAQ programme, the MoH is currently focusing on sampling and monitoring air quality in its premises (Ministry of Health Malaysia, 1992).

7.2.1.6 The National Environmental Health Action Plan (NEHAP)

The NEHAP is a set of strategies jointly developed by relevant agencies and selected non-governmental organizations (NGOs) for improving environmental health in the country by specifying the roles and responsibilities of all parties. The WHO has encouraged all countries to embark on developing and implementing NEHAPs. The Malaysian Cabinet endorsed the NEHAP as a government policy in December 2012, and implementation is underway, with state governments assuming responsibility for formulating and implementing their respective State Environmental Health Action Plans (SEHAPs) (Tuan Mat, 2016). Some states, such as Sabah, Pahang, Perak and Melaka, have already started finalizing their SEHAPs, and the momentum is growing among other states (Tuan Mat, 2016). States' adoption of the SEHAPs will be followed by the development of Local Environmental Health Action Plans (LEHAPs).

In order to be effective, NEHAP has to be given priority at all levels, including full participation and commitment from relevant agencies and NGOs, appropriate resource allocation and the enforcement of laws and regulations. The Engineering Services Division of the MoH facilitates and monitors the process by assuming the role of secretariat for the NEHAP, its steering committee, technical committee and the thematic working groups (TWGs). Eleven TWGs address various areas of concern such as vector-borne diseases, urban drainage and air quality as well as emerging issues such as climate change (National Environmental Health Action Plan, n.d.; Tuan Mat, 2016). The Division is also working with the Malaysian Space Agency (MYSA), formerly known as the Malaysian Remote Sensing Agency, to develop a geospatial risk map. This will be an invaluable tool for pre-empting adverse environmental health incidents.

Health impact assessments (HIA) have been incorporated as part of the Environmental Impact Assessment (EIA) process. The MoH undertakes the review of the components of EIA related to environmental HIA. Its importance is further emphasized by its inclusion as a TWG under NEHAP.

7.2.2 Factors Contributing to Success

The MoH rightly invested in environmental health programmes early on, which is believed to have significantly contributed to the country's elevated health status. Other than investment, the hallmarks of the developmental process included leadership from the MoH in initiating and sustaining inter-agency collaboration and co-operation, human resource development and selective organizational strengthening, enactment of legislation and development of guidelines, and strategic involvement of the private sector while the public sector retained responsibility for policy and oversight.

Inter-departmental co-operation/organizational shift of responsibilities: From the beginning, the MoH recognized that inter-departmental collaboration was vital, given that so many aspects of the human environment and activities have an impact on health. The MoH adopted two distinct modalities. In the case of rural water supply, the MoH took over the role that had traditionally rested with state governments and the PWD. In other cases, the MoH took the lead in spearheading the required changes and subsequently handing over authority to the relevant government departments (see Section 7.2.1.3). Spearheading change involved building technical and managerial capacity in other organizations and providing technical guidance and advice in various forms, including research, guidelines, formulation of legislation and creation of appropriate infrastructural capacity, for example, for chemical testing. However, the MoH maintained its responsibility for health by insisting that health matters be referred to it where relevant, for example, HIA in EIA for development projects. It continues to provide advice via the Environmental Quality Council (The Commissioner of Law Revision Malaysia, 2006).

Building human resource capacity: Initially the MoH had to build its own capacity for environmental health. This was done by acquiring two engineers seconded from the PWD in the 1970s. They went on to develop a pool of public health engineers, some of whom were subsequently seconded to the DOE, MHLG, SSD, Solid Waste Department (SWD) and so on to spearhead change in those agencies and to help them recognize that their responsibilities encompassed not merely engineering perspectives but needed to expand to include environmental health perspectives. An outstanding outcome of this initiative is the formulation of the EQA and its subsidiary regulations, which provided for licensing and establishing standards for preventing, abating and controlling environmental pollution primarily from industries and shipping. Other outcomes include the enactment of the Sewerage Services Act 1993 and the Solid Waste and Public Cleansing Acts 2007.

Community participation: In rural areas in particular, EHS succeeded by incorporating community involvement and participation in all programmes. Community participation helped to reduce the cost of projects and resulted in speedy implementation because the community leaders were motivated and wanted results quickly. There was shared ownership, and communities maintained the sanitation and water systems. The leadership structure in villages, such as the village action committee established under the government's integrated rural development programme, helped with proper project planning and implementation. The series of health education campaigns by the district health offices also helped to mobilize the community. The support of local politicians further boosted effective community participation (Suleiman & Jegathesan, n.d.).

Private sector involvement: The private sector complemented the role of the public sector in several ways. In the early years, the private sector was engaged to develop plastic pour-flush latrines for the RESP and later in developing Malaysian home-grown plastic hand pumps, water tanks and other accessories. The mass production of these essential items brought the cost to affordable ranges. Later, when the national privatization policy was introduced, the private sector played greater roles (Japan International Cooperation Agency (JICA), Malaysia Office, 1999). The public sector outsourced to the private sector the programmes for national sewerage development, including the urban solid waste management programme, clinical waste management and the monitoring of air quality throughout the country. The privatization policy helped to strengthen and further develop EHS in a systematic manner, as it allowed the government to focus on its primary functions of policy and oversight while the private sector delivered services. Under the privatization policy, the required funding mechanisms were also put in place with revenue generation opportunities. Various laws and regulations were enacted to delineate responsibilities among the various agencies and to set standards for service delivery (Japan International Cooperation Agency (JICA), Malaysia Office, 1999).

With outsourcing, the oversight function for ensuring that the private sector achieved good outcomes still rested and continues to rest with the government and its agencies. For example, when the clinical waste management service was privatized, the MoH engaged specialists to monitor the performance of the private concessionaires (Suleiman & Jegathesan, n.d.) against standards and guidelines and even introduced a fee deduction mechanism for non-performance or poor performance of the service. Similarly, when sewerage service was privatized, a new Sewerage Services Department was created to enforce the legislation. The government had to create standards, codes of practices and guidelines as well. Privatization does not absolve the government of its responsibilities.

Outsourcing has worked well in Malaysia and has fast-tracked many EHS programmes. Other countries seeking to privatize should carefully consider the selection of the privatization model and take into consideration that once a service is privatized, it is difficult to reverse it.

7.3 Key Messages from Malaysia's Experience

7.3.1 What Went Well?

- Basic rural interventions for water and human waste disposal used
  - simple technology,
  - strong community participation, and
  - allied health staff delivered them effectively using established community structures.
- Higher technological interventions requiring appropriate competencies were
  - possible for concentrated urban populations (water, solid and liquid waste management);
  - needed for complex issues (clinical waste, radiation);
  - under the jurisdiction of authorities outside the health sector and needed inter-sectoral co-ordination.
- The health sector successfully
  - acquired and empowered staff with the appropriate competencies;
  - provided leadership and assisted, then mentored, other agencies to develop the required competencies and exercise their powers through governance, outsourcing and oversight;
  - mobilized private sector finance through outsourcing; and
  - gained experience and expertise in outsourcing.

7.3.2 What Did Not Go So Well?

Several issues outside the jurisdiction of the health sector remain problematic, for example, occupational health, air pollution and road traffic accidents.

7.3.3 Trends and Challenges

Climate change is expected to increase the frequency and severity of conditions that will stretch the capacity of the health system

References

The Commissioner of Law Revision Malaysia. (2006). *Act 127: Environmental Quality Act 1974. Laws of Malaysia.* Kuala Lumpur: Commissioner of Law Revision Malaysia.

Economic Planning Unit (EPU). (1981). *Master Plan and Feasibility Study for Sewerage and Drainage Systems in Kuantan and Kuantan Port Inception/ Progress Report.* Kuala Lumpur: Minconsult.

Federation of Malaysia. (n.d.). *Report of the Medical Department 1960.* Kuala Lumpur.

Hashim, J. H. and Hashim, Z. (2009). *Guidance Document on Health Impact Assessment (HIA) in Environmental Impact Assessment (EIA).* Putrajaya: Department of Environment Malaysia.

Japan International Cooperation Agency (JICA), Malaysia Office. (1999). *Privatisation of Water, Sanitation and Environment-Related Services in Malaysia.* Kuala Lumpur: Japan International Cooperation Agency, Malaysia Office.

Japan Sanitation Consortium (JSC). (2011). *Country Sanitation Assessment in Malaysia.* Tokyo: Japan Sanitation Consortium.

Ministry of Health Malaysia. (1988). *Annual Report 1986.* Kuala Lumpur: Ministry of Health Malaysia.

Ministry of Health Malaysia. (1989). *Annual Report 1987.* Kuala Lumpur: Ministry of Health Malaysia.

Ministry of Health Malaysia. (1990). *Annual Report 1988.* Kuala Lumpur: Ministry of Health Malaysia.

Ministry of Health Malaysia. (1991). *Annual Report 1989.* Kuala Lumpur: Ministry of Health Malaysia.

Ministry of Health Malaysia. (1992). *Annual Report 1990.* Kuala Lumpur: Ministry of Health Malaysia.

Ministry of Health Malaysia. (1993). *Annual Report 1991.* Kuala Lumpur: Ministry of Health Malaysia.

Ministry of Health Malaysia. (1997). *Annual Report 1995.* Kuala Lumpur: Ministry of Health Malaysia.

Ministry of Health Malaysia. (2002). *Annual Report 2000.* Kuala Lumpur: Ministry of Health Malaysia.

Ministry of Health Malaysia. (2003). *Annual Report 2001.* Kuala Lumpur: Ministry of Health Malaysia.

Ministry of Health Malaysia. (2017). *Annual Report 2015.* Putrajaya: Ministry of Health Malaysia.

Ministry of Housing and Local Government, Malaysia. (2005). *National Strategic Plan for Solid Waste Management.* Kuala Lumpur: Ministry of Housing and Local Government Malaysia.

National Environmental Health Action Plan (n.d.). *Areas of Concern*. Online report. http://nehapmalaysia.moh.gov.my/about-nehap/areas-of-concern

National Water Services Commission. (2019). *The Commission's Role: National Water Services Commission*. Online webpage. www.span.gov.my/article/view/the-commission-s-role

Pillay, M. S., Sinha, K. and Talha, M. Z. M. (2003). Water quality and health. *Environmental Health Focus: Managing the Environment for Health in the Asia Pacific*, 1(2), 8–11.

Pillay, M. S., Sinha, I. K. and Talha, M. Z. M. (n.d.). *Providing Reliable Drinking Water Supply to Remote Communities in Malaysia*. Putrajaya: Ministry of Health Malaysia.

Sahani, M., Khan, M. F., Mahiyuddin, W. R. W., Latif, M. T., Ng, C. F. S, Yussof, M. F. et al. (2016). Air pollution and health in Malaysia: case studies from Asia. In D.-C. Shin, ed., *Hazardous Air Pollutants*. Boca Raton, FL: CRP Press, pp. 97–114.

Sewerage Services Department, Ministry of Housing and Local Government. (2001). *Sewerage Services Report*. Kuala Lumpur: Ministry of Housing and Local Government.

Suleiman, A. B. and Jegathesan, M. (eds.). (n.d.). *Health in Malaysia: Achievements and Challenges*. Ministry of Health Malaysia.

Tuan Mat, E. A. (2016). Significance of NEHAP Malaysia. Paper presented at Persidangan NEHAP Malaysia 2016, PICC Putrajaya.

Ujang, Z. (2006). Strategy and planning of sewerage infrastructures for developing countries: experience of Malaysia. In Z. Ujang and M. Henze, eds., *Municipal Wastewater Management in Developing Countries*. London: IWA, pp. 46–69.

WHO Western Pacific Region. (1977). *Western Pacific Regional Centre for the Promotion of Environmental Planning and Applied Studies (PEPAS) (Resolution)*. Manila: WHO Regional Office for the Western Pacific.

System Analysis Case Study 7.1: Rural Water Supply and Sanitation

Mukundan Sugunan Pillay, Debbie Siru and David T. Tan

Introduction

Adequate water supply and sanitation are basic requirements for ensuring safety from waterborne diseases such as cholera and typhoid. A gap in adequate water supply for rural communities caused major disease outbreaks among this population. In response, the MoH Malaysia launched a major nationwide initiative, the Rural Environmental Sanitation Programme (RESP), which resulted in the reduction of waterborne diseases. The initiative relied on introducing engineering principles and practices coupled with health education and community participation to attain success. This case study elaborates on the programme in further detail.

The Problem

The Malaysian government prioritized water and sanitation infrastructure as a health and development strategy to curb the spread of waterborne diseases. This function was the traditional role of the state governments and the federal Public Works Department (PWD). However, limitations in personnel and finance meant that the PWD adopted a big-project, cost-efficiency approach, focusing on population centres and working outwards towards semi-urban areas. They were not equipped to deliver smaller, intermediate solutions to rural areas because their workforce was small and lacked connections to rural communities.

Thus there were long delays before rural communities could be served. Indeed, a landmark survey in 1968 by the MoH showed that only 3.6% of the rural population received a treated piped water supply, with 85.3% depending on water supply from unprotected wells and 11.1% relying on untreated surface waters (Suleiman & Jegathesan, n.d.). There were many outbreaks of waterborne disease in rural areas. The PWD was unable to respond to these negative health outcomes (Figure 7-A, B1 loop dotted line).

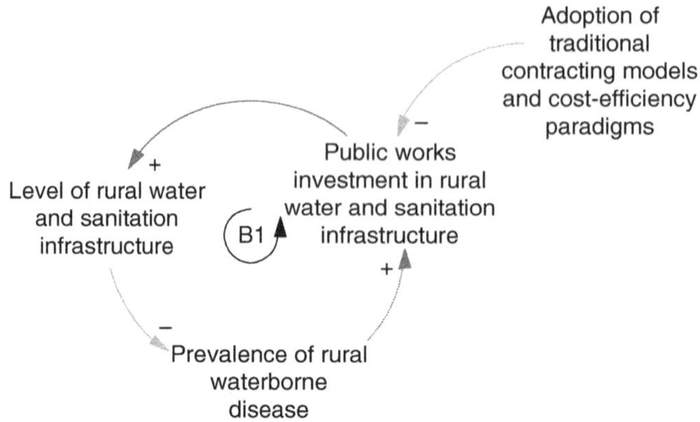

Figure 7-A The PWD strategy for expanding the water and sanitation network was unable to respond to rural disease burdens in a timely manner.

The MoH attempted to address the spread of waterborne disease through educational efforts on sanitation practice (Figure 7-B, B2 loop). However, communities were unresponsive to these efforts, particularly as trust in government actors was low due to the absence of visible government investment in their communities.

Addressing the Problem

In response to the survey findings and considering the grave health consequences, the federal government commissioned environmental sanitation pilot projects in mid-1968. Through these pilot projects, the intention was to achieve safe water supply, sanitary disposal of excreta using sanitary latrines, safe disposal of solid waste and sullage, and improvement of the general cleanliness of the village environment. The pilot projects had four basic elements: community participation, health education, appropriate technology and training.

However, there was a strong paradigm that infrastructure work was outside MoH's mission of healthcare delivery. This generated internal resistance to the additional work and external resistance sceptical of the ministry's endeavours. The initiative required an extensive change in mindset among health personnel. Training was prioritized for the health staff, mainly health inspectors and health overseers, and incorporated the four elements used in the pilot projects. The approach successfully overcame resistance as described in

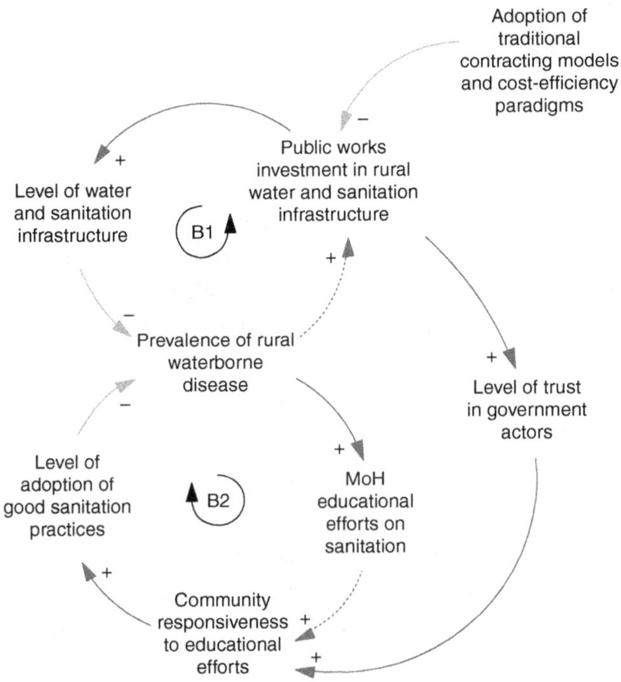

Figure 7-B Inadequate rural infrastructure investment in sanitation undermined community trust in government actors, hindering educational efforts that attempted to address the sanitation issues.

this case study, enabling scaling up of the programme, leading to the institutionalization of the National Rural Environmental Sanitation Programme by the federal government in 1973 under the mid-term review of the Second Malaysia Plan. This programme was later called the BAKAS programme or the Water Supply and Environmental Sanitation Programme (Pillay et al., n. d.).

The BAKAS (Bekalan Air dan Kebersihan Alam Sekeliling) Approach

Programme execution became the responsibility of the state public health departments, which provided funds and supplies to the various district health offices. At ground level, the district health officer, often assisted by the senior health inspector and health overseers, interacted with the village heads and village committees to organize health education, community participation and project initiation activities. State public health engineers provided technical input related to engineering (see Box 7-A for more details).

The communities responded with overwhelming support, with projects being executed within weeks of initiation. This success also encouraged many local politicians to lend their support and contribute to these community participation activities. State governments welcomed the programme initiated by the federal government and in time extended their full co-operation through their network of district administrative officers, who helped to identify needy communities and provided assistance to the district health officers.

By 2000, the coverage of rural households with safe water supplies was 93.5%, and it was 98.2% for sanitary latrine coverage (Ministry

Box 7-A Details of the BAKAS approach

It was always clear from the onset that the technology utilized must be low-cost and appropriate. For sanitary latrines, the pour-flush toilet, which was connected to pits dug behind the toilets, was selected. Wherever available and feasible, small dams were constructed in hills, and water was piped to each household using PVC (polyvinyl chloride) and HDPE (high-density polyethylene) pipes. Each house was provided with one standpipe. Engineering surveys were done to ensure appropriate pressures were maintained. Open sanitary wells were constructed in areas with no hill sources; in other areas, tube wells were constructed and fitted with hand pumps or motor pumps.

The MoH supplied all materials needed, while the community provided the labour needed to instal the facilities. The villagers were also trained in maintaining these facilities. The villagers were repeatedly advised to boil the water before consumption. These small projects were completed within a few weeks and were a great relief for the communities, who had been waiting for a long time for a cleaner, more accessible water supply.

In summary, the key features that made BAKAS a success were the government's commitment to funding for all materials, the combined approach of addressing latrine construction and water supply, and the provision of technical staff with basic engineering knowledge, health education and training, while the community provided labour support and took ownership and undertook maintenance of the projects.

Box 7-B Leadership and commitment of state public health engineers

Pilot projects started with educational talks on the importance of clean water supply and sanitation and its impact on health. It was soon realized that these talks were insufficient to get the community to participate. An innovative move by a public health engineer – turning up at the house of the village head with all the materials required – convinced the village head that this was not just more government propaganda and mere lip service. This led to the co-operation of the entire village. News soon spread, which led to local politicians coming on board and requesting similar projects to be set up in their constituencies. This single move led to a reversal of situations – instead of the MoH having to convince villagers of the need for water supply and sanitation facilities, the demand came from the villagers themselves, with a commitment to community participation. The results of the programme were gratifying, seen in the joyous faces of the rural population getting clean water on their doorsteps after years of waiting.

of Health Malaysia, 2002). This success could be attributed to leadership and commitment (see Box 7-B), available front-line health personnel who were based in the rural areas, the adoption of health as the paradigm for improved sanitation and water supply, and the four basic elements of the BAKAS programme. The mobilization of large numbers of auxiliary front-line staff in rural areas to engage local communities, supported by engineers with technical expertise, and enabled lower-cost solutions in which rural communities could participate and take ownership. This created rapid, cost-effective and locally sustainable solutions not possible under the traditional PWD approach, which relied on engaging contractors to construct large engineering projects (Figure 7-C).

The BAKAS programme was successful, and the delivery of infrastructure re-established trust in the government, enabling not only educational efforts on sanitation but also increasing responsiveness to other health initiatives. Apart from the low-cost water supply and sanitary latrines, other components were added, such as the disposal of solid waste and sullage water and the general cleanliness of the village environment. This programme complemented the other health programmes implemented at the district

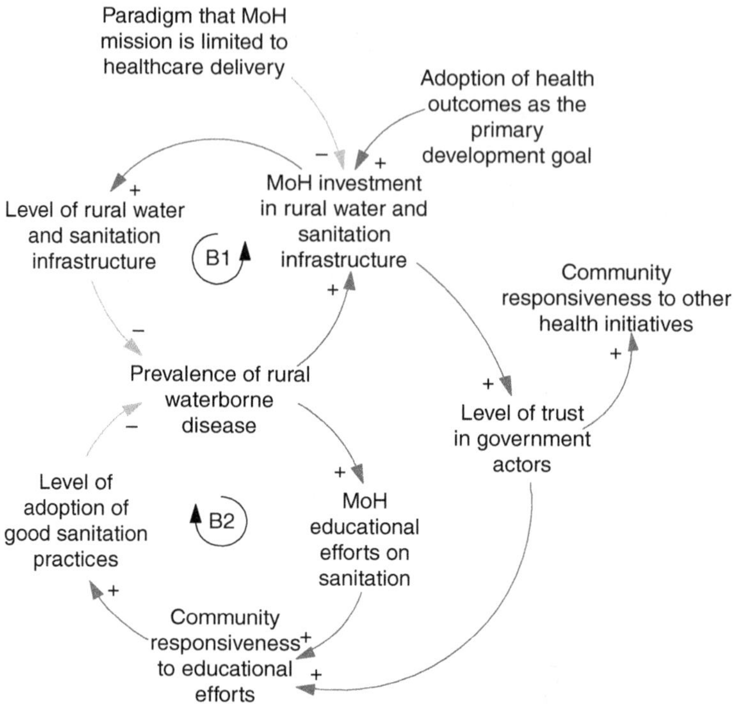

Figure 7-C The paradigm that the MoH mission is limited to healthcare delivery created internal and external barriers to its involvement in rural water and sanitation. However, once those barriers were overcome, its large personnel base and ability to prioritize health outcomes enabled community trust and responsiveness to rural water and sanitation interventions.

level, such as health education, communicable disease control, food hygiene and vector control.

Systems Lessons

Systems analysis illustrates that health authorities need to venture out of their traditional roles to address social and environment determinants of health. In this case study, the MoH had to undertake responsibility for rural water and sanitation, acquire engineering expertise, provide leadership to upgrade the basic engineering skills of front-line health workers, solicit community support, successfully convince the federal government to allocate the needed funds, and acquire administrative support from state governments and district officials. The analysis also highlights how a practical demonstration of government commitment can earn community trust and active partnership in environmental health initiatives.

References

Ministry of Health Malaysia. (2002). *Annual Report 2000*. Kuala Lumpur: Ministry of Health Malaysia.

Pillay, M. S., Sinha, I. K. and Mohd Talha, M. Z. (n.d.). *Providing Reliable Drinking Water Supply to Remote Communities in Malaysia*. Putrajaya: Ministry of Health Malaysia.

Suleiman, A. B. and Jegathesan, M. (eds.). (n.d.). *Health in Malaysia: Achievements and Challenges*. Ministry of Health, Malaysia.

System Analysis Case Study 7.2: Clinical Waste Management

Debbie Siru, Mukundan Sugunan Pillay and David T. Tan

Overview

Careful handling of clinical waste is essential for mitigating adverse health and environmental consequences and is thus a crucial component of environmental health protection. While many governments recognize that integrating a systematic and multifaceted framework for clinical waste management into healthcare services is essential, this is often difficult to achieve because of competing priorities for limited government funding. This case study describes the strategies the Malaysian government adopted to achieve this.

Background: The Problem

Up until the 1980s, there was no proper system for managing clinical waste in Malaysia. With the emergence of HIV, the MoH revised the policies and guidelines for preventing and controlling infectious diseases to include clinical waste handling. However, these guidelines and policies only addressed the handling of waste at the hospital level, providing guidance on what categories of waste should be disinfected and how sharps should be handled. There were no comprehensive guidelines, policies or infrastructure for the 'cradle to grave' management of clinical waste.

Likewise, no department within the MoH took the lead to drive the many institutional and infrastructural changes required to ensure that clinical waste was properly managed. Thus each hospital managed clinical waste in its own fashion. Attempts at implementing piecemeal policies and guidelines on waste segregation were futile efforts, as waste was either burned in incineration kilns on hospital grounds or merely dumped in a hole in the ground and covered or burnt. In many other hospitals, clinical waste was simply discarded into the general waste stream and disposed of together with other solid waste in landfill dump-sites. Attempts by some more diligent personnel to segregate sharps saw innovative but ineffective use of all manner of non-puncture-proof containers, from used saline bottles to soda cans.

These poor levels of clinical waste management in hospital and clinic settings and the improper disposal of clinical waste created adverse societal and health outcomes, such as the misappropriation of used needles by drug users. Such incidents should have led to greater investment in resources and personnel for clinical waste management (Figure 7-a, B1 loop). However, the relevant investment was persistently inadequate due to limited resources, slow government processes and the high capital investment required for procuring the necessary facilities. Compounding this problem was the low priority hospital staff gave to clinical waste management. Assigned staff had other duties, and duties that directly related to patient care were routinely given priority at the expense of waste management duties.

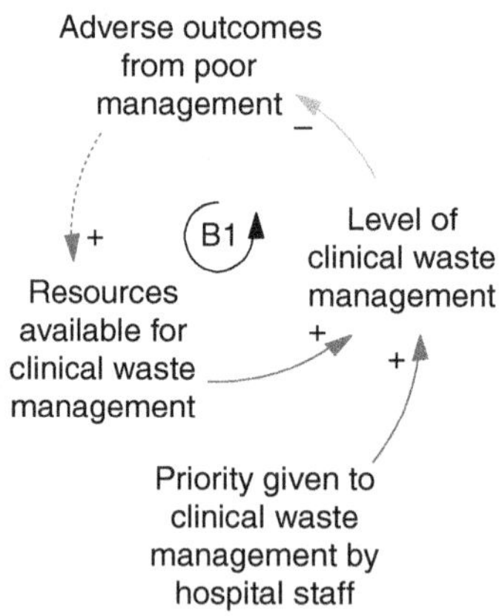

Figure 7-a Factors that led to poor clinical waste management. Limited government budgets prevented capital investment necessary for appropriate clinical waste management (dotted arrow). Adequate clinical waste management also requires prioritization by hospital staff; however, this was typically a low priority, with tasks directly related to the delivery of health services taking precedence.

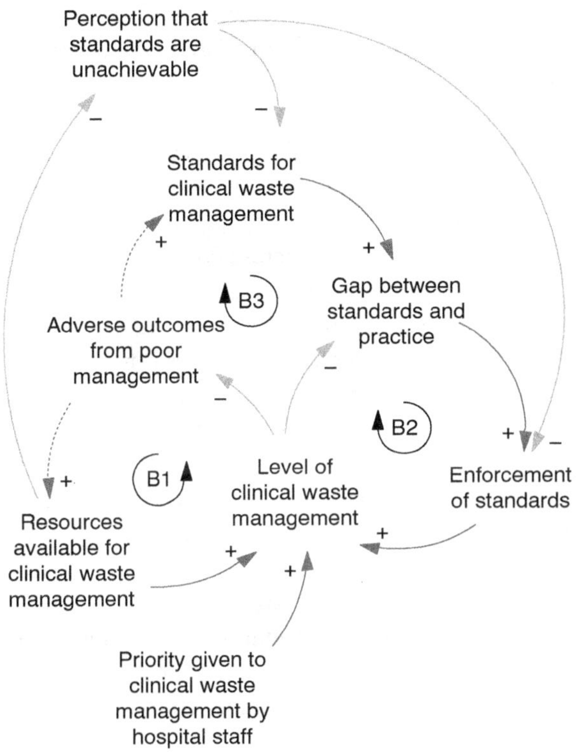

Figure 7-b Inability of the government to allocate sufficient resources for clinical waste management undercut both the enforcement of standards that did exist and the development of further standards necessary for 'cradle-to-grave' management.

The unavailability of facilities, both within and outside of hospitals, necessary for complying with DOE legislation for clinical waste management created the paradigm that these standards were unachievable, rendering legislation unenforceable (Figure 7-b, B2 loop). Furthermore, the lack of forthcoming resources to address the existing shortcomings in practice made any efforts to improve on the existing MoH guidelines seem futile (Figure 7-b, B3 loop).

Addressing the Problem

While the MoH was aware of these problems, the financing bottleneck was a major barrier to any practical solution. The impetus for action finally arrived when the clinical waste problem entered public awareness through media reports of dogs scavenging body parts from hospital waste. Thus the MoH made the unprecedented decision to outsource clinical waste management. This was a controversial move that faced opposition from within the government and from large segments of the public and was possible only because of the urgency of the problem and a policy by the then prime minister on the privatization of government services.

Private investment in clinical waste infrastructure created the potential for the feedback loops that enable good clinical waste management to function properly (Figure 7-c). Indeed, the MoH took on the task of developing a set of detailed and comprehensive guidelines (Figure 7-c, B3 loop), including the Policy on Hospital Waste Management, the Guidelines for the Management of Clinical and Related Wastes in Hospitals and Healthcare Establishments, and the Action Plan for Waste Management in Hospitals and Healthcare Establishments, that identified the hospital's management responsibilities, the main components of clinical waste management and the protocols required. However, successful implementation required well-designed governance systems to create the right incentives for private sector contractors and hospital administrators, together with the information systems necessary to enable this. The details of the implementation are described in the following section.

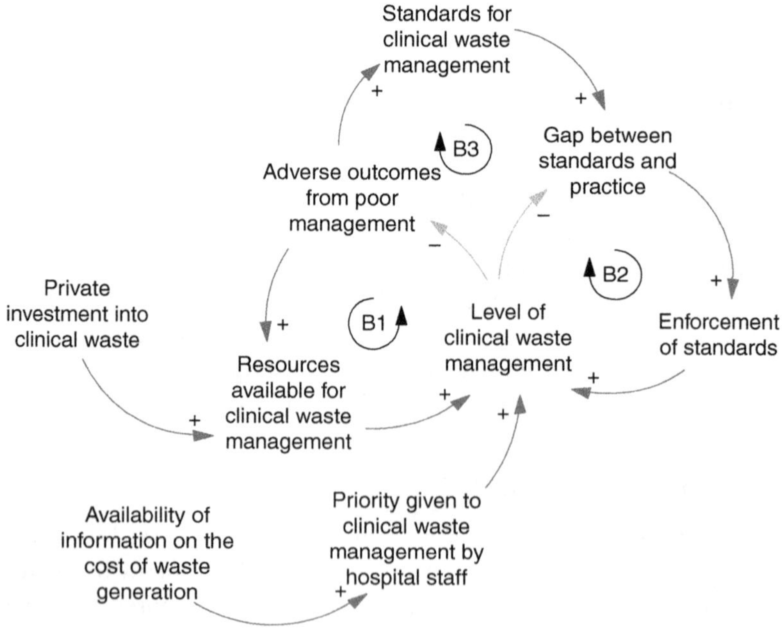

Caption for Figure 7-c (cont.)

Figure 7-c Outsourcing of clinical waste services enabled necessary capital investment for clinical waste management, enabling the B1, B2 and B3 loops to function properly. Well-designed governance and information systems were critical to successful implementation.

Creation of the Outsourced Clinical Waste Management System (CWMS)

Outsourcing (privatizing) what is essentially a component of healthcare services was unique and a paradigm shift, as it involved the private sector working in collaboration and in close proximity with the government sector. To ensure success, the following features and structure were incorporated:

Financing and Development of CWMS

- Capital costs were shifted to the private sector, removing the bottleneck, as operating costs were more easily approved in government budgetary process. Contracts with private sector operators (PSOs) locked in the amount the government had to appropriate for operating costs. This counteracted the tendency to underfund waste management.
- The private sector became responsible for the human resources, institutional development and infrastructure development required for a comprehensive CWMS. Thus the private sector was required to undertake all aspects of clinical waste management, with the exception of segregation. This also involved procuring the necessary equipment and vehicles for segregating, collecting and transporting waste to treatment facilities and constructing and maintaining storage and treatment facilities, as well as compliance with emission and all other environmental standards.
- The availability of resources overcame the perception that creating and enforcing standards would be futile – paving the way for the development and enforcement of guidelines complying with the 'cradle to grave' principle (see 'Creation of Standards').

Assurance of Project Viability and Sustainability

- To encourage private sector involvement, a fifteen-year contract was signed with selected PSOs. The long-term contract made it easier for the PSOs to secure financing. The amortization of capital costs over this period allowed for the determination of a reasonable and affordable service fee. The long-term contract also enabled the planning of upgrades and continuous improvement.
- At the time of signing the contract, a total of 127 existing MoH hospitals and institutions were included as part of the privatization package, with the potential for the addition of other new MoH hospitals in the future. This economy of scale not only benefited the PSOs but also meant that the service fee would be more affordable for the government.
- The fee structure based on Malaysian ringgit (MYR)/kg waste further ensured sustainability and profitability, as it was expected that the generation of clinical waste would increase with time, which proved to be true.
- To further ensure viability and sustainability, it was packaged with four other hospital support services as part of the privatization package: cleansing services, linen and laundry services, facilities engineering maintenance services and the biomedical engineering maintenance service.
- The PSOs were also allowed to generate additional revenue by extending their clinical waste management services to private hospitals.

Non-monopoly

- Based on experiences of other privatization exercises, the MoH awarded the privatization package to three companies instead of just one. This not only generated a healthy competitive environment for continuous improvement among the selected PSOs but also allowed the PSOs to utilize each other's treatment facilities in the event of shutdown for maintenance or other contingencies.

Balancing Profitability and Public Good Service

- While profitability was recognized as an important motivation for the private sector, the MoH ensured that its environmental health objectives would be met by:

- **Creation of standards:** The privatization contract incorporated a detailed scope of works, procedures, performance indicators and standards:
  - Technical Requirements and Performance Indicators (TRPI): Specify the scope of service and performance indicators.
  - Master Agreed Procedures (MAP): Specify detailed procedures for the service.
- **Quality assurance and implementation mechanisms:**
  - The privatization contract required PSOs to obtain the relevant certificates and licences, for example:
    - ✓ ISO 9001 certification.
    - ✓ Certificates of compliance with standards for bags and sharps containers.
    - ✓ Detailed EIAs for incinerator installation.
    - ✓ Compliance with various regulatory requirements and valid licences, for example, licence to operate incinerator, licence to transport waste, commercial vehicle licence, etc.
  - In addition, the PSOs were required to develop the following for approval and implementation:
    - ✓ QAP: Sets out key performance indicators of the service at the zone and hospital levels.
    - ✓ Computerized central management information system (CMIS): Provides almost real-time data and information on various aspects of the service, such as waste generation, waste collection, waste consignment tracking, etc. The CMIS[1] is also accessible anywhere and anytime with a secure ID and password.
    - ✓ Hospital-Specific Implementation Plan (HSIP): Details the operationalization of the TRPI and MAP at a specific hospital.
- **Penalty mechanisms:** To further ensure that services would be delivered to the required standards, the contract included the following:
  - Deduction formula: Allows the MoH to deduct fees for non-performance or unsatisfactory performance by the PSOs. The CMIS also incorporated a module for automatic capture of certain unsatisfactory performance, for example, non-

compliance with collection and transportation schedules, validity of licences, emission standards, etc.

- Third-party clauses: Allow the MoH to engage alternative PSOs or other vendors in the event that any aspect of the service is not delivered in a timely manner.

- **Monitoring and auditing mechanisms:**
  - A regulatory unit was set up within the MoH to monitor and enforce the contractual requirements.
  - This unit was assisted by a third-party consulting company. In addition to verifying the accuracy of the CMIS data, these consultants monitored aspects of the service that could not be captured in the CMIS, for example, correct procedures and supply of correct receptacles for segregation. They also advised hospital staff on their roles and responsibilities on verifying the work by the PSOs as well as various aspects of the service.

The transformation brought about by privatization is summarized in Table 7-A. Apart from this transformation, privatization yielded information and resulted in accountability. The cost of waste management, which was previously hidden (e.g. by tasking hospital staff with clean-up responsibilities in addition to other duties), became clear. Paying the private sector per kilogram of waste also incentivized the system to reduce waste generation. Payment for services to a third party also created the rationale for a monitoring system to hold contractors and hospitals accountable to the MoH. For the first time too, data on waste generation was available to provide information on status and to enable the assessment and planning of future needs.

Table 7-A *Comparison of scope of services before and after privatization*

No.	Scope of services	Before privatization	After privatization
1.	Yellow bags for non-sharps clinical waste	No	Yes
2.	Blue bags for autoclaving microbiological waste	No	Yes
3.	Dedicated waste receptacles with lids and pedals to hold bags	No	Yes
4.	Sharps containers for sharps segregation	Partial	Yes

Table 7-A (*cont.*)

No.	Scope of services	Before privatization	After privatization
5.	Dedicated collection containers and trolleys	No	Yes
6.	Dedicated vehicles for waste transportation	No	Yes
7.	Regular washing and disinfection of receptacles and trolleys	No	Yes
8.	Secured and covered stores, refrigerated if necessary	No	Yes
9.	Washing facilities at store with connection to sewers	No	Yes
10.	Tagging and identification: date, time and source of generation	No	Yes
11.	Personal protective equipment	No	Yes
12.	Collection and transportation schedules: frequency and time	Partial	Yes
13.	Weighing of waste and consignment note system for 'cradle to grave' waste tracking	No	Yes
14.	Clinical waste incinerators with air pollution controls, stores, washing facilities, etc.	No	Yes
15.	Continuous emission monitoring for selected parameters	No	Yes
16.	Ash disposal at secured hazardous waste disposal sites	No	Yes
17.	Compliance with all other regulatory requirements and valid certificates and licences	No	Yes
18.	Computerized data management system	No	Yes

Other Benefits of Privatization

The knock-on effect of the CWMS outsourcing is the development of local industry and competency. Examples include:

1. **Manufacturing industry:** Clinical waste bags, on-site storage receptacles and sharps containers imported at the start of the privatization

exercise are now locally manufactured and conform to international standards.

2. **Laboratory services:** The DOE requirement for incinerators to comply with various environmental standards, for example, effluent, air emissions, ambient air and noise standards as well as incinerator performance standards, have created opportunities for local laboratories. The increased demand for such testing services has also spurred the development of local competency. Dioxin and furan sampling and testing capability, which were once sourced from foreign laboratories, are now locally available. This has in turn resulted in savings in testing costs and foreign exchange.
3. **Human resource development and job opportunities:** Approximately 2,300 personnel employed by the MoH were absorbed by the companies under the privatization exercise. Staff strength has increased since then to more than 10,000, with approximately 2,000 people directly employed for the outsourced CWMS. In addition to these job opportunities was the development of skills and expertise among personnel.
4. **Export of expertise and services:** The development of local competency within the government and private sector has now put Malaysia in a position where its services and expertise are exportable.
5. **Expansion of privatization scope:** The scope of waste management has been expanded to include all other hazardous wastes in hospitals, such as chemical waste.

Challenges

As with any project, especially one that has never been attempted before, there were challenges. Examples encountered at the hospital level included:

1. Changing the mindset of hospital personnel, for example:
   - Discarding waste without segregation had to be unlearned.
   - Unrealistic expectations that, with privatization, hospital personnel were absolved of all responsibilities relating to clinical waste management. Thus verification of waste collection, weighing of waste, etc. were considered as competing with their core responsibilities, that is, patient care.

- Hospitals are typically space-constrained, hence there was reluctance to give up what was considered valuable space for the placement of dedicated clinical waste receptacles.

2. Some hospital personnel made unwarranted and impractical demands in the name of infection control. Examples are:
   - Requiring collection to be done three times a day even from wards or departments that generated only small amounts of clinical waste.
   - Not allowing the use of service lifts for collection trolleys.
3. Misuse of equipment and services by hospital personnel.
   - As the bags and sharps containers were of high quality, hospital personnel found other incorrect uses for these, for example, storing tissue samples.
   - Discarding other hazardous waste into the clinical waste stream.
4. Non-compliance by PSO personnel.
   - Poor verification by hospital personnel led to some non-compliance with schedules, and these non-compliances were not accurately captured in the CMIS.
   - Aspects of the service that could not be captured in the CMIS were sometimes not complied with, for example, collection procedures, receptacle-washing procedures, etc.
5. Ambiguous standards and incorrect interpretation of standards. Some aspects of clinical waste management were not sufficiently detailed in the MAP, while some were ambiguous, leading to incorrect and non-uniform practices.

These challenges were overcome via:

1. User training by the PSOs, which was a requirement in the privatization contract.
2. Audits by the MoH regulatory unit as well as audits and training by the third-party consultant engaged by the MoH.
3. Development of guidelines by the third-party consultant.

At the regional level, there were delays on a few occasions by a PSO to:

1. Repair or upgrade air pollution controls, leading to shutdown of the incinerator by the DOE.

2. Upgrade the incineration capacity or instal additional facilities to meet increasing clinical waste generation, leading to a pile-up of clinical waste at the treatment facility and hospitals.

One factor contributing to the delay was the difficulty in finding suitable sites for the installation of an incinerator due to different priorities of different government agencies and land-zoning issues at the local municipal level. The lack of commitment by new company shareholders in investing was another possibility. Thus the initial suggestion for the contract to stipulate a minimum period of the shareholding of the PSO should have been considered.

The non-monopoly strategy was keenly realized as an advantage during these times, as the other PSOs were able to assist. Realizing the need to resolve this problem, the DOE also relaxed the licence conditions, enabling the PSOs to transfer waste to other treatment facilities during this period.

Systems Lessons

Systems analysis demonstrates how inadequate financial resources could create and sustain several interconnected vicious circles of poor management and negative attitudes, resulting in poor health outcomes. A hitherto untried approach of mobilizing private sector funding converted the vicious circles into virtuous ones.

While privatization through outsourcing may not be the solution for every country, it seems clear that this was the right path to take in Malaysia. The experience gained from 15 years of implementation enabled the MoH and its consultants to refine the system further to improve the efficacy of service delivery. It has been 22 years since clinical waste management was first privatized, and Malaysia has a system that remains functional and with an expanded scope that covers other types of healthcare waste. Enforcement by the DOE in private hospitals and clinics is also possible now. Thus potential health risks are not only minimized but a potentially massive and expensive environmental clean-up has been averted, which would have been required if the pre-privatization situation had been allowed to continue.

References

Borongan, G., Siru, D. and Hassan, M. N. (2015). Review on the status of healthcare waste management in selected countries of the Western Pacific Region. *Journal of the Indian Society of Hospital Waste Management*, 13&14(1), 22–41.

Pillay, M. S. (June 1999). Privatization of Support Services in Medical and Healthcare Setting: Evaluation and Cost Implication. Proceedings of the Directors' Conference 1999, Ministry of Health Malaysia.

Siru, D., Pillay, M. S. and Sinha, K. (2006a). A national approach to clinical waste management. *Journal of Solid Waste Technology and Management*, 32(4), 199–205.

Siru, D., Pillay, M. S. and Sinha, K. (February 2006b). *Health Care Waste Management in Malaysia*. Proceedings of the International Seminar on New Trends in Hazardous and Medical Waste Management.

Siru, D., Pillay, M. S. and Sinha, K. (February 2006c). *Health Care Waste Management in Malaysia*. Proceedings of the International Workshop on Reasons and Remedies for Sustainable Healthcare Waste Management.

World Health Organization. (2015). *Status of Health-Care Waste Management in Selected Countries of the Western Pacific Region*. Geneva: World Health Organization.

Note

[1] This has since been upgraded and is now called the Asset and Services Information System (ASIS).

8 *Health Workforce*

INDRA PATHMANATHAN

8.1 Introduction

This chapter explores how the Malaysian health workforce evolved over a 60-year period. It analyses the dynamic interactions between various forces in the health system and explores how broader societal elements such as education levels and economic growth; evolving epidemiological, demographic and behavioural patterns; and macroeconomic policies contributed to the dynamic interactions and influenced the subsequent outcomes for the health system.

This chapter does not attempt to provide a detailed profile of the Malaysian health workforce, as such information is available on the websites of the Malaysian Ministry of Health (MoH) (Ministry of Health Malaysia, 2016b) and the World Health Organization (WHO) (World Health Organization, 2014).

8.2 Post-independence: The Early Phase (1960s and 1970s) – Focus on Improving Access

During the years immediately after independence, the Malaysian population was largely rural and had relatively low literacy and high rates of maternal and infant mortality, vaccine-preventable diseases, malaria, tuberculosis, water- and soil-borne disease and malnutrition (see Chapter 3). The economy was doing well, with a steadily increasing gross domestic product (GDP). Guided by strong political considerations, the government implemented policies for rapid integrated rural development, focusing on infrastructure, education and healthcare (see Chapter 3). A nationwide rural health service developed rapidly (see Chapter 4), together with vertical disease control programmes for malaria, tuberculosis, filariasis, yaws and various food-, water- and soil-borne diseases (Chapter 6). Community mobilisation was a key feature of the development process. Table 8.1

Table 8.1 *Summary of interacting influences on the evolution of the health workforce, 1960s and 1970s*

	Population behaviour and demographic profile	Morbidity and mortality profile	**Economy and macro policies**
Socio-economic ecosystem	Largely rural population Low literacy Low health literacy	High rates of • maternal and infant mortality • vaccine-preventable diseases • malaria • tuberculosis • water- and soil-borne diseases • malnutrition	Steady increase in GDP Rapid integrated rural development
	Health services	Education sector	Governance and financing
Health and education sectors	Development of rural health service and vertical disease control programmes Demand for staff for maternal and child healthcare (MCH), disease control and sanitation Competence for community mobilisation for health	Rapid expansion of primary and secondary schools Rising education level of school leavers	Production of health personnel *only* in public sector Policy to focus on training of nurses, midwives, medical assistants and public health assistants, and less emphasis on producing doctors
	Production of health workforce	Health workforce: key features	Outcomes
Health workforce	Rise in training institutions in MoH Rapid production of basic allied health staff Standardised management protocols; supervisory training	Comprised of public and private sector providers Rapid increase in public sector health workforce, particularly nurses and midwives	Increased access to and use of basic health services in rural communities

Box 8.1 Key features of the rapid production of allied health personnel

1. Basic pre-service courses were of 1–3 years' duration.
   a. The WHO and international agencies provided assistance for developing basic curricula, training trainers and establishing standards for qualifying exams, thereby contributing to quality standards.
   b. All health programmes delivered through the rural health service had standardised clinical and management protocols and standard packages of equipment and drugs. Frequent in-service training ensured that all staff acquired competence in these protocols.
   c. The training incorporated basic concepts of community mobilisation. This subsequently enabled rural health staff to recruit from village development committees in health projects, particularly for sanitation, immunisation and safe motherhood.
2. Some of the more competent and experienced staff received additional training in supervisory techniques and became supervisors who lived and worked close to the front-line staff.

summarises key drivers shaping the development of the workforce at this time.

The rapidly expanding rural health programmes needed large numbers of healthcare workers close to rural communities. The interventions they needed to deliver were not too technically complex. The MoH concentrated on rapidly producing large numbers of allied health personnel (mainly nurses of different categories) to populate the rural health services. At this juncture, the government did not attempt to rapidly increase the number of doctors (Table 8.2). Several considerations underpinned this policy. First, entry competence for basic training was lower for allied health personnel than for doctors, so allied health candidates were more readily available, given the literacy levels at that time. Additionally, allied health personnel were more affordable. The challenge was to ensure the production of sufficient numbers of health personnel

Table 8.2 ***Production of allied health personnel (selected categories), 1956–1995***

Category	1956–1965	1966–1975	1976–1985	1986–1995
Nurse	2,900	3,350	5,200	9,900
Community nurse	n.a.	n.a.	1,229	1,794
Assistant nurse[1]	2,000	2,152	3,800	1,800
Midwife[1]	n.a.	790	1,700	180
Medical assistant	No intake yet	899	1,137	1,913
Health inspector	No intake yet	68	866	791
Public health assistant	30	143	355	810
Pharmacist assistant	No intake yet	200	746	930
Radiographer	49	192	224	338
Medical laboratory technologist	No intake yet	No intake yet	853	907
Medical laboratory assistant	110	469	720	80
Physiotherapist	No intake yet	22	129	184
Occupational therapist	No intake yet	No intake yet	41	141
All	5,089	8,263	17,000	19,768

Source: Suleiman and Jegathesan, 2000.
[1] Phasing out.
n.a. – not available

with the skills and competence to provide safe and effective care. To address this, training institutions for allied health personnel were placed under the control of the MoH rather than in universities under the Ministry of Education (MoE). At that time, the sentiment was that universities were too distant from the front-line of healthcare delivery and would focus on academic measures of excellence rather than the practical skills needed at the front-line. Box 8.1 summarises the critical features of the training programmes. Training institutions were confined to the public sector, enabling the MoH to co-ordinate production with subsequent employment and deployment in the rapidly expanding public sector services. Another feature was that domestic funding, and not foreign aid, supported the training programmes. Foreign assistance was mainly of a technical nature (Box 8.1).

Training programmes expanded rapidly for allied health personnel, namely midwives and health nurses (for MCH and nutrition), public health overseers and health inspectors (for environmental sanitation), and medical assistants and pharmacy assistants (for treating common illnesses) (Table 8.2).

In contrast, during this phase of development, the production of doctors, dentists and pharmacists was limited. For example, during the 20-year period 1955–1975, the number of nurses and assistant nurses/midwives increased at a much faster rate than that of doctors (Table 8.3).

Table 8.3 *Evolution of the composition of the health workforce (selected categories) 1955–2015*

Category	1955[1]	1974/1975	1995	2015
Doctor	736	2,374	9,608	46,491
Pharmacist	n.a.	52	1,537	10,511
Medical assistant/assistant medical officer	1,075	1,379	4,261	14,724
Nurse	1,065	3,963[2,3]	1,3647[2]	99,925
Assistant nurse and midwife	1,132	4,740[2,4]	5,495[2]	25,175
Sanitary engineer	0	5	n.a.	n.a.
Sanitary inspector/health inspector/ assistant environmental health officer	168	398[2]	1,425	4,517
Assistant health inspector	n.a.	526[2,3]	n.a.	n.a.
Medical laboratory technologist	n.a.	428[2]	1,698	6,324[5]
Laboratory technician	78	542[2]	980	
Occupational therapist	n.a.	n.a.	n.a.	1,054
Physiotherapist	n.a.	n.a.	n.a.	1,361

Sources: Government of the Federation of Malaya, n.d.; World Health Organization, 1977; Ministry of Health Malaysia, 1995a; 1995b; 2016b.

[1] Excludes Sabah and Sarawak.

[2] Government only.

[3] Excludes Sabah.

[4] Data for 1974.

[5] Public sector only: data for 2013.

n.a. – not available

Courses that provided the basic qualification for doctors were available only in three local universities, and the number of places was severely limited. No post-graduate training was available, and there was a limited number of scholarships for specialist training in foreign countries (mostly in the UK). During these earlier years, expatriate staff on short-term contracts filled key vacancies in medical officer and specialist positions until local staff became available and replaced them.

As a result of the rapid recruitment and training of nurses and midwives, the number of people per nurse/midwife declined about four-fold from 2,488 in 1964 to 570 in 1980 (see Chapter 3: Supplementary Table 3.L). The number of people per doctor also declined by about half from 7,145 in 1960 to 3,563 in 1980 (see Chapter 3: Supplementary Table 3.K).

Several governance mechanisms controlled the quality of health personnel (World Health Organization, 2014). First, legislation mandated that qualified personnel in core categories such as doctors, dentists, pharmacists, nurses and midwives had to be licensed to practice and were placed on registers. This served to control unqualified, illegal practitioners. Second, as the public sector was by far the largest employer of health personnel, their employment conditions were governed by civil service rules and regulations that also defined their financial and non-financial benefits such as medical care, travel subsidies, highly subsidised housing, employment security and pension benefits. Thus the public sector was able to control the composition and quality of the health workforce.

The health system outcomes relevant for assessing this early phase of development include availability of and access to health staff, utilisation of services, and selected mortality and morbidity indicators closely associated with the performance of the health workforce. Data for nurses/midwives suggests that increased availability was associated with utilisation and health status (Table 8.4) (trend data for other categories were not available).

8.3 The Second Phase of Development (1980s–1990s)

Several overarching features influenced development during the 1980s and 1990s. Rapidly rising female literacy and rural-to-urban migration contributed to the evolving morbidity and mortality patterns (see Chapter 3). Communicable diseases (CDs) declined, while non-

Table 8.4 *Selected health staff, utilisation rates and health outcomes*

	Maternal mortality ratio (MMR)	Live births per midwife[1] (LB)	Percent births with skilled attendance	Number of people per nursing staff[2]	% infants with DPT3 immunisation[3]	Incidence of diphtheria
1961	200	320	41	2488	n.a.	
1970	148	149	67	1879	15	11.10[4]
1980	63	101	n.a.	570	72	0.97
1990	20	102	89	481	92	0.05

Sources: Calculations by the author derived from data from Pathmanathan et al. (2003) and Suleiman and Jegathesan (2000).
[1] Includes nurse-midwives and certified trained midwives.
[2] Includes nurses, assistant nurses, midwives and community nurses.
[3] Diphtheria, tetanus and pertussis.
[4] In 1975.
n.a. – not available

Box 8.2 System observations: stocks and flows of personnel

Stocks and flows explain inertia in a system; that is, the delay between actions and their outcomes. The importance of this systems thinking concept to health system strengthening is perhaps most clearly seen in human resources due to the length of time required to train medical personnel and the number of personnel that can be trained at any one time (flows). Such considerations contributed to the choice to emphasise the production of allied health personnel over doctors (and task shifting) in the early stages of the Malaysian health system. System inertia is also seen in the pool of existing personnel (stocks). Indeed, medical personnel may be part of a health system for decades, enabling and constraining health strategies and imposing financial obligations on the health system.

communicable diseases (NCDs) became more common (see Chapter 6). As long-established vertical disease control programmes (malaria, tuberculosis, leprosy) merged with primary care (Chapter 4), their staff were absorbed and, where necessary, re-trained to provide a broader range of services. Larger hospitals that offered treatment facilities were overcrowded while smaller district hospitals were underutilised, catering mainly for normal childbirth and ambulatory care for less complex conditions (Public Health Institute, 1983). The bypassing of clinics and district hospitals by patients in favour of larger or more sophisticated facilities for inpatient and ambulatory care was a significant pattern in health care utilisation at this time (Chapter 5). This phenomenon illustrated the growing demand for higher levels of clinical and technical services that came with rising socio-economic and educational status in the population. Table 8.5 summarises the interactions that influenced the evolution of the health workforce at this time.

Staff with higher levels of competence were needed. Several new categories of personnel were recruited. For example, public health engineers were recruited to complement health inspectors (Chapter 7) and pharmacists to complement pharmacy assistants (Chapter 10).

Categories of staff such as nurses, medical assistants and health inspectors attending training programmes in the public sector received

Table 8.5 *Summary of interacting influences on the evolution of the health workforce, 1980s and 1990s*

	Population behaviour and demographic profile	Morbidity and mortality profile	Economy and macro policies
Larger ecosystem	• Increased rural–urban migration • Rapid rise in female literacy • Good access to basic services, and demand for more sophisticated clinical care	• Decline in CDs • Rise in NCDs	• Budget constraints • Private sector as engine of growth • Improve efficiency to counter budget constraints • In the public sector, nationwide quality improvement initiatives • Address imbalance between regions • Poverty reduction programmes
	Health services	Education sector	Governance and financing
Health and education sectors	• Provision of more complex services: o clinical o technical • Improved management aimed at better quality and efficiency • Increase in private sector clinics and hospitals in response to public demand	• Better-qualified candidates demanding tertiary education • Expanded tertiary education including local production of doctors and various allied health professionals • Increasing demand for medical education	• Allow production in the private sector of selected categories of personnel • Increase in scholarships for training in foreign institutions

	Production of health workforce	Health workforce: key features	Outcomes
Health workforce	• Transfer of MoH training institutions to MoE (universities and colleges) • Rapid increase in private sector training institutions • Strengthened governance structure (Malaysian Qualifications Authority (MQA))	• Brain drain from public to private sector • Upgrading of entry levels and exit competencies of pre-employment training • Employment of higher-level categories of staff • Improved management skills • Efforts to redress geographic imbalances	• Disparities between geographic regions for access to care were reduced

living allowances and accommodation during their training period. The health personnel training programmes profile of 1975 provides an insight into the evolutionary process of the workforce. The training of nurses and assistant nurses was at a peak; midwives were being converted into community nurses, health inspector training was upgraded and pharmacist training had just begun (Table 8.6).

Meanwhile, growing prosperity encouraged the growth of private sector healthcare. This was associated with the continuing challenge of the brain drain of doctors, particularly those who

Table 8.6 *Profile of health worker training programmes*

Category[1]	Programme duration (years)	Schools (no.)	Expected annual output
Medical doctor	5	2	250
Pharmacist	4	1	Intake of 50. No output yet
Nursing professions			
Staff nurse	3	9	570
Assistant nurse	2	23	583
Midwife	2	16	205
Community nurse (basic course)	2	2	No output yet
Community nurse (conversion course)[2]	0.5	3	108
Other health worker			
Hospital assistant	3	2	166
	1 (existing)	1	58
Health inspector[3]	3 (new)	1	No output yet
Radiographer	2	1	21
Physiotherapist	3	1	4

Source: Ismail & Martinez, 1975.

[1] Universities provided training of medical doctors and pharmacists as a degree programme; training of nursing professionals and other health workers was via an MoH certificate programme.

[2] For trained, certified midwives to enable them to perform a wider role.

[3] In 1975, two types of training programme for health inspectors co-existed as the training was transitioning from the one-year programme, which was being phased out, to the new three-year programme.

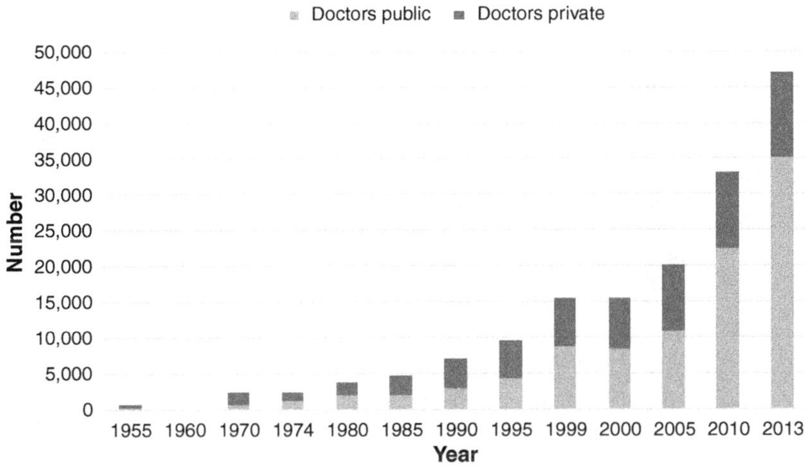

Figure 8.1 Malaysian doctors in the public and private sectors, 1955–2013.
Sources: Calculations by the author derived from data from the Ministry of Health Malaysia (1971; 1974; 1982; 1983; 1984; 1986; 1995a; 2000; 2010) and the Government of the Federation of Malaya (n.d.).

were more experienced and specialist, from the public sector to the private sector (Ministry of Health Malaysia, 2016b). Although the production of doctors increased during the 1980s and 1990s, a sizeable proportion moved from the public to the private sector after the mandatory period of public sector service. Thus the ratio of public-to-private sector doctors remained about 50:50 (Figure 8.1). According to an analysis by Hameed Musafar (2014), the major contributory factors of this brain drain were the slowing of wage growth in the public sector combined with the rapid increase of private hospitals and beds, where doctors had better remuneration and working conditions.

The shift of doctors from the public to the private sector also created regional disparities. The West Coast states of Peninsular Malaysia experienced much faster socio-economic development than the East Coast states and the states of Sarawak and Sabah[1] (see Chapter 3), thus private sector healthcare was concentrated in the West Coast states, where patients could pay for these services (Figure 8.2). Consequently, the health sector faced the dual challenge of addressing brain drain to the private sector and inequitable access to healthcare between the regions.

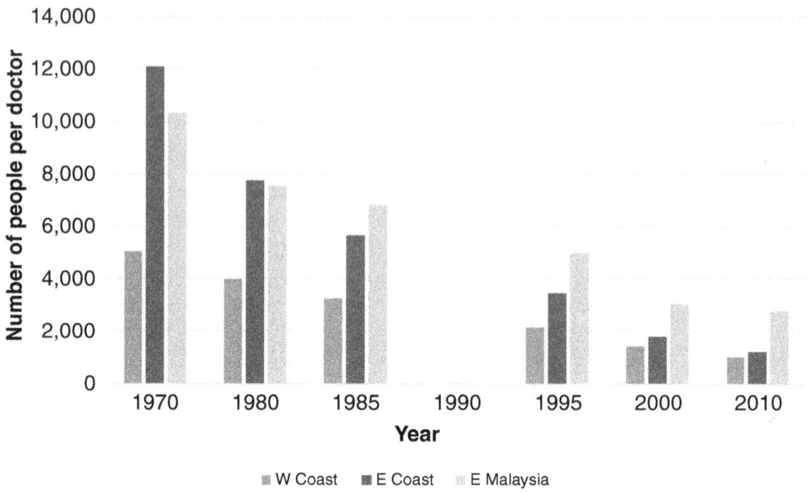

Figure 8.2 Regional disparities in availability of doctors, 1970–2010.
Sources: Calculations by the author derived from data from the Ministry of Health Malaysia (1971; 1974; 1982; 1983; 1984; 1986; 1995a; 2000; 2010) and the Government of the Federation of Malaya (n.d.).

Several policy responses targeting health sector development emerged to address these challenges. One was the national drive to balance the inequitable development that had seen the West Coast states progress much faster than the other states (Prime Minister's Department, n.d.b). Faster development of the less-developed states was expected to facilitate the growth of the private sector, including the private healthcare sector. Another policy was to improve managerial skills in the public sector for better efficiency (obtaining more and better outputs for the inputs) (Prime Minister's Department, n.d. a). Better in-house personnel management was expected to address some of the frustrations of the higher-level categories in the public hospitals. A third approach was to leverage the scarce resources of skilled clinical specialists in the public sector by upgrading the competencies of healthcare workers and encouraging the adoption of a team approach by clinical specialists working together with other categories of healthcare workers. Internal MoH policies on staff placement continually struggled to increase numbers in the less-developed states. These policies resulted in changes in the health workforce profile.

Clinical competencies were upgraded through curricula changes. Some allied health professional categories were upgraded to acquire broader competencies and better remuneration, while others were phased out (Box 8.3). Simultaneously, nursing training was broadened and opened to private sector training institutes. These strategies resulted in a rapid increase in the nursing workforce. As a result, the number of people per nursing personnel was reduced from 1,879 in 1970 to 481 in 1990 (Table 8.7).

The local production of physiotherapists, occupational therapists and radiographers also increased rapidly (Table 8.2). Improved school enrolment and positive discrimination measures enabled rural students to acquire secondary education and resulted in larger numbers of better-qualified candidates for these courses. To improve managerial efficiency, doctors who occupied managerial positions at district and state levels received specialist postgraduate training in public health, while those with managerial positions in hospitals attended purpose-designed in-service management courses (Box 8.3). The establishment of new medical schools accelerated the production of doctors (Table 8.3); specialist training for doctors and for nurses was enhanced.

Various measures were introduced to redress the geographic imbalance in distribution (e.g. special allowances and housing, access to specialist training) and also to stem the brain drain to the private sector (e.g. compulsory public sector service for specified periods). However, as illustrated in Figure 8.1, the proportion of doctors in the public and private sectors did not change until the end of this period. The flow to the private sector was merely contained and not reversed. Also,

Table 8.7 ***Number of people per doctor and per nursing staff, 1970–2000***

	People per staff			
Year	1970	1980[1]	1990	2000
Nursing personnel	1,879	570	481	599
Doctors	4,263	3,800	2,553	1,490

Source: Calculations by author based on data from MoH annual reports from various years.

[1] Data from Suleiman and Jegathesan (2000).

Box 8.3 Examples of key initiatives to upgrade health staff competencies during the 1980s and 1990s

Allied Health Personnel

- Rural midwives were converted to community nurses.
- Junior hospital assistants were replaced by medical assistants.
- Medical laboratory assistants were replaced by medical laboratory technologists.
- Trained nurses were given in-service training to become health staff nurses.
- Curriculum for health inspectors was upgraded and converted from a one-year to a three-year programme that included competency-based practical training.
- Nurse training included a strong management component.
- Local production of physiotherapists and radiographers was expanded.
- Training of health education officers was initiated in the MoH and subsequently transferred to universities.

Doctors and Other Professional Staff

- Doctors and relevant teams were given in-service training in hospital management.
- This training included team training in conducting local-level research and using such information for decision-making (health systems research) and quality improvement (see Chapter 10).
- Post-graduate training in local universities was established for several specialities for doctors.
- Post-graduate training in public health for doctors and engineers included strong management components.

Notable: Most courses included strong components of:

- Cultural and behavioural determinants of health and health-seeking behaviour.
- Practical exercises that enhanced the appreciation of how such determinants applied in the Malaysian context.

although the availability of doctors improved steadily, the gap between the West and the East Coast states of Peninsular Malaysia narrowed only after 1995, while the gap with East Malaysia remains challenging even today (Figure 8.2).

Systemic factors driving individual and collective choices have contributed to the persistence of the gap. Doctors in East Malaysia face more difficulties in accessing facilities such as education for children and entertainment, as well as distance from extended families (Ministry of Health Malaysia, 2016b). Additionally, both public and private hospitals are in places with higher population density for economies of scale; with doctors and medical staff of other higher categories concentrated in hospitals, the pursuit of efficient resource use inadvertently contributes to inequalities. Finally, private hospitals are concentrated in more prosperous regions, where the community has the ability to pay for services. These factors jointly create conditions for the inequitable distribution of human resources, and especially of doctors.

The challenges of regional inequalities notwithstanding, overall access to healthcare has increased, with a significant proportion of this increase resulting from private sector expansion (Table 8.8), and utilisation has increased along with access (Figure 8.3).

Table 8.8 *Access to health facility (with doctor, medical assistant or community nurse)*

Percent within 3 km of nearest facility	1986[1] Population	1996[1] Living quarters
Public[2]	24	50
Private[3]	18	80
Both	32	
Peninsular Malaysia	74	89
Sarawak	n.a.	48
Sabah	n.a.	66
All		81

Sources: Institute for Public Health, 1986; 1996.

[1] Peninsular Malaysia only in 1986; including states in Borneo in 1996.

[2] Staff might have been a community nurse, medical assistant or doctor.

[3] Staff was a private medical doctor.

n.a. – not available

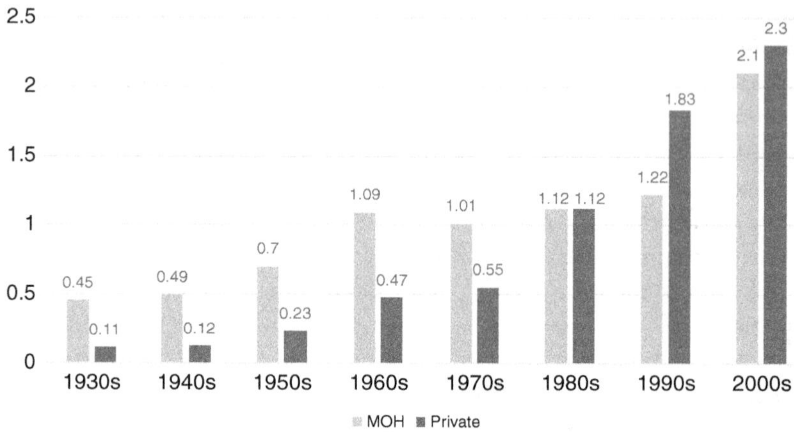

Figure 8.3 Utilisation of outpatient services in Malaysia.
Source: Reproduced from Health Policy Research Associates et al. (2013).

8.4 The Third (Most Recent) Phase of Development (2000s through to 2017)

After the turn of the century, macroeconomic policies focused on achieving 'developed country status' by 2020, which included eradicating poverty and redressing imbalances, building a knowledge-based society and strengthening human resource development with higher levels of knowledge, technical and thinking skills (Economic Planning Unit, n.d.). Globalisation and information communication technology increased, as did urbanisation (62% in 2000) (Department of Statistics, 2001). Lifestyles changed, particularly in relation to food and exercise habits (Lim, 2016; Koh et al., 2015), and migration increased (an estimated 0.23% of the population) (Department of Statistics Malaysia, 2019), with a sizeable proportion of undocumented migrants. All these forces impacted on the health status of the community (see Chapter 3). While the prevalence of NCDs was rising rapidly, some CDs re-surfaced (tuberculosis and dengue) while new threats emerged (HIV/AIDS, severe acute respiratory syndrome (SARS)) (see Chapter 6). Meanwhile, public expectations of health services also increased, influenced not only by rising economic and education levels but also by readily accessible information through electronic connectivity (see Chapter 3).

Medical technology in clinical, imaging and laboratory sciences developed rapidly, bringing with it demands for more varied and higher levels of competencies in the health workforce. These demands on the health services were mirrored by demands from the health workforce for better recognition, higher levels of education and better wage scales. Table 8.9 illustrates how different socio-economic changes at that time influenced the evolution of the health workforce.

A confluence of pressures from socio-economic forces, population behaviour, technological advances, and demands from health service delivery and the health workforce resulted in changes in three related but distinct developments in human resources for health, namely:

1. Basic (pre-employment) education programmes for health and allied health professionals increased their entry requirements and became more focused on achieving defined exit competencies, replacing the earlier implicit and often vague academic standards. A wide range of education programmes for health personnel that hitherto had been under the purview of the MoH were transferred to universities and colleges under the purview of the MoE so that they could have diploma- or degree-level qualifications that commanded higher remuneration packages.
2. A wider range of categories of health personnel, particularly allied health personnel, was produced and employed. By 2014, there were 31 categories of allied health professionals employed by the MoH (Ministry of Health Malaysia, 2016b). They required relevant governance mechanisms (qualification standards, practice regulations, remuneration packages, career pathways) (World Health Organization, 2014).
3. Demand for specialists increased, bringing with it challenges in ensuring standards of quality, appropriate remuneration, distribution and access. This in turn gave rise to the need for managing standards for quality (specialist registers, accreditation, credentialing and continuing education) and remuneration packages (World Health Organization, 2014).

Dichotomies between the health and education sectors and between the public and private sectors in education and health were major structural challenges that affected all the above three aspects of development, which in turn constrained health service delivery. The education sector produced health personnel, while the health sector utilised

Table 8.9 *Summary of interacting influences and the evolution of the health workforce, 2000s and 2010s*

	Population behaviour and demographic profile	Morbidity and mortality profile	Economy and macro policies
Larger ecosystem	• Growing urban population with changing lifestyle around food and physical activity • High social connectivity (electronic and mobile phone) and globalisation • Ever-increasing health literacy, misconceptions and expectations • Increasing migrant labour force (many undocumented)	• Epidemic of NCDs (hypertension, diabetes) • Re-emerging CDs (tuberculosis, dengue) and emerging CDs (HIV/AIDS, etc.) • Increased awareness of problems of mental health, ageing, environment and need for rehabilitation and long-term care	• Building knowledge-based society • Strengthening human resource development with higher levels of knowledge, technical and thinking skills • Rapidly increasing demands on limited public funds • Health tourism as an income-generating activity
	Health services	Education sector	Governance and financing
Health and education sectors	• Rapid increase in private hospitals and facilities – with changing focus to include profit motives • Increased demand for, and rapid increase of, specialist services both public and private • Efforts in public sector to improve equitable access to more sophisticated services to meet more complex disease picture	• Continued high demand for tertiary education • Policy to establish Malaysia as an international education hub • Political pressures to increase educational opportunities by relaxing standards and governance mechanisms	• Failure of information and co-ordination systems between education and health sectors resulting in excessively rapid production of new graduates • Belated application of governance and financing measures to cool excessively rapid production

	• Continued emphasis in the public sector on: o client satisfaction o effective outcomes of care • Equitable access, particularly for lower socio-economic groups		
	Production of health workforce	Health workforce: Key features	Outcomes
Health workforce	• Rapid increase in public and private training institutions and foreign training • Inadequate monitoring and enforcement of quality control measures in tertiary education • Rapid increase in new graduates of varied quality seeking pre-registration training and subsequent employment (consequent to rapid increase in output of training facilities) • Insufficient clinical training facilities and experienced clinical supervisors for training	• Continued brain drain from public to private sector, especially of experienced senior staff • Improved benefits packages to retain specialist doctors and support better deployment • Unanticipated increase in new graduates exceeded the absorption capacity of the health system • Rapid increase in types and numbers of allied health professionals to meet the demands of increasingly diverse and specialised services	• Satisfaction with care providers was good (for public and private clinics) • Outcomes of care for some conditions was good, while quality was less than expected for conditions requiring long-term follow-up

them. There was a dichotomy in the vision and motivations of education and health between the public and private sectors. In both education and health, the public sector focused on societal expectations within tightly controlled budgets and the private sector on commercially viable and competitive enterprises. Box 8.4 summarises the Malaysian experience.

Box 8.4 Malaysian experiences on moving basic training of health personnel from the health to the education sector

Positive

- Establishment of the MQA with adequate legislative, administrative and financial authority to regulate quality of tertiary education.
- Good co-ordination mechanism between health and education specialists for setting criteria and standards for curricula based on competencies required in the health service and for approving training programmes.
- Standardised system for recognition of qualifications linked to remuneration in the public sector.

Negative

The education sector at that time had only one teaching hospital, and all other universities depended on MoH clinical facilities for clinical teaching, resulting in too many students for the available resources.

The strategic planning mechanism for human resources for health in the MoH was dismantled, and there was a lack of clarity regarding responsibility for strategic planning for the health sector as a whole.

As a result:

- There was poor information exchange between the education and health sectors.
- Intakes to education programmes outstripped the capacity of the health sector to provide clinical and practical training, which were almost entirely in the MoH.

- The health sector was unable to absorb the graduates of training programmes in medicine, nursing, dentistry and pharmacy at the pace they were being produced.
- Political and commercial factors drove extremely rapid growth of programmes offering diplomas and degrees in health sector disciplines, undermining the quality control measures and resulting in varied quality of graduates.

Sources: World Health Organization, 2014; Buchanan, 2015; Hambali, 2015.

Basic (pre-employment) training. The training of almost every category of allied health professional was upgraded to college or university level and therefore transferred out of the MoH to the MoE. Within the MoH, structural re-organisation resulted in the MoH changing its focus from strategic planning for the entire health sector to merely planning for its own workforce. Thus a strategic vision for human resource development for health was forfeited. Existing training institutions were re-vamped to become research institutions under the umbrella of the new National Institutes of Health (NIH).

Meanwhile, in the education sector, the number of training programmes for health personnel expanded at an explosive rate, driven by demand from the public as well as by commercial and political forces (Ministry of Health Malaysia, 2016b). Additionally, there was an increase in graduates returning from foreign training programmes, many of them funded by scholarships from the public and private sectors. The demand for nursing had escalated with the growth of hospitals in the private sector as well as demand from other countries, particularly in the Middle East, while the unmet demand for medical doctors was a long-standing issue. The quality of graduates varied greatly (Noorliza et al., 2012). This was particularly apparent in nursing and medicine. The health sector had inadequate capacity to absorb the rapidly increased number of new graduates, with insufficient public health service posts to provide placements for the requisite pre-registration and supervised training of doctors (house officers (HOs)), dentists and pharmacists. Meanwhile, the private sector health services were unprepared to employ fresh, inexperienced nursing graduates. The illustrative case study in this chapter explores the dynamics and impact of the structural challenge in relation to the production and utilisation of medical doctors.

Two underlying systemic issues contributed to the genesis of the problems. Medical, dental and pharmacy education programmes are relatively long (4–6 years). Hence there is a significant time lag between entry into training programmes and graduates seeking entry into the workforce. There was no institutional mechanism for regular timely exchange of critical information between the education and health sectors that would have facilitated pro-active planning taking into account the numbers of entrants and expected graduates. Additionally, institutional mechanisms for joint strategic planning and decision-making are unstable and personality-dependent (Box 8.4) (Buchanan, 2015).

For the first time, doctors and nurses in the public sector outnumbered those in the private sector. However, a large majority of those in the public sector were younger and inexperienced, and difficulties arose in providing them sufficient supervision and guidance (Ministry of Health Malaysia, 2016b).

Several strategies were employed to address the situation, including a moratorium on the establishment of new training programmes for doctors, dentists, pharmacists and nurses; rationalising and consolidating existing programmes; and capping the annual intake in each school. Universities were encouraged to offer post-graduate training of doctors in specialist areas instead of focusing solely on basic undergraduate programmes (see Case Study 8.1 and the later sub-section on 'Issues related to the growing trend of specialisation'). For nurses who had graduated from substandard nursing programmes, special re-training programmes were implemented in both public and private colleges. This facilitated their subsequent employability, particularly in the growing private hospital sector. Pharmacy graduates were allowed to perform their requisite pre-registration training in the private sector.

Expansion of categories of staff. The shift of basic training to the education sector and the establishment of the MQA served well in providing standards for training, recognition of qualifications and establishing remuneration criteria for a large and growing number of allied health professionals. By 2012, the MoH was employing 31 different categories of allied health professionals who had graduated from accredited diploma or degree programmes in colleges and universities. Both public and private sector hospitals began to establish units and programmes that required the skills of these personnel. Practice modalities within health service delivery changed from a heavy focus on the doctor towards a team approach that reflected the growing competence levels of the allied health and other professional groups. In turn, this team approach was integrated into teaching–learning situations in human resources development.

Box 8.5 System observations: stocks and flows of personnel

System inertia complicates decision-making, generating outcomes that under- or overshoot targets. In human resources planning in health systems, this is further complicated by different decision-making loci that shape the flows of human resources, which include education, the public and private health sectors and medical personnel. Several practices can improve the management of system inertia in human resources for health systems, including: (1) closely co-ordinated planning of service delivery strategies with human resource development strategies, (2) using a whole-pipeline approach that cuts across sectors and organisations, and (3) a robust information system that can recognise upcoming trends and needs.

Box 8.6 Rapid and effective implementation of programmes

The Malaysian health workforce is known for its capability for rapid implementation of programmes. An outstanding recent example is the achievement of coverage of the human papillomavirus (HPV) vaccination in the eligible population of adolescent girls – within years of the programme being introduced, higher coverage had been attained than that achieved in many 'first world' countries (Buang e al., 2018).

Who is responsible for implementing health programmes?

- Supervisory categories of nurses manage many front-line services.
- Doctors specialising in public health manage state health departments and health districts and several hospitals.

Their training includes significant emphasis on programme management. This probably contributes to the impressive capacity for rapid and effective implementation of health programmes, particularly those largely delivered through the MCH services.

Similarly, other categories of the health workforce, especially those including senior managerial positions, attend mandatory management courses designed for all civil service officers as part of their career development, while other people who occupy managerial positions in any programme in the MoH attend purpose-designed in-service courses on management.

Continuing education. Participation in continuing education and access to regularly updated practice guidelines is one of the strengths of the Malaysian health workforce. For those in the public sector, the employing agencies (the MoH and other ministries) organise and fund continuing education activities through the various training institutions, hospitals and the NIH. In the private sector, professional bodies take on this role, often in association with pharmaceutical agencies. The MoH also takes the lead in assembling teams of specialists to develop practice guidelines using systematic reviews and other relevant information produced by the health technology unit.

Governance structure and procedures that had served the earlier established medical, dental, nursing, medical assistant and pharmaceutical professions well were replicated to cover several newer categories (Box 8.7).

Specialist competencies. Healthcare services delivery required increasingly complex skills from its workforce to address the growing numbers of patients with complex and multiple disease presentations. They had to use new medical technologies that became available every year. This resulted in a trend toward specialisation, where a small section of the workforce gained much higher competencies in selected fields of medical care.

Issues related to the growing trend of specialisation. The number of such specialised fields is growing steadily. Table 8.9 gives examples of the fields of specialisation and the relevant governance mechanisms established to control quality and safety of practice. This growth presents the continuing challenge of producing sufficient trained personnel for each

Box 8.7 Governance structures (legislation, boards, registration and annual licensing) to ensure quality and safety of practice of healthcare professionals

- Nursing and midwifery: since 1950 and 1966, respectively
- Pharmacists: since 1951
- Medical and dental: since 1952 and 1948, respectively
- Assistant medical officers: since 1977
- Opticians and optometrists: since 1991
- Food analysis: since 2011
- Traditional and complementary medicine: since 2013
- Allied health professionals: since 2016
- Traditional and Complementary Medicine Act: since 2016

The regulatory authority and governance structures described in detail elsewhere (World Health Organization, 2014) have served well in the past to control the practice of these professions by unqualified persons and to set standards of practice for each profession.

However, with the growing number and size of the professions, the evolution of the health system has brought to prominence the need to modernise legislation and governance structures. A recent review by Wraight (2015), a WHO consultant, recommended:

- Harmonising the regulation of all professional groups for 'consistency of purpose to achieve consistent, transparent and fair regulation that protects the public'.
- Strengthening 'arrangements for governance and accountability ... and the relative autonomy of councils and boards' (currently, all councils and boards are under the purview of the MoH, although all have elected representation from the respective professions).
- Establishing sufficiently resourced standalone secretariats with clear demarcation of the roles between the secretariats and the respective divisions in the MoH.
- Alignment of processes to establish standards, procedures, requirements and codes of conduct across all regulated professions to ensure they 'do not compromise the Regulators' ability to protect the public'.

This range of recommendations illustrates the challenges of responding to new circumstances.

> The critical impediments are: (a) the time taken to amend legislation, with some changes taking more than 15 years, and (b) the capacity and political will required to establish standalone secretariats and clear demarcation between the roles and authority of the regulatory bodies vis-à-vis the MoH.

field and distributing them equitably in the health system. Additionally, as the number of specialities increases and the field of each specialisation narrows, particularly for doctors, there are concerns that this could lead to the management of specific manifestations of diseases and health conditions rather than holistic treatment of the patient. Team approaches mostly focus on multi-disciplinary teams of health professionals and allied health professionals but less on teams of senior clinical specialists.

Doctors and dentists undergo specialist training in university-based training programmes. However, as with basic training programmes, specialist training depends on MoH hospitals to provide the very large component of clinical and practical training. Such training requires supervision from specialists in MoH hospitals. As specialists capable of providing supervision are frequently limited in number, there is insufficient capacity to produce specialists at the rate they are needed (the case study illustrates the dynamics of this situation). Consequently, it is difficult to achieve the desired distribution between the geographic regions. Several strategies have been formulated to improve access in the face of the inequitable distribution.

This developmental process has also created new tensions. For example, nursing education has progressed from certificate-level training within the MoH to diploma and degree status in universities. However, the majority of nursing positions in the MoH, the major employer of nurses, are for certificate- or diploma-level candidates. The nursing profession continues to struggle to attain professional status commensurate with degree holders. The role of nursing degree holders in the health sector is as yet unclear, illustrated by the fact that speciality training is limited to credentialing existing nurses with experience rather than requiring further training and qualifications as is the case for doctors. Meanwhile, a dilemma arises from the need for personnel who perform the simpler tasks of bedside nursing. These tasks used to be performed by assistant nurses, a category that no longer exists. Interestingly, more 'developed' countries are eyeing

Table 8.10 ***Examples of specialisation and the relevant governance mechanisms***

Category of staff	Fields of speciality training	Governance mechanism
Nurses Medical assistants (assistant medical officers)	• Perioperative care • Ophthalmology • Emergency medicine • Trauma care	**Credentialing** for two-year periods Authority: MoH Two years' prior experience in the field followed by training and demonstrated competence in specified procedures
Doctors	Thirty speciality areas, e.g.: • Anaesthesiology and critical care • Emergency medicine • Internal medicine • General surgery Each speciality area has a number of sub-speciality areas, e.g.: • Internal medicine has 14 sub-speciality areas such as cardiology, dermatology, endocrinology, etc. • General surgery has six sub-speciality areas such as breast, endocrine, colorectal etc.	**Post-graduate degrees** that are recognised by the Malaysian Medical Council (MMC) in accordance with explicit criteria Placement on the National Specialist Register established under the Medical Act 2012 and managed by the MMC.

Sources: World Health Organization, 2014; National Specialist Register, n.d.

Malaysia's expertise in training assistant nurses as a possible solution to nursing needs arising in their own countries. Another issue is whether the health workforce is sufficiently prepared to address the changing epidemiological picture, with high rates of non-communicable disease together with the ability to mobilise communities to empower individuals and families to take responsibility for their health.

8.5 Workforce Performance

The performance of the health workforce is intimately related to its equitable distribution and utilisation, client satisfaction and quality of healthcare. This sub-section provides information on selected indicators of the performance of the workforce.

8.5.1 Equitable Distribution

Specialist doctors are the most expensive category of healthcare worker and the category for which equitable distribution is the most difficult to achieve. The distribution of selected illustrative key specialist doctors in 2013 was, as expected, highest in the West Coast states of Peninsular Malaysia, but there was a much smaller difference between the Peninsular East Coast states and East Malaysia (Figure 8.4).

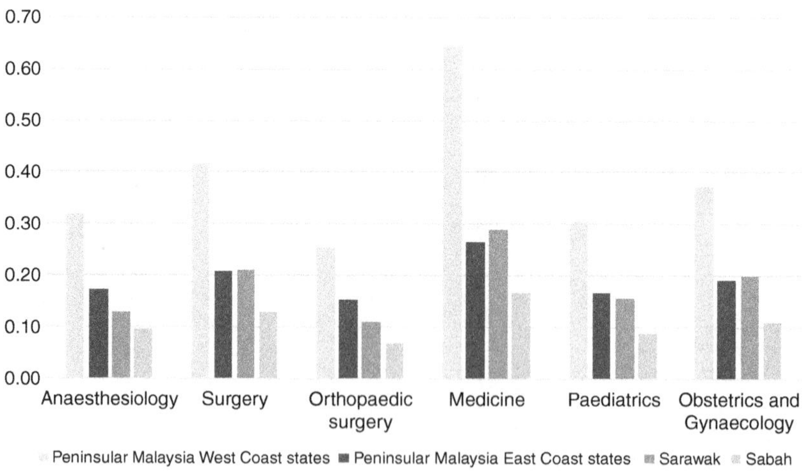

Figure 8.4 Distribution of selected specialist doctors in Malaysia, 2013.
Source: Ministry of Health Malaysia, 2016b.

8.5.2 Utilisation: Level of Utilisation and Equitable Utilisation

The Malaysian Health Care Demand Analysis in 2013 noted that the per capita outpatient visits to doctors in Malaysia 'are comparable with the lower end of the range of levels seen in OECD economies, and about average for countries in the Asia Pacific region with available estimates'. It also found that utilisation had increased from one consultation per capita in the 1930s to >4 consultations in the 2000s. This came from increased utilisation of the public sector starting from the 1960s and 1970s and the rapid increase in utilisation of the private sector after 1980 (Health Policy Research Associates et al., 2013) (Figure 8.4). In terms of equitable utilisation, the study found that 'the poorest 50% of the population used almost two-thirds of ... visits to public facilities, whilst the richest 50% of the population account for two-thirds of visits to private providers'. Similar patterns were observed for the utilisation of inpatient services. Unfortunately, the study did not report on differentials in utilisation in the three geographic regions.

8.5.3 Satisfaction

Human resources play a large role in determining client satisfaction with healthcare services. The community perception module of the 2015 National Health and Morbidity Survey obtained user satisfaction scores on several aspects of services in clinics and hospitals in the public and private sectors. In terms of provider behaviour, more than 70% of users of clinics and hospitals recorded satisfaction levels of 'good' or 'excellent' in terms of 'ability to give diagnosis and treatment', 'give clear explanations' and 'courtesy and helpfulness'. There was little difference between the satisfaction levels reported by users of public and private facilities (Figures 8.5 and 8.6). However, among the other aspects of care, the main source of dissatisfaction regarding public sector clinics and hospitals was waiting time, whereas that for the private sector was treatment charges (Figures 8.5 and 8.6).

8.5.4 Quality of Care

While many factors contribute to quality of care, provider competence and behaviour is a crucial factor therein. During the 1980s, Malaysia was a leader among the developing nations in developing systematic

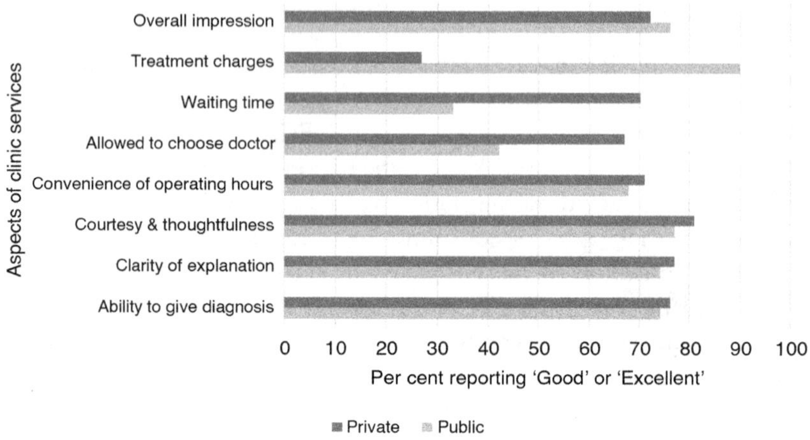

Figure 8.5 Reported satisfaction with public and private clinics, 2015. Source: Institute for Health Systems Research, n.d.

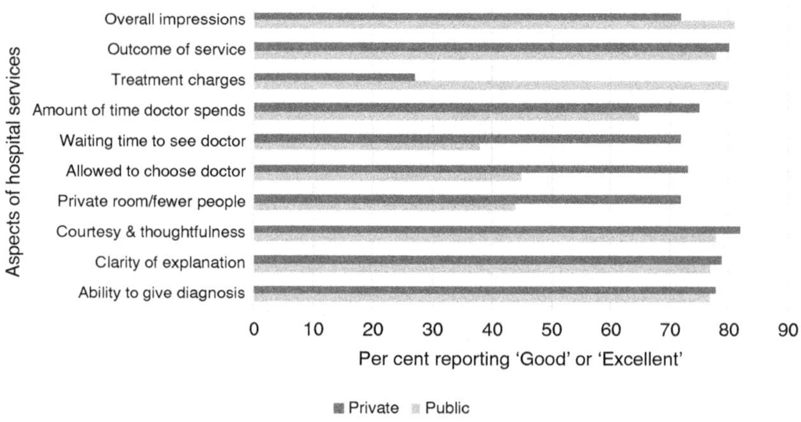

Figure 8.6 Reported satisfaction with public and private hospitals, 2015. Source: Institute for Health Systems Research, n.d.

monitoring and improving quality of care in the health sector. The aim has been to encourage the adoption of a mindset for quality and care that ensures good monitoring and improvement practices among healthcare providers. Although there is a wealth of data from the public sector, data from the private sector are limited, thereby limiting the overall estimate of quality of care.

A 2016 study by an international group from the Harvard T. H. Chan School of Public Health and the MoH (Ministry of Health Malaysia & Harvard T. H. Chan School of Public Health, 2016) used data from the National Medical Care Surveys (NMCS 2012 and 2014) (Clinical Research Centre, 2014) to replicate 66 indicators to analyse the quality of primary care. They found that 'patients received around 57% of recommended care' and that 'these estimates are close to the aggregated quality of care estimates found in the United States and Australia, which range from 55 to 57% although the estimates are not strictly comparable due to differences in the set of indicators used and patient case mix'.

Systematic data for hospital care were limited (Ministry of Health Malaysia & Harvard T. H. Chan School of Public Health, 2016). However, based on mortality rates for common acute conditions, they found that

> 30-day mortality rates for acute myocardial infarction and haemorrhagic and ischaemic stroke (admissions calculated according to actual deaths both in and outside hospitals) were high in 2008 compared to most OECD countries (but comparable to Korea) but have been declining in the past decade with convergence towards rates observed in OECD countries … Hospital case management has been improving and approaches OECD countries for these conditions. (Ministry of Health Malaysia & Harvard T. H. Chan School of Public Health, 2016).

It could be concluded that the quality of clinical care provided by the Malaysian health workforce is generally within acceptable standards.

8.6 Conclusion

In the Malaysian experience, the evolution of the health workforce was determined by the demands of the evolving service delivery system and the capacity of educational institutions, both local and foreign, to produce health workers. As noted in earlier chapters, the evolution of service delivery patterns was influenced by evolving socio-economic status, demographic profile and morbidity and mortality in a community. In parallel, educational status and evolving socio-economic status influenced the evolution of educational institutions. This interaction between demand and supply was moderated by financing and governance measures that evolved over time in recognition of the competing pressures from the larger ecosystem on the demand for and supply of health workers.

Governance and financing mechanisms flexibly shaped the health workforce in response to demands from the health services as they evolved in response to population and health demands.

Legislation required registration and annual licensing for practice key professions, resulting in:

- control of unqualified practitioners, and
- standards for practice defined by recognised qualifications and sources of qualification.

Education standards for curriculum and quality were enforced during:

- the earlier phases – through licences and recognition only of institutions only in the public sector (mainly the MoH), and
- the later phases – through a regulatory authority (the MQA).

Financing of students for training has mostly been from the government for study at local public and private institutions and foreign institutions. This largely facilitated the government's management of the composition, numbers and quality of the health workforce.

Employment: Being the major employer, the public sector can set standards regarding wage structure and benefits packages. However, in the case of specialist doctors, where demand exceeds supply, pressures from the private sector created the necessity for the public sector to upgrade its benefits package.

Foreign inputs have been used strategically to develop and support local resources:

- Monetary aid has been negligible.
- Technical input is used strategically to design curricula, train trainers and set standards.
- Expatriate staff have been very few, mainly for working in rural areas during the earlier years and to provide specialist skills while awaiting the development of local expertise.

The **composition of the workforce** contributed to the development of an affordable health system.

- Nurses were the backbone of the rapidly developing rural health service that responded effectively to conditions of high maternal and infant mortality (Pathmanathan et al., 2003) and remain the dominant category in the health workforce. They far outnumber doctors.
- 'Task shifting', although not acknowledged formally, has been practised throughout all phases of development in accordance with specific service needs. Anecdotal evidence suggests that it was associated with focused on-the job training (e.g. procedures in and anaesthesia by medical assistants, emergency obstetrics by nurse-midwives in hard-to-reach locations, and renal dialysis by nurses).
- Education programmes aim to build competence, particularly among nurses and doctors specialising in public health, to manage health programmes and respond to health behaviour that is influenced by the patient's cultural and personal beliefs.

Alignment of educational curricula with the competencies required in the health sector has been achieved through effective institutional mechanisms. However, the reliance on the public sector to provide almost all facilities for acquiring clinical skills is a major impediment.

The major challenges that persist include:

- **The structural divide between the public and private sectors,** where the health workforce in the public sector is tax-funded and salaried, and in the private sector it is largely fee-for-service self-employed. This has contributed to:
  - experienced and more highly skilled staff moving from the public sector to the private sector, and
  - the consequent difficulty in achieving geographic equity in staff distribution.
- **The gap between the education and health sectors,** whereby:
  - healthcare workers are produced in the education sector, and
  - graduates are utilised in the health sector.

The higher categories of healthcare workers undergo relatively long and expensive training. The time lag between entry to an education programme and entry into the workforce could range from 4 years for courses of shorter duration to as long as 10–12 years for doctors. The health sector is unable to predict and prepare for large changes in the quantity or quality of entrants into the workforce, because institutional mechanisms are weak in terms of:

- providing timely information on the numbers and types of graduates the health sector can expect in forthcoming decades, and
- joint strategic planning between the two sectors to adjust production to the capacity for utilisation.

The result is an imbalance between production and absorption capacity and between production and health sector requirements. When the health sector had control over both production and utilisation, the two could be managed through relatively simpler governance mechanisms. With the evolution of systems, much more sophisticated and time-sensitive mechanisms are needed to generate information and co-ordinate policies and policy implementation tools.

The outcomes of this interaction between the supply and demand of healthcare workers impacts on the access, quality, satisfaction and safety of healthcare, which in turn impacts on the morbidity and mortality in the community.

8.7 Key Messages from Malaysia's Experience

8.7.1 What Went Well?

- The composition of the workforce was crucial in the development of an affordable healthcare system. Key features were:
  - The availability and competence of staff to deliver key tasks at the sites where they were required.
  - Nurses, midwives and medical assistants formed the backbone in the early years.
  - 'Task shifting', although not acknowledged formally, was practised in accordance with specific service needs.
  - Educational curricula for all categories were closely aligned to explicitly defined competencies required in healthcare services.
- The health workforce was shaped flexibly to respond to demands from the health services:
  - through recognition of opportunities and threats in the larger ecosystem and the appropriate use of:

  - governance (e.g. registration, annual licensing, defined standards for eligibility to practise, wage and benefits packages), and
  - financing mechanisms (such as publicly funded training).
- Foreign inputs were used strategically to develop and support local resources.

8.7.2 *What Did Not Go So Well?*

- The structural divide between the public and private sectors contributed to:
  - brain drain from the public sector to the private sector, and
  - a consequent difficulty in achieving geographic equity in distribution of staff.
- There were gaps in co-ordination between production (education) and utilisation (health) due to weak institutional mechanisms.

8.7.3 *Trends and Challenges*

- Rising expectations of the workforce and the public create the risk of mismatch between workforce competencies and the community's healthcare requirements.
- Rapid development of technology will require new competencies and render some competencies redundant.

References

Buang, S., Jaafar, S., Pathmanathan, I. and Saint, V. (2018). Human papillomavirus immunisation of adolescent girls: improving coverage through multi sectoral collaboration in Malaysia. *British Medical Journal*, 363(k4602), 74–82.

Buchanan, J. (2015). *HRH Governance, Strategic Planning and Analysis: Support to HRH Strategic Planning in Malaysia, Office for Malaysia.* Brunei and Singapore: World Health Organization (unpublished).

Clinical Research Centre. (2014). *National Medical Care Survey.* Kuala Lumpur: Clinical Research Centre.

Department of Statistics. (2001). *Population Distribution and Basic Demographic Characteristic Report, Population and Housing Census 2000.* Online report. www.statistics.gov.my/english/census/pressdemo.htm

Department of Statistics Malaysia. (2019). *Migration Survey Report, Malaysia, 2016*. Online report. https://dosm.gov.my/v1/index.php?r=column/cthemeByCat&cat=125&bul_id=RldLdXFnQUppeGM5Yk1HODlTMVl6UT09&menu_id=U3VPMldoYUxzVzFaYmNkWXZteGduZz09

Economic Planning Unit. (n.d.). *Rancangan Malaysia Kelapan (Eighth Malaysia Plan) 1986–1990*. Online report. https://web.archive.org/web/20070323094806

Economic Planning Unit. (2004). *Malaysia: 30 Years of Poverty Reduction. Growth and Racial Harmony. A Case Study from Scaling Up Poverty Reduction*. Shanghai: World Bank.

Government of the Federation of Malaya. (n.d.). *Annual Report, Malaya, 1955*.

Hambali, Z. B. (2015). *Kajian Perlaksanaan Polisi KMP dan KKM: Keberkesanan Pelaksanaan terhadap Permintaan and Pengeluaran Doktor Perubatan IPT di Malaysia 2014* [Study of the implementation of policies of the Ministries of Higher Education and Health: Effectiveness of implementation regarding demand and production by Medical Institutions in Malaysia 2014] (unpublished study).

Hameed Musafar, L. B. (2014). *An Enquiry into Privatisation's Impact on Healthcare Services in Malaysia*. Kuala Lumpur: University of Malaya.

Health Policy Research Associates (HPRA), Institute for Health Systems Research (IHSR) and Institute for Health Policy (IHP). (2013). *Malaysia Health Care Demand Analysis: Inequalities in Healthcare Demand and Simulation of Trends and Impact of Potential Changes in Healthcare Spending*. Putrajaya: Ministry of Health Malaysia.

Institute for Health Systems Research. (n.d.). *Community Perceptions Module of the National Health and Morbidity Survey 2015*. Setia Alam: Institute for Health Systems Research.

Institute for Public Health. (1986). *National Health and Morbidity Survey 1986*. Kuala Lumpur: Institute for Public Health.

Institute for Public Health. (1996). *National Health and Morbidity Survey*. Kuala Lumpur: Institute for Public Health.

Ismail, A. M. and Martinez, E. J. (1975). *Our Health Services in the Seventies*. Kuala Lumpur: Ministry of Health Malaysia.

Koh, P. C. and Abdul Rahman, Z. A. (2015). Tracking the past: the local culture of Malaysian eating and lifestyle. International Conference on Local Knowledge: Axis of Global Knowledge. Online paper. www.academia.edu/37630568/Tracking_the_Past_The_Local_Culture_of_Malaysians_Eating_Habit_and_Lifestyle

Lim, K. G. (2016). A review of adult obesity research in Malaysia. *Medical Journal Malaysia*, 71(Supplement1), 1–19.

Ministry of Health Malaysia. (1971). *Annual Report*. Kuala Lumpur: Ministry of Health Malaysia.

Ministry of Health Malaysia. (1974). *Annual Report*. Kuala Lumpur: Ministry of Health Malaysia.

Ministry of Health Malaysia. (1982). *Annual Report*. Kuala Lumpur: Ministry of Health Malaysia.

Ministry of Health Malaysia. (1983). *Annual Report*. Kuala Lumpur: Ministry of Health Malaysia.

Ministry of Health Malaysia. (1984). *Annual Report*. Kuala Lumpur: Ministry of Health Malaysia.

Ministry of Health Malaysia. (1986). *Annual Report*. Kuala Lumpur: Ministry of Health Malaysia.

Ministry of Health Malaysia. (1995a). *Annual Report*. Kuala Lumpur: Ministry of Health Malaysia.

Ministry of Health Malaysia. (1995b). *Health Facts 1995*. Kuala Lumpur: Planning Division, Ministry of Health Malaysia.

Ministry of Health Malaysia. (2000). *Annual Report*. Kuala Lumpur: Ministry of Health Malaysia.

Ministry of Health Malaysia. (2010). *Annual Report*. Putrajaya: Ministry of Health Malaysia.

Ministry of Health Malaysia. (2016a). *Health Facts 2016*. Putrajaya: Planning Division, Ministry of Health Malaysia.

Ministry of Health Malaysia. (2016b). *Human Resources for Health, Country Profiles 2015 Malaysia*. Putrajaya: Ministry of Health.

Ministry of Health Malaysia and Harvard T. H. Chan School of Public Health. (2016). *Malaysian Health Systems Research Volume 1: Contextual Analysis of the Malaysian Health System March 2016*. Putrajaya: Ministry of Health Malaysia.

National Specialist Register. (n.d.). *National Specialist Register*. Online document. www.nsr.org.my/index2.htm

Noorliza, M. N. et al. (2012). *Report: House Officer Performance in Malaysia 2009–2011*. Setia Alam: Institute of Health Systems Research, Ministry of Health.

Pathmanathan, I., Liljestrand, J., Martins, J. M., Rajapaksa, L. C., Lissner, C., de Silva, A. et al. (2003). *Investing in Maternal Health: Lessons from Malaysia and Sri Lanka*. Washington, DC: World Bank.

Prime Minister's Department. (n.d.a). *Rancangan Malaysia Kelima (Fifth Malaysia Plan) 1986–1990*. Online report. http://pmo.gov.my/dokumenattached/RMK/RMK5.pdf

Prime Minister's Department. (n.d.b). *The Fourth Malaysia Plan (FMP) 1981–1985*. Online report. www.pmo.gov/dokumenattached/RMK/RMK4.pdf

Public Health Institute. (1983). *Study of Hospital Utilization in Peninsular Malaysia*. Kuala Lumpur: Ministry of Health.

Suleiman, A. B. and Jegathesan, M. (eds.). (2000). *Health in Malaysia: Achievements and challenges*. Putrajaya: Ministry of Health Malaysia.

World Health Organization. (1977). *World Health Statistics Annual, 1973–77*. Geneva: World Health Organization.

World Health Organization. (2014). *Human Resources for Health Country Profiles: Malaysia*. Online report. https://iris.wpro.who.int/handle/10665.1/10530

Wraight, B. (2015). *Strengthening Health Professionals Regulation in Malaysia: Key Observations and Policy Options*. Putrajaya: Ministry of Health.

System Analysis Case Study 8.1: Unexpected Influx of New Medical Graduates Threatens to Overwhelm the Health System

Indra Pathmanathan and David T. Tan

This case study illustrates the interactions between the health and education sectors and the interactions between the health workforce and service delivery, health sector governance (administrative and legislative) and health sector financing (payment of providers and budgetary allocations). It also provides insights into the dynamics between the broader ecosystem (public perceptions and demands and political responses) and the health workforce.

Background

Like all developing countries, Malaysia struggled for decades to have sufficient doctors for its growing population and increasingly complex healthcare requirements. During the first decade of the 21st century, there was an unforeseen three-fold increase of new medical graduates seeking to enter the workforce (Figure 8-A). The health system

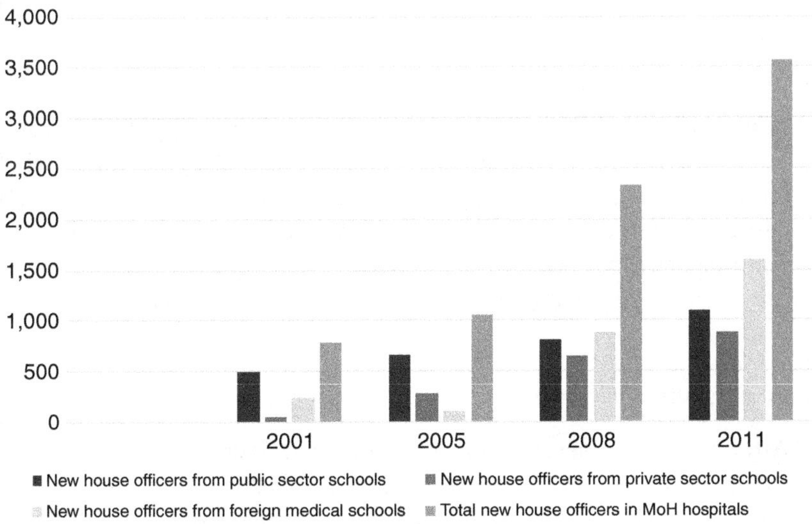

Figure 8-A New graduates entering the workforce as HOs.
Source: Ministry of Health Malaysia, 2016, p. 73.

struggled to provide sufficient HO positions for the new graduates, and questions arose as to whether Malaysia had too many doctors. A mini crisis was in the making.

A quick review showed that Malaysia's number of doctors per 1,000 population was relatively low compared to OECD (Organisation for Economic Co-operation and Development) countries and regional neighbours. The issue was not too many doctors but the inability to cope with the rapid increase in the production of new doctors. This case study analyses the genesis of the situation, its subsequent impact on the health system and the health system's responses.

Box 8-A The career pathway for doctors in Malaysia

Production of Doctors

The average duration of a medical programme is five years. Malaysian doctors are produced in public and private (for-profit) Malaysian universities and in several foreign universities. Most students are supported by scholarships and loans provided largely by the government.

House Officers

Every medical graduate is required to complete an internship as a house officer, which is a supervised apprenticeship in public sector hospitals. During this period, HOs are governed by stringent criteria, including sufficient specialist doctors to serve as supervisors, clinical material (patients) and clinical facilities (hospitals, beds, equipment). On successful completion of this stage of their training, the doctor is registered as a medical practitioner (or general practitioner – GP).

Post-graduate Training

After a period of service as medical officers, doctors undergo up to four years of post-graduate (PG) training to become specialists. This training requires supervision by competent specialist doctors, and it requires patients or practice settings and equipment relevant to the speciality (Figure 8-B). Such training is available only in hospitals in the public sector – very largely those under the MoH.

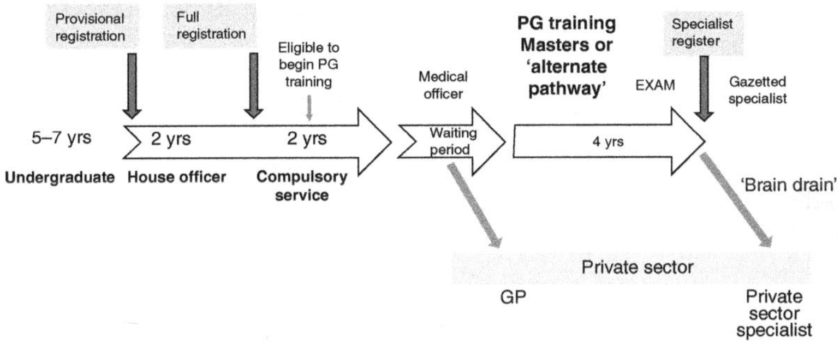

Figure 8-B Doctors' average career path in Malaysia.

Genesis of the Mini Crisis

Historically, the annual supply of new medical graduates was far below the number of available HO positions and the numbers required for the objective of having one doctor per 400 population (Prime Minister's Department, Malaysia, 2015). Towards the end of the 20th century, economic and educational growth had resulted in a rapid increase in school leavers eligible for tertiary education. Thus demand for medical education grew rapidly – a positive development in light of the need for more doctors. This created a gap between supply and demand for medical education, which the Malaysian government responded to via two major actions (Figure 8-C).

First, the liberalisation of education policies opened the tertiary education sector to the private sector. This was part of a broader privatisation policy by the Malaysian government and led to the establishment of many new medical schools, which rapidly escalated the production of medical graduates (Table 8-A and Figure 8-C, B1 loop). However, the limited availability of experienced academic clinical staff and inadequate clinical training facilities severely limited the quality of training in several of these institutions.

Concurrently, responding to public demand, the government rapidly increased loans (Figure 8-C, B2 loop) for Malaysian students to study at foreign universities. Political pressures contributed to large numbers

Table 8-A *Rapid increase in medical schools and new medical graduates*

	1995	2001	2005	2008	2011
Medical schools in Malaysia[a]	6	13	19	21	30
New HOs from public sector medical schools[b]		496	659	808	1,088
New HOs from private sector medical schools[b]		43	286	641	877
New HOs from foreign medical schools[b]		241	104	877	1,600
Total new HOs in MoH hospitals[b]		780	1,049	2,326	3,565

Sources: (a) https://en.wikipedia.org/wiki/List_of_medical_schools_in_Malaysia (b) Planning Division. 2016. Human Resources for Health country profiles 2015: Malaysia. Ministry of Health.

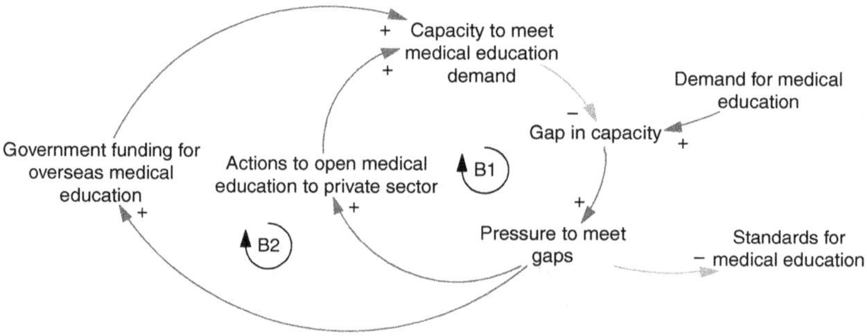

Figure 8-C Meeting the demand. Pressure to meet the gap between supply and demand for medical education led the government to make policy changes that rapidly increased the capacity for medical education, with potential compromises in education standards.

of foreign medical degrees being recognised for registration and subsequent medical practice in Malaysia. While the country had a mechanism for recognising both local and foreign medical qualifications using fairly stringent criteria, the rapid increase in applications for recognition outstripped the system's capacity to apply the recognition criteria with diligence, creating a negative impact on education standards. (Figure 8-C, 'Standards of Medical Education').

Both these actions reduced the gap between demand for and provision of medical education. Two balancing loops (Figure 8-C, loops B1

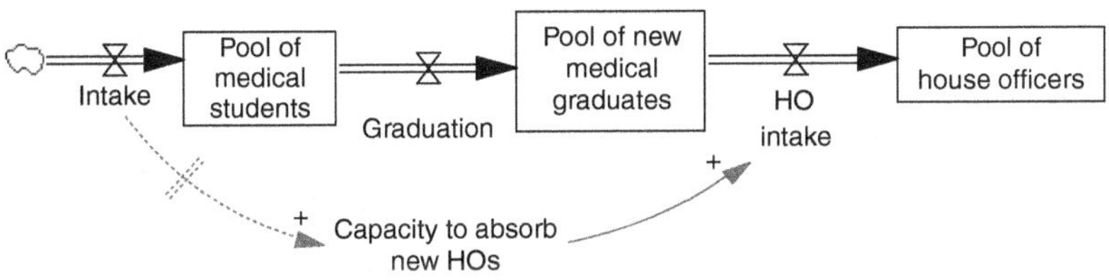

Figure 8-D Lack of capacity planning. Employment planning did not reflect student intake rates. The dotted arrow indicates this lack of information flow and the missed opportunity to adjust the capacity of the health system to receive new medical graduates. The delay mark on the dotted arrow reflects the time required for the system to adapt to increase capacity.

and B2) had been set in motion, albeit with some potential compromises in the standard of education delivered.

By 2008, the scene was set for the large cohorts who had entered medical school during 2000–2003 to graduate and seek employment as HOs. Their competence was highly varied, depending on the quality of their medical education. However, the MoH was unprepared for the sudden surge in HO numbers. Neither the Ministry of Higher Education nor the MoH had used the medical student intakes to plan future employment capacity. Instead, the MoH had based its planning on previous trends. This approach had worked well in the past but was unable to detect and respond to changes outside the established pattern. Thus the extent of the employment challenge surfaced only when the number of applications for house officer positions became overwhelming (Figure 8-D).

The First Bottleneck: An Imbalance between the Pool of Graduates Awaiting Employment and the Capacity to Provide House Officer Placements

The health system had insufficient specialist doctors to supervise and clinical facilities to absorb all the new graduates. In 2014, only 3,602 places were available for 4,740 graduates. This resulted in an increasing pool of graduates awaiting employment (Figure 8-E, 'Pool of New Medical Graduates'), which generated frustration and anxiety among

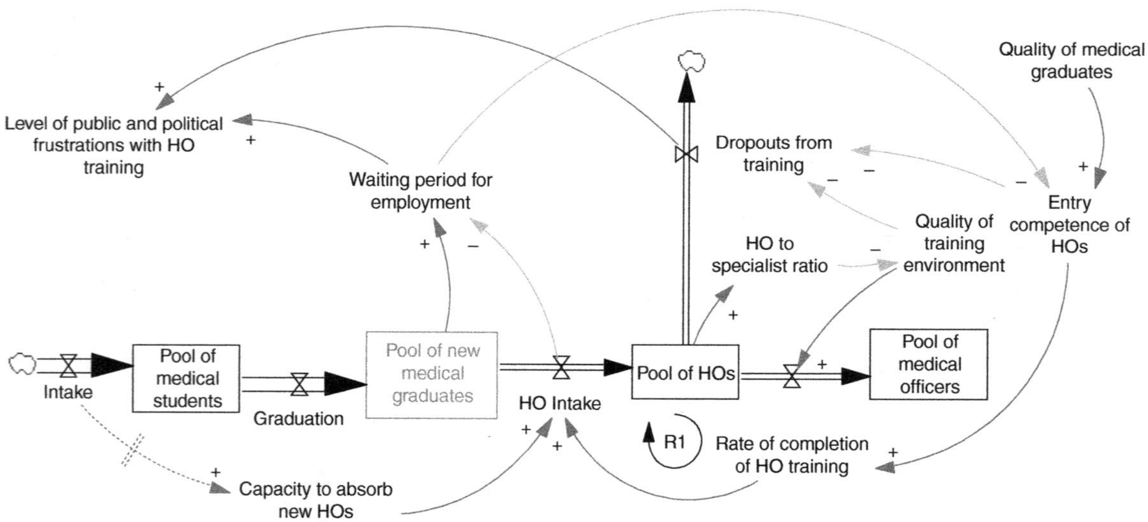

Figure 8-E Impact of the bottleneck on the HO experience. Mismatch in graduation and HO intake rates created long waiting periods for employment. Inadequate entry competence of HOs and high HO-to-specialist ratios extended their training period, further reducing the availability of HO posts and reinforcing the longer waiting time for employment.

graduates and their parents, loss of skills in the new graduates and increased public and political pressures.

The reduced standards for medical education (described earlier) lowered the average skill level of the incoming house officers such that a significant proportion of new entrants into the HO programme had inadequate entry competence. This resulted in extension of the HO period beyond the specified 2 years, as seen in 2014, when only 58.8% of HOs completed their training in the allotted time, thereby clogging up available posts and exacerbating the waiting times. Additionally, the waiting period for employment deteriorated the skill levels of the incoming house officers, creating a reinforcing feedback loop that further contributed to longer waiting periods (Figure 8-E, R1).

Initial attempts to accommodate the increased demand for HO positions placed pressure on the training environment. For example, instead of 14 beds per trainee, the ratio was reduced to 2.8 beds per trainee. Only internal medicine had the desired ratio of five trainees per specialist (Lim, 2017). The supervisory load on existing specialists escalated. Inadequately prepared HOs and their overworked and frustrated supervisory specialist doctors showed many signs of stress: the symptoms included illness, complaints and even dropouts from HOs, and complaints, frustration and lowering of supervision standards among specialists. Thus the quality of HO training was compromised.

The Second Bottleneck: An Imbalance between Applicants (Medical Officers) and the Capacity to Provide Post-graduate (Specialist) Training

Experienced practising specialist doctors are critical for the training of HOs and potential specialists. As described earlier in this chapter, an ongoing challenge for the health system is the loss of specialist doctors from the public to the private sector. This limits the rate at which HO and specialist training can be carried out, creating reinforcing feedback loops (Figure 8-F, loops R2a and R2b) that exacerbated the limited absorption of HOs from the waiting pool.

The MoH was aware of this challenge. Advocacy over several previous years resulted in new policies being implemented in 2011, which coincided with the height of the house officer bottleneck crisis. Salaries and other perks were given to public sector specialists. However, this also generated an unintended consequence: it

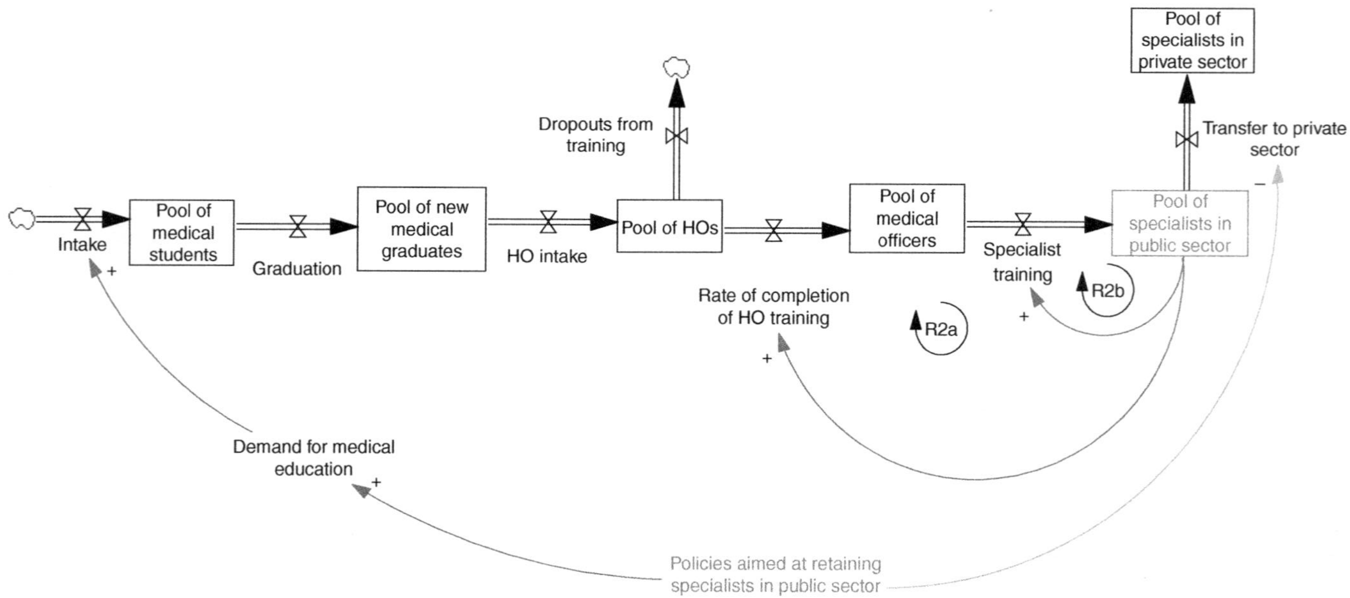

Figure 8-F The specialist bottleneck. The pool of public sector specialists limits the capacity to train HOs and medical officers and further their career progression, which in turn limits the pool of public sector specialists.

enhanced the prestige of the medical specialist, thereby reinforcing the latent demand for medicine as a career among students and their parents, thereby adding pressure to the already engorged pipeline of would-be doctors (Figure 8-F, 'Demand for Medical Education').

As the enlarged cohorts of medical graduates advance through their career paths, a second bottleneck is emerging. The career path of medical officers requires post-graduate training in speciality areas (Figure 8-B). The existing number of public sector specialists available to provide this training limits the system's capacity, creating another crucial feedback loop (Figure 8-F, R2b).

In 2013, 4,500 new graduates entered the workforce, compared to only 240 doctors (Ministry of Health Malaysia, 2016) who completed post-graduate training. These larger cohorts will substantially increase the pool of medical officers awaiting post-graduate training, creating much longer waiting times. This will result in frustration and loss of skills and motivation and will create strong pressure for expanded opportunities for specialist training. In the long term, resolving the specialist training bottleneck and retaining specialists in the public sector is crucial for increasing MoH capacity to train house officers and medical officers.

System Responses

An analysis of the health system's response shows the capacity for self-correction but also reveals that the structural flaws that allowed the emergence of the HO crisis have not been addressed (Figure 8-G).

Increase Capacity for Training House Officers

Public sector. First, the MoH addressed public expectations regarding waiting time for HO appointments. The MoH went on to revise the structure of HO training by expanding HO postings beyond the four traditional core postings to include a further four specialities. The details of the training and service delivery systems had to be co-ordinated, such as criteria for rotations, duration of shifts and contact

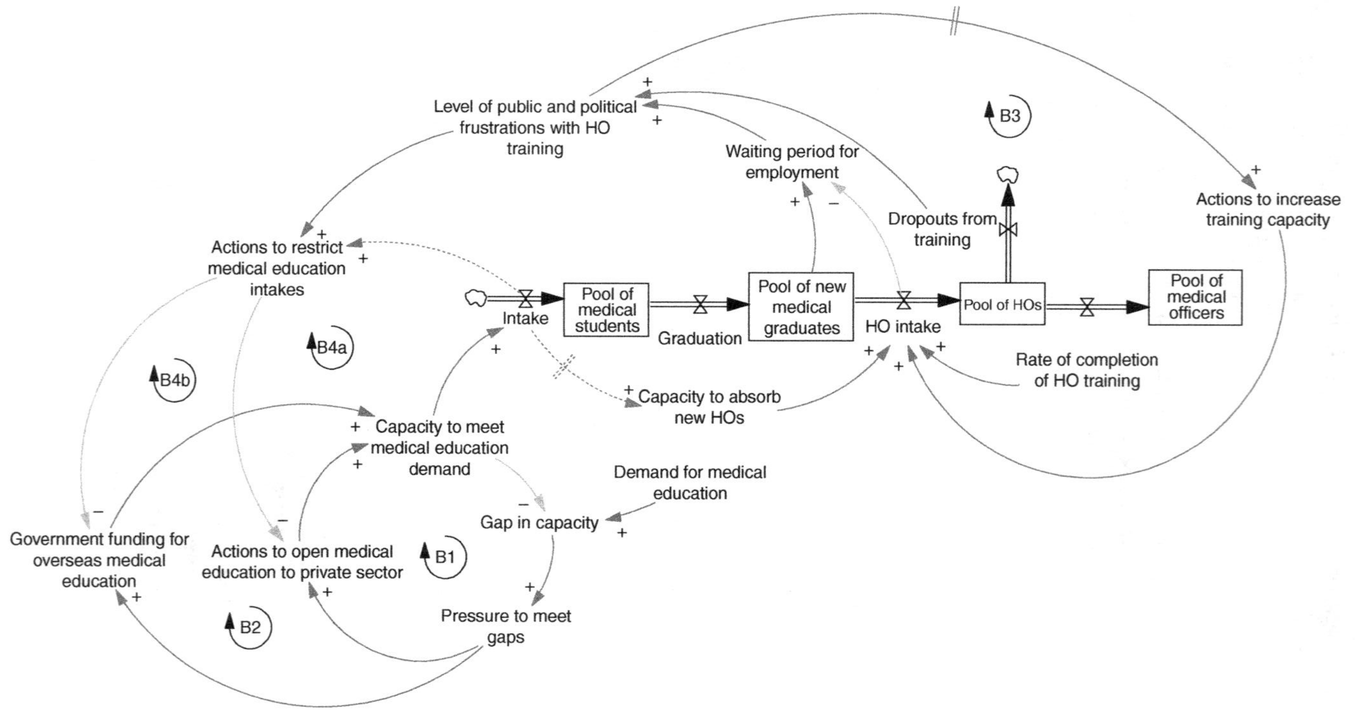

Figure 8-G Systems responses to the crisis. New measures were taken to increase training capacity (B3) and to restrict medical education intakes to prevent continued escalation of the HO crisis (B4a and B4b). However, the gaps in the flows of information that prevented anticipation and proactive response to the change in the number of medical graduates has not been addressed. Thus the health system remains vulnerable to future shifts in the production of medical graduates.

hours with supervising specialists, to ensure quality of training while preserving quality of service delivery. To address the varied entry competence of new graduates, additional basic training had to be created for weaker HOs, while a fast-track system was introduced to enable competent HOs to reduce their training duration. Emphasis shifted from duration of training to demonstration of competence. The use of clinical skills laboratories was enhanced so that HOs acquired basic clinical skills without overburdening the patients. These measures improved the training output within the existing limitations but took time to design and implement (B3 loop, delays mark) and were insufficient to fully address the large increase in demand for HO training.

Private sector. Efforts to recruit the private sector to provide HO training proved unsuccessful. A variety of issues contributed to the barriers. The governance and financing structure of private hospitals posed barriers. Private hospitals would have to absorb the cost of the HO and their training with little financial benefit. In the private sector, most specialists had a contractual relationship with private hospitals. There would be complex financial, administrative and legal implications regarding the responsibilities for supervising HOs. Few private hospitals had the required case mix to provide adequate HO training.

Regulate the Numbers of New Medical Graduates The MoH engaged successfully in intersectoral dialogue at policy level to restrict the intake of medical students. A moratorium was placed on new medical schools, the number of entrants per school was capped and existing schools were required to rationalise through mergers to limit production and improve quality (Figure 8-G, loop B4a). Local medical schools required sufficient numbers to ensure financial viability; therefore, regulations were eased regarding the percentage of non-Malaysian students (not eligible for local HO training) permitted in each school. The dialogue also resulted in the limitation and rationalisation of public sector funding for medical training in foreign institutions (Figure 8-G, loop B4b). This situation created dismay among new cohorts of would-be students, aggrieved at not receiving the same benefits as their predecessors, and has the potential for negative political fallout.

Increased Post-graduate Training for Specialist Doctors (Education and Health Sector Interaction)

The training of specialists is the purview of public universities, who themselves are under the MoE. Public sector medical schools have been encouraged to change focus from under-graduate training to specialist training. However, the number of available supervising specialists and clinical facilities (beds, equipment, patients) limits the capacity for increasing the production of specialists. A parallel pathway for specialist training was established under the MoH, whereby candidates completed their clinical training at MoH hospitals and sat for examinations conducted and accredited by UK-based boards such as the Royal College of Physicians. This initiative proved effective only for specialities that had limited requirements for gaining competency in interventional procedures, due to the limited access to facilities and equipment for such procedures. Various smaller initiatives were also established for twinning programmes with foreign universities that had campuses in Malaysia. Whether these measures will be sufficient to address the upcoming second bottleneck remains to be seen.

The Persistence of the Information Gap

The health system was able to respond to the causes and consequences of the HO crisis with varying degrees of success. However, systems that would enable the collection and use of information that would allow the health system to adjust the intake of medical graduates and to prepare to receive HOs have not been implemented. This effectively creates a set of balancing loops with very long delays (Kim, 1992), which tends to generate a pattern of under-responsiveness followed by overcorrection. As the time between entry into medical school and production of doctors and the consequent system delays are largely fixed (Figure 8-B), early indicators such as medical student intake are all the more critical for the health system to respond to changes in the health workforce pipeline in a proactive, timely and sufficient manner.

While the Malaysian experience illustrates several successful policy interventions, it also demonstrates shortfalls. The most critical is the inability to establish a system that would provide timely information on future graduates to enable strategic planning. Efforts to create integrated information on human resources for health, through co-ordination between education, health, finance and other sectors, have failed because of the absence of incentives for such information. A strategy that would shift the control of information to the health sector would be useful. Such a strategy would require entrants to medical schools to register their interest in obtaining HO positions.

Systems Lessons

Systems analysis demonstrates that human resource (HR) management in health systems needs to apply lessons from the science of management logistics to avoid imbalances between the production and the utilisation of the health workforce, especially as the long training periods for most healthcare workers restrict the ability of health systems to detect and respond to these imbalances. Without strong mechanisms to ensure two-way information flows between producers who control the evolving status of future HR stocks and the managers and users of those stocks, 'feast or famine' scenarios will result for various categories of healthcare workers.

References

Kim, D. H. (1992). *System Archetypes I: Diagnosing Systemic Issues and Designing Interventions*. Online report. https://thesystemsthinker.com/systems-archetypes-i-diagnosing-systemic-issues-and-designing-interventions

Lim, C. H. (July 2017). *Housemanship Programme in Malaysia: Availability of Positions and Quality of Training*. Online report. https://penanginstitute.org/wp-content/uploads/jml/files/research_papers/HousemanshipIssue_LCH20July2017-Final.pdf

Ministry of Health Malaysia. (2016). *Human Resources for Health. Country Profiles, 2015. Malaysia. Ministry of Health*. Putrajaya: Ministry of Health Malaysia.

Prime Minister's Department, Malaysia. (2015). *Eleventh Malaysia Plan 2016–2020: Anchoring Growth on People*. Putrajaya: Economic Planning Unit, Percetakan Nasional Malaysia Berhad.

Note

1. West Coast states: Perils, Kedah, Penang, Perak, Selangor, Kuala Lumpur, Negri Sembilan, Melaka and Johor. East Coast states: Kelantan, Terengganu and Pahang. East Malaysia: Sabah, Sarawak and Labuan.

9 *Financing Health Care*

CHIU-WAN NG

9.1 Introduction

How a country chooses to finance health care for its people is an important indicator of the value it places on health as a public good. A country that relies predominantly on public funding for health care reveals a strong commitment by the state to ensure its people's access to care.[1] The growth of private funding for health care, particularly when it results in out-of-pocket payments (OOPPs)[2] for households, is a real risk for financial impoverishment.

A country's history plays a major role in shaping its health system (Phua, 1989). Some former British colonies in Asia, for example, have retained many welfare-oriented features of the British National Health Service. These include minimal user fees or even free services at the point of use. However, history cannot be the sole reason for current systemic failures in health. Health systems do not remain static but evolve in response to challenges to their resilience. The state is beholden to ensure through good governance that such transformations meet the changing health needs of its people.

What, then, is the situation in Malaysia? Reliable historical estimates of national health expenditure are not fully available. However, it is known that although health care in the country has been mainly financed using public funds since 1997, the share of public funding just barely exceeded that of private funds for health (Ministry of Health Malaysia, 2019, p. 26). This is in contrast to the situation in 1983, just slightly more than a decade earlier, when the share of public funding was more than 75% of the country's health expenditure (Westinghouse Health Systems, 1985, p. 4).

By 1997, not only had private funding of health care reached almost half of the country's health expenditure, this private funding was also mainly composed of OOPPs (Ministry of Health Malaysia, 2019, p. 40).

Coincidentally, the 1980s also marked the start of the period when the private provision of health care in the country began a rapid upward trajectory (Chee & Barraclough, 2007, p. 23). Malaysia's current hybrid health system is one in which the financing and delivery of health care follow the public–private divide – publicly funded public health care providers exist alongside privately funded private health care providers. Over the past few decades, the private health system has expanded at a faster rate than its public counterpart, with consequences not just on the trends but also on the composition of health financing in the country.

However, the *raison d'être* of any country's health financing system is not merely to pay for health care. The system should also ensure that the burden of payment, independent of use, is fairly distributed among the population in a country. In many welfare-oriented countries like Malaysia, this translates to a progressive health payment system where richer households contribute proportionately more from their income than poorer ones (Yu et al., 2008). In addition, the system should also ensure that health funds, especially public funds, are allocated in a manner that can meet population health needs. Like many other middle-income countries, Malaysia is undergoing an epidemiological transition from communicable to non-communicable diseases (NCDs). To curtail the epidemic of these chronic lifestyle diseases effectively, adequate funding should be allocated to preventive and promotional services, early disease identification, early treatment initiation and, most importantly, sustained delivery of needed care. In the case of NCDs, most of these services can be provided efficiently at the primary care level.

This chapter will tell the story of Malaysia's changing health financing landscape. It starts with a description of the trends in health financing since the 1980s; not just overall expenditure figures but also an analysis of the different financing sources that comprise public and private health financing. This section will also include a brief review of allocative efficiencies in terms of spending patterns according to the categories of services. As financing sources are intricately linked to how health care providers are paid in Malaysia, the narrative will also outline a discussion on the changes within the health care delivery system, the forces at work behind these transformations and the eventual impact on health care financing in this country. The chapter will end with a review of the challenges facing health care financing and a discussion of the way forward for Malaysia.

9.2 Trends in Health Care Financing in Malaysia

The work involved in estimating national health expenditure is not only data-intensive but also has to be conducted in a systematic manner following internationally accepted accounting frameworks to facilitate comparability across time and countries. Efforts to develop the Malaysia National Health Accounts (MNHA) (Box 9.1) to routinely capture the totality of financing flows within the Malaysian health system only started in 2001, and to date, MNHA has produced a series of national health expenditure estimates spanning 1997 to 2017 (Ministry of Health Malaysia, 2019, p. 24). Despite the lack of such accounting systems in the years prior to this, it is still possible to obtain an understanding of the public–private mix of health financing in the country from government documents and reports.

The Malaysian government disseminates policy directions for national development in a series of reports known as the Malaysia Plans, reviewed and updated every five years. The First Malaysia Plan, covering from 1966 to 1970, focused on national priorities during the early years after the birth of Malaysia, and the country is currently in the Eleventh Malaysia Plan period (2015–2020). These reports detail achievements in various economic or social sectors,

Box 9.1 Establishment of the MNHA

The Malaysian government collaborated with the United Nations Development Programme in 2001 to initiate the MNHA Project (Ministry of Health Malaysia, 2006, p. ii). The MNHA Project was eventually institutionalised within the Ministry of Health (MoH) as the MNHA Unit in 2005 (Ministry of Health Malaysia, 2008, p. 1).

The estimation framework adopted by the MNHA was based on the System of National Accounts developed by the Organisation for Economic Co-operation and Development, which allowed for the systematic capture of health expenditure data from multiple sources and the reporting of a rich array of expenditure information along three dimensions, namely financing sources, health providers and health care functions (Ministry of Health Malaysia, 2006). Essentially, the MNHA information system permits the tracking of health funds from the funding source to the health care provider and finally to the purpose for which the health funds have been used.

including health, in the preceding five years before going on to lay down the government's policies for the following five years. The reports also detail the financial allocations that the government has committed towards the implementation of the policies. The health chapter contained in the Fifth Malaysia Plan (1986–1990) was pivotal. While the first four reports were essentially a re-telling of government priorities to increase public investment in the public health sector, especially to expand access to rural health services (Malaysia, 1966; 1970; 1976; 1981), the Fifth Malaysia Plan was the first to acknowledge the growing financial burden on the government such that 'programmes for health services under the Fifth Plan will take into account the limited financial capacity of the public sector as well as the need to expand the health care system', and it noted the need to seek out new sources of health financing, including increased cost sharing with the community to ensure that 'those who can afford to pay bear a larger share of the cost burden' (Malaysia, 1986, p. 514).

It was apparent that concerns over the government's ability to sustain public funding of health care using revenues from general taxation grew in the period of the Fourth Plan. This led the government to initiate the Health Services Financing Study (HSFS)[3] in 1983 to review the performance of the overall Malaysian health system and to provide recommendations for alternative financing methods for Malaysia (Westinghouse Health Systems, 1985, pp. 1–10). As part of the work, the HSFS estimated that, in 1983, Malaysia spent $1.8 billion[4] or 2.8% of the gross national product (GNP) on health (Westinghouse Health Systems, 1985, p. 165). The HSFS noted that 76.6% of this amount was spent on public health care services delivery and that these funds came mainly from general taxation. Full understanding of the estimated private sector expenditure has been difficult, as a full description of the funding sources was not provided. However, the report noted a 'direct payments'[5] component that may refer to OOPPs in households (Westinghouse Health Systems, 1985, p. 165). The OOPPs for households in 1983 was estimated at 18.8% or nearly a fifth of the entire country's health expenditure.

In his classic review of the Malaysian health system of 1984, Roemer (1991, pp. 395–412) also included an estimate of Malaysia's health expenditure. He had gathered the available information about the country's health expenditure from various sources and concluded that the country's health expenditure in 1983 totalled $1.7 billion, or

2.6% of the GNP, of which 74.3% was from public sources and 25.7% was spent on purchases of care from private providers (Roemer, 1991, p. 408). He was unable to provide an estimate of OOPPs.

Thus, although comprehensive estimates of Malaysia's national health expenditure in the early years are scarce, both the HSFS's and Roemer's accounts appear to concur in that, at least in 1983, about three-quarters of the health funding in Malaysia came from public sources and that possibly nearly a fifth of health funding in the country had come from private household OOPPs.

The MNHA yielded more contemporary estimates. The available information showed that total expenditure on health (TEH) in Malaysia increased more than three-fold in real terms from Malaysian ringgit (RM) 17.1 billion to RM 57.4 billion over the 21 years from 1997 to 2017[6] (Table 9.1). However, this increase is less apparent after taking into consideration population expansion over this period. The increase in health expenditure per person was just two-fold – from RM 790 in 1997 to RM 1,790 in 2017. During this time, health expenditure as share of gross domestic product (GDP) had fluctuated within a narrow range, from a low of 3.0% in 1997 to a high of 4.3% in 2015.

Public funding of health care predominated throughout 1997 to 2017, but public shares did not exceed 61% of TEH (Figure 9.1).

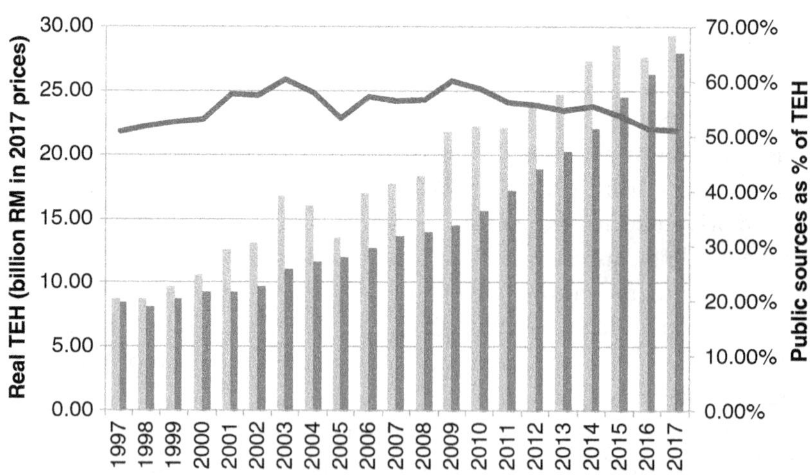

Figure 9.1 Public and private health financing sources, Malaysia, 1997–2017.
Source: Ministry of Health Malaysia, 2019.

Table 9.1 ***Total and per capita expenditure on health, Malaysia, 1997–2016***

Year	TEH[1] (billion RM in 2017 prices)	Per capita TEH[1] (RM in 2017 prices)	TEH as % GDP
1997	17.10	790.09	3.03
1998	16.88	755.86	3.23
1999	18.34	799.74	3.31
2000	19.88	846.41	3.30
2001	21.85	906.45	3.60
2002	22.75	920.65	3.56
2003	27.78	1,096.30	4.11
2004	27.72	1,070.70	3.84
2005	25.50	963.95	3.35
2006	29.70	1,107.35	3.70
2007	31.32	1,152.02	3.67
2008	32.26	1,171.44	3.61
2009	36.30	1,301.74	4.12
2010	37.89	1,325.34	4.00
2011	39.29	1,352.41	3.94
2012	42.76	1,449.43	4.07
2013	44.98	1,489.05	4.09
2014	49.38	1,608.21	4.23
2015	53.11	1,703.04	4.33
2016	54.00	1,706.76	4.23
2017	57.36	1,790.00	4.24

Source: Adapted from Ministry of Health Malaysia, 2019.

[1] Total expenditure on health. TEH and per capita TEH are reported in RM in 2017 prices.

The MNHA categorises sources of health expenditure by the institutions directly incurring expenditure on health care, with the understanding that these institutions can control and finance such expenditure (Ministry of Health Malaysia, 2006, pp. 14–15). Financing sources are then further divided into public and private sources (Box 9.2).

Most of the public funding for health comes from government agencies, to which the MoH contributed the largest share – exceeding 80% of the total public funding of health annually (Table 9.2). Among the

Box 9.2 Sources of health care financing as captured in the MNHA

The public sources of health care financing are mainly government agencies at the federal, state or local authority levels, as well as social security agencies in Malaysia. These include:

- The MoH as the main provider of health care in the country.
- The Ministry of Education with its teaching hospitals.
- The Ministry of Defence with its health facilities for providing care mainly to military personnel and their dependents.
- State and local authorities providing services mainly related to sanitation, food quality control and vector control services in larger towns.
- The EPF, a fund providing retirement benefits for its members that also permits withdrawals for members' health care needs.
- The SOCSO, a workers' compensation scheme that provides financial benefits when workers suffer disabilities due to work-related injuries and illnesses.

The main private sources of health care financing are:

- Private health insurers that pay health care providers for the care consumed by those insured under their programmes.
- MCOs, which are not risk takers but function mainly to administer the health benefits of those who are enrolled in their health schemes. These companies purchase third-party insurance coverage, which is then bundled into the health schemes they sell to individuals as well as to companies.
- Private corporations that pay for the health care consumed by their employees as part of their employment benefit plans.
- Private household OOPPs for health, which refers to the portion of health care payments not paid for by any third-party payers and which are thus borne directly by households.

Source: Ministry of Health Malaysia, 2006.

public sources of health financing, the two main social security organisations in Malaysia, the Employees' Provident Fund (EPF) and the Social Security Organisation (SOCSO), are minor contributors. Although these organisations do incur health expenditures because they finance some health care for their members, health care is not the primary component of their benefit packages. Consequently, health funds from these organisations do not feature prominently in the estimates of TEH in Malaysia. In 2017, the combined health funding from the EPF and SOCSO amounted to only 0.7% of TEH or 1.3% of financing from public sources (Ministry of Health Malaysia, 2019, p. 30). In 1997 – 2017, on average, the annual social security contributions to TEH accounted for only 1.2% of overall public funding.

Over the years, funds from private health insurers have gradually increased, reflecting the uptake of private health insurance in Malaysia. In 2005, about 15% of the population had some form of health insurance cover (Central Bank of Malaysia, 2005, p. 58). By 2014, the coverage had increased three-fold to 45% of the population, or about 14.7 million people (Malaysian Productivity Corporation, 2016, p. 112).[7] In 1997, private health insurers financed 4.0% of the nation's TEH, and this share increased to 8.8% in 2017 (Table 9.2). In contrast, the financing component from private corporations dropped from 7.2% of total health financing in 1997 to 2.3% in 2017, perhaps as a result of corporations purchasing third-party health insurance cover for their employees instead of self-insurance or obtaining the services of managed care organisations (MCOs). The predominant private financing source in Malaysia from 1997 to 2017 remained private household OOPPs, which made up on average 74.7% of the annual private health expenditure or 37.6% of the annual TEH in Malaysia. In fact, private household OOPPs is one of the main financing sources for health care in Malaysia, second only to the MoH (Table 9.2).

From the perspective of household welfare, private funding of health care is not desirable. Services provided by government agencies, including the MoH, are mainly funded through general taxation (Rozita, 2000). As in most countries, taxation in Malaysia has been structured to ensure that the wealthy are required to pay more in taxes as a proportion of their income than the poor. The progressive nature of taxes in Malaysia is reflected in the funding of health care partially from general taxation (Yu et al., 2008). Regardless of contribution, entitlement to care remains the same. This makes for a fairer distribution of the burden of health funding. In addition, this form of public funding has several welfare-enhancing features, including fund pooling and pre-payment (Box 9.3), which protects households from financial catastrophe resulting from health payments.

Table 9.2 *Public and private health expenditure, Malaysia, 1997–2017*

	Public sources of financing in billion RM[1] (% of TEH)			Private sources of financing in billion RM[1] (% of TEH)			
Year	MoH	Other government agencies[2]	Social security[3]	Private insurance	OOPPs	Private corporations	Other[4]
1997	7.23	1.37	0.11	0.69	6.33	1.23	0.13
	(42.29)	(8.03)	(0.67)	(4.03)	(37.02)	(7.20)	(0.75)
1998	7.27	1.36	0.12	0.80	6.02	1.18	0.13
	(43.06)	(8.05)	(0.71)	(4.73)	(35.67)	(7.01)	(0.76)
1999	8.03	1.48	0.13	0.91	6.44	1.21	0.13
	(43.79)	(8.06)	(0.73)	(4.96)	(35.14)	(6.61)	(0.71)
2000	8.91	1.52	0.14	1.01	7.07	1.08	0.16
	(44.84)	(7.64)	(0.72)	(5.06)	(35.55)	(5.42)	(0.78)
2001	10.56	1.87	0.16	1.17	6.68	1.24	0.16
	(48.34)	(8.56)	(0.75)	(5.38)	(30.56)	(5.68)	(0.73)
2002	10.92	2.01	0.17	1.35	6.88	1.24	0.17
	(47.98)	(8.85)	(0.76)	(5.94)	(30.26)	(5.45)	(0.76)
2003	14.33	2.23	0.19	1.73	7.98	1.13	0.19
	(51.60)	(8.02)	(0.68)	(6.22)	(28.72)	(4.07)	(0.69)
2004	13.34	2.51	0.21	1.79	8.63	1.04	0.20
	(48.14)	(9.06)	(0.76)	(6.46)	(31.12)	(3.74)	(0.72)
2005	11.04	2.32	0.22	1.69	8.93	1.10	0.21
	(43.30)	(9.08)	(0.86)	(6.62)	(35.01)	(4.32)	(0.81)
2006	14.34	2.44	0.20	1.86	9.61	1.03	0.22
	(48.27)	(8.21)	(0.68)	(6.27)	(32.37)	(3.47)	(0.72)
2007	14.16	3.32	0.22	2.01	10.16	1.22	0.24
	(45.21)	(10.59)	(0.69)	(6.41)	(32.45)	(3.90)	(0.77)

2008	14.89	3.27	0.16	2.18	10.56	0.95	0.25
	(46.16)	(10.15)	(0.49)	(6.76)	(32.72)	(2.94)	(0.77)
2009	17.84	3.84	0.17	2.68	10.48	0.99	0.29
	(49.14)	(10.59)	(0.48)	(7.39)	(28.87)	(2.73)	(0.80)
2010	18.38	3.69	0.20	2.85	11.43	1.04	0.31
	(48.50)	(9.73)	(0.52)	(7.53)	(30.16)	(2.73)	(0.82)
2011	18.04	3.87	0.21	3.12	12.76	0.94	0.34
	(45.90)	(9.85)	(0.55)	(7.95)	(32.47)	(2.40)	(0.88)
2012	19.74	3.91	0.23	3.33	14.07	1.09	0.40
	(46.17)	(9.14)	(0.54)	(7.79)	(32.89)	(2.54)	(0.92)
2013	20.57	3.84	0.28	3.46	15.63	1.11	0.09
	(45.74)	(8.54)	(0.63)	(7.70)	(34.74)	(2.46)	(0.19)
2014	22.97	4.09	0.33	3.84	17.01	1.10	0.05
	(46.51)	(8.29)	(0.66)	(7.77)	(34.44)	(2.23)	(0.09)
2015	24.00	4.23	0.33	4.61	18.63	1.23	0.08
	(45.18)	(7.97)	(0.62)	(8.68)	(35.08)	(2.32)	(0.15)
2016	23.07	4.24	0.38	4.92	20.05	1.24	0.09
	(42.73)	(7.85)	(0.70)	(9.11)	(37.13)	(2.30)	(0.17)
2017	24.72	4.24	0.39	5.07	21.57	1.31	0.07
	(43.09)	(7.38)	(0.67)	(8.84)	(37.61)	(2.29)	(0.12)

Source: Adapted from Ministry of Health Malaysia, 2019.

[1] Reported in RM in 2017 prices.

[2] Including the Ministries of Education and Defence, state and local authorities.

[3] EPF and SOCSO.

[4] Including non-governmental organisations providing health care to the public.

Box 9.3 Pre-payment and fund pooling features in health financing sources

Pre-payment for health care describes a situation in which payment for health care is made in advance of the need for care. As a person's health, and thus their need for health care, is uncertain (Arrow, 1963), it would be difficult for anyone to have enough savings to cover all health care eventualities. Pre-payment circumvents this problem by ensuring that care is paid for in advance and will be made available when needed.

Fund pooling refers to the pooling of collected health funds before payments are made to providers (World Health Organization, 2010, p. 4). This is intended to distribute the financial risks of ill health among a pool of people. Once a person contributes to the pooled funds, they are entitled to health care paid for from the pool. However, restrictions may apply to such payments and may be related to the types of services to be funded, levels of co-payments and other financial limits.

Are these lauded pre-payment and fund pooling features absent in private funding sources? Not quite, as these features are also present, albeit to a limited extent, in some private funding sources, including private health insurance and private corporations. However, the financial risk protection these mechanisms confer is restricted to those who have bought private insurance cover or those with formal employment that provides health benefits. Unfortunately, in the case of Malaysia, funding of health care from these private sources pales in comparison to private household OOPPs for health care, a financing source that has neither pre-payment nor fund pooling features (World Health Organization, 2010, pp. 5–6).

Private household OOPPs for health care is the one source of health financing with the highest potential to impact household welfare adversely, especially for poorer households (World Health Organization, 2010, p. 5). A multi-country assessment has shown that household financial catastrophe caused by OOPPs for health care can only drop below negligible levels if that country's OOPPs are below 15–20% of TEH (Xu et al., 2010). In 1997 to 2017, during which health expenditure has been reliably estimated, the levels of

OOPPs for health in Malaysia have consistently exceeded this threshold (Ministry of Health Malaysia, 2019, p. 24). Despite this, the levels of financial catastrophe arising from health care payments in Malaysia have been surprisingly low. In 1998, when OOPPs for health made up 35.7% of TEH, only 0.8% of households paid OOPPs for health care exceeding 25% of their non-food expenditures (van Doorslaer et al., 2007).

These large OOPPs were concentrated in the richer households. In 2009, OOPPs made by only 0.2% of households in the poorest quintile exceeded the 25% of non-food expenditure threshold as compared to 0.55% of households in the richest quintile (Health Policy Research Associates et al., 2013, p. 37). Thus the situation in Malaysia appears to defy the conventional wisdom that high levels of OOPPs for health in a country lead to high levels of household financial catastrophe (Box 9.4).

The explanation may lie in the fact that, for most households in the country, health care remains affordable. In 2009, on average, OOPPs for health made up only 1.1% of the average household expenditures, with the poorest quintile of households committing only 0.7% of household expenditures to pay for health care and the richest households a 1.5% share (Health Policy Research Associates et al., 2013, p. 32). The situation in Malaysia supports the findings from recent

Box 9.4 System observations: intuition and systems surprises

The observation that high OOPPs in Malaysia have not appeared to create household financial catastrophe or differences in utilisation across income is surprising and points towards the importance of checking intuition with data and disaggregating populations when attempting to model health systems. While this finding is welcome, it should not be assumed that this state of affairs will automatically persist if current arrangements between the public and private sectors remain the same. Indeed, systems often have both zones of stability and tipping points outside of these zones, where change can be swift and dramatic. As such, continued close monitoring of public and private health care spending and the development of causal models that predict impact on household financial security are important.

international comparative work on financial risk protection for health (Wagstaff et al., 2018a; 2018b). These studies suggest that the levels of financial risk protection offered to the population may not depend on health expenditure as share of a country's GDP but on shares of TEH that are pre-paid, especially through taxes and other mandatory contributions. In 2009, pre-paid sources of financing[8] made up 69.7% of TEH, with government agencies funding up to 59.7% of TEH, most of which came from taxation (Ministry of Health Malaysia, 2019, p. 25). It would seem that the high levels of pre-payment inherent in the taxation-funded Malaysian health care system have conferred protection against financial catastrophe for most of the population in the country.

Financial risk protection aside, there are arguments to suggest that health care resources in Malaysia may not have been allocated in a manner that yields maximum health benefits (Ministry of Health Malaysia & Harvard T. H. Chan School of Public Health, 2016, pp. 87–91). Partially due to lifestyle changes in the Malaysian population, NCDs are emerging as a major health issue in the country. In 2015, the prevalence of hypertension and diabetes among the adult population in Malaysia was 30.3% and 17.5%, respectively (Institute for Public Health, 2015, p. 22). More alarmingly, about half of the adults with these conditions were unaware of them and thus did not seek treatment. NCDs such as hypertension and diabetes should be identified and managed in a primary care setting (Varghese et al., 2019). However, the strength of Malaysia's well-established public primary care delivery system lies mainly in the provision of acute care services related to communicable diseases, minor ailments and maternal care (Mustapha et al., 2014). Some re-orientation of thinking would be required for the expansion to the country's primary care system to manage the increasing burden of chronic NCDs effectively.

Strengthening the primary care system in Malaysia would require substantial financial investment. However, the patterns in TEH show otherwise. It has been estimated that Malaysia spent 49% of TEH on secondary and tertiary care and only 17% on primary care (Ministry of Health Malaysia & Harvard T. H. Chan School of Public Health, 2016, p. 87). The pattern of government spending was even more skewed, with only 11% of the expenditure allocated to primary care as opposed to 65% to secondary and tertiary care services. However, more disconcerting is that shares of health expenditure for primary care services declined from 13% in 2008 to 10% in 2010.

This brief review of the available national expenditure for health appears to indicate the increasing prominence of private funding of health care, particularly the OOPPs component, in Malaysia. Malaysia's situation is different from that of many other countries, such as South Korea, Taiwan and Japan, where public funds are used to pay private health care providers. In this country, public funding is mainly channelled to the public health system; likewise, private sources fund the private health sector. Thus the rise of private health funding in Malaysia is likely to be mirrored by a similar rise in private provision of health care.

9.3 The Expansion of the Private Health Sector in Malaysia and Its Impact on Health Care Financing

Public and private provision of health care have long co-existed in Malaysia. However, the size of these two sectors, as well as the composition of health care providers, have changed over the years.

In the early days, private health care providers did not feature prominently in the health landscape and consisted mainly of single-doctor clinics in the larger towns. Roemer (1991, pp. 402–4) noted that in 1984, the public health care system, of which MoH facilities made up the largest component, was the backbone of health care delivery in the country in terms of geographic coverage and health infrastructure. However, rapid development of the private health sector started in the 1980s, and this was more apparent in the hospital sector (Chee, 2008). In 1980, there were only 50 private hospitals with 1,171 beds, or 5.8% of all acute hospital beds in the country (Chee, 2008). Over the next 5 years, the number of private hospitals more than doubled to 133 with 3,666 beds, or 14.5% of the country's acute hospital beds. Since then, the capacity of private hospitals has continued to increase at a faster pace than that of public hospitals such that by 2017, the share of private hospital beds had increased to 27.3% of all acute hospital beds in the country (Ministry of Health Malaysia, 2018a). In the same year, approximately 30% of all acute hospital admissions were in private hospitals (Ministry of Health Malaysia, 2018a).

Growth of the private health sector was not just evident from the numbers of hospital beds alone but also from the diversity of health

Table 9.3 *Licensed private health care facilities, Malaysia, 2007–2017*

Facility	2007	2010	2017
Medical clinic	2,992	6,442	7,571
Dental clinic	937	1,512	2,137
Hospital (beds)	195 (11,291)	217 (13,186)	200 (14,799)
Maternity home (beds)	21 (175)	22 (97)	16 (50)
Nursing home (beds)	10 (228)	12 (263)	22 (700)
Hospice (beds)	3 (28)	3 (30)	2 (17)
Ambulatory care centre (beds)	n.a.	36 (125)	100 (186)
Blood bank	n.a.	5	4
Haemodialysis centre (chairs)	n.a.	191 (2,195)	450 (484)
Community mental health centre (beds)	n.a.	1	1
Combined ambulatory care centre and haemodialysis centre (beds/chairs)	–	–	1 (14/21)

Source: Ministry of Health Malaysia, 2007; 2010; 2018a.
n.a. – not available

care facilities in the country. The MoH is the main regulator of the private health sector. Prior to 1998, the ministry regulated only three categories of private health facilities: hospitals, maternity homes and nursing homes. Since then, this list has expanded to include psychiatric hospitals, ambulatory care centres, psychiatric nursing homes, blood banks, haemodialysis centres, hospices, community mental health centres and medical and dental clinics. The MoH currently regulates a total of 12 distinct categories of private health care facilities in Malaysia (Table 9.3).

The expansion of the private health sector in Malaysia has had a direct impact on the public–private mix in health financing. The provision of public health care is mainly financed by general taxation. Other minor funding sources for public health care are private household OOPPs, employer-sponsored care, private health insurance and EPF and SOCSO. In 2017, 97.6% of funding received by MoH hospitals came from general taxation, 1.9% was from OOPPs, 0.3% was private health insurers and 0.2% was from EPF and SOCSO (Ministry of

Health Malaysia, 2019, p. 78). The main reason these sources play a much less significant role in financing public health care is because public funds from taxation have been used to keep user fees[9] low for most services provided in public health facilities (Rohaizat, 2004). The government legislates user fees for MoH facilities (Ng, 2019). Although these fees are meant as a tool for cost recovery in public health facilities (Malaysia, 1990, p. 353), they are much lower than the actual cost of delivering the services. It was estimated that the cost of an outpatient visit to a MoH hospital in 2009 ranged from RM 77.46 to RM 129.11 (Institute for Health Systems Research, 2013, p. 6). The comparable legislated fees for the first specialist outpatient visit to a MoH hospital would have been RM 30.00 if the patient had been referred by a private clinic and free if the referral had come from a public clinic (Government of Malaysia, 1982). The fees for subsequent visits were RM 5.00 for each visit. In 2014, medical fees billed to patients amounted to only 1.4% of the ministry's operating expenditure (Ministry of Health Malaysia, 2015, pp. 32–6). The shortfall was made up using general taxation.

In contrast to the public sector, private health care providers do not receive direct government funding to provide health care services to the public. In consequence, fees in the private sector are set at cost plus profits and are thus higher than those in the public sector. As a measure to ensure that such services remain affordable, the government regulates professional medical fees charged by doctors practising in private facilities (Government of Malaysia, 1998).[10] In 2013, a patient would have had to pay RM 80 to RM 235 for the first specialist outpatient visit to a private hospital and RM 40 to RM 105 for subsequent visits (Government of Malaysia, 2013). This excludes fees for drugs, investigations and other administrative charges. In 2012, the average household monthly income per person was RM 1,451 (Department of Statistics Malaysia, 2013, p. 12). Payment of fees for private health care services comes from a variety of sources. As part of their employment benefit packages, employees' health care may be paid in full or partially by employers. The health care for persons who have purchased private health insurance may be paid in full or partially by their health insurers. Some EPF members may also withdraw funds to pay for health care. Unlike the public health sector, which receives the bulk of its funding from general taxation, the major funding source for private care is private household OOPPs.

Changing consumer preferences could have accounted for the changes in the public–private mix of health care providers. Over time, increasing consumer purchasing power has allowed at least the rich to purchase the more expensive, yet at the same time perceived to be of higher quality, private care (Chee & Barraclough, 2007). However, the expansion of the private health sector in the 1980s could also be partially attributed to enabling government policies that encouraged private sector participation in all sectors of the Malaysian economy, including the health sector. The British welfare philosophy on health care, which emphasised public provision and funding of care for all, had guided the early development of the health sector in this country (Barraclough, 1999; Chee & Barraclough, 2007; Rasiah et al., 2011). Mirroring developments in the United Kingdom itself, where government commitment to these noble sentiments has also been watered down over time, the Malaysian government has gradually changed its stance on public provision and financing of health care to meet the health needs of the country.

In 1983, the government unveiled its privatisation policy to actively increase private sector participation in the development of the country's economy (Institut Tadbiran Awam Negara Malaysia, 1994, pp. 62–3). This move was aimed at reducing the presence of the government in the economy and at lowering the level and scope of public spending. In the realm of health care, the government encouraged private provision of care, stating that 'the private sector, including NGOs, will be encouraged to expand and complement the Government's effort in providing a comprehensive range of health care services for all income groups' (Malaysia, 1996, p. 549). To aid the public's ability to purchase expensive private care, the government re-structured the main social security agency for private sector workers, the EPF, in 1994 to allow for a medical savings account mechanism to enable EPF members to withdraw their savings for the purchase of health care (Ng, 2005). The government also provided tax deductions for medical expenses and for the purchase of private health insurance (Chee & Barraclough, 2007).

The government has not only promoted the development of the private health sector but has also invested in private care. Many private hospitals are fully or partially owned by government-linked companies (GLCs)[11] but operate as commercial for-profit enterprises (Chan, 2014). These GLCs include IHH Health Care Berhad, a subsidiary of

Khazanah Nasional Berhad, the federal government sovereign wealth fund, and KPJ Healthcare Berhad, a public-listed company belonging to Johor Corporation, the investment arm of the Johor state government. Other state governments, including those of Terengganu and Malacca, are also involved in providing private health care. Sime Darby, another GLC, owns hospitals through Ramsay Sime Darby, a joint venture with Ramsay Health Limited, an Australian company. Currently, the proportion of private hospital beds owned by GLCs exceeds 50% of the total private hospital beds in the country (Ng, 2019). The provision of private health care by GLCs indicates the extent of the reversal in the government's attitude towards the provision of health care. Early post-independence efforts that focused on expanding publicly funded health care to the whole country, especially the underserved rural areas, which is a welfare-motivated ideal, had by the 1990s given way to the view that private provision of health care could be a socially acceptable manner of distributing health care, especially to the rich, as well as an acceptable manner of generating government revenue.

Towards the end of the 20th century, the government embarked on an additional avenue to support the expansion of private care in the country. Health tourism, the business of providing health care to foreigners, was born in the aftermath of the 1997 Asian financial crisis as an answer to financially ailing private hospitals in the country (Chee, 2007). During this time, private hospitals had to turn from the diminishing pool of local patients who were no longer able to afford private care to foreign patients, for whom favourable currency exchange made it financially attractive to enter the country for health care. Initial government support included the MoH setting up the National Committee for the Promotion of Medical and Health Tourism in 1998 to develop strategies to attract foreign patients (Chee, 2007). The responsibility of promoting health tourism in the country has now been taken up by the Malaysia Healthcare Travel Council, a public–private collaborative agency housed under the Ministry of Finance (MoF) Malaysia.[12] Continued government support of private sector expansion has now been linked to the support for health tourism, as has been made clear in the Eighth Malaysia Plan, which stated that 'further development of the health sector, particularly tertiary medical care in private hospitals, will provide a conducive environment for the promotion of health tourism'(Malaysia, 2001, p. 495).

The HSFS conducted in 1985 had foreseen that the private health sector in Malaysia was 'on the verge of dramatic and explosive potential expansion' (Westinghouse Health Systems, 1985, p. 3), and in a sense this prediction has come true. However, as seen in the above narrative, the expansion of private health care has generally been welcomed. Private provision of care is seen to complement public provision of care. The government stated its intention to reduce its role in the provision of health care services and instead to concentrate efforts on regulating the health sector (Malaysia, 1996, p. 544). Fears were raised that this would lead to a two-tier health system, with public services, which are perceived to provide a lower quality of care in return for lower fees, being relegated to the poor while the rich can afford expensive, higher-quality private care (Ng et al., 2016, p. 187). To date, the pattern of health care utilisation, especially for inpatient care, does not appear to support these sentiments.

In 2011, it was estimated that on average, each person in Malaysia had 4.3 outpatient consultations and that there were 111 inpatient discharges per 1,000 population in the country (Health Policy Research Associates et al., 2013, p. 20). The outpatient consultations were equally distributed between public and private health care providers. However, inpatient admissions were predominantly public. Admissions to public hospitals made up 74% of all admissions. However, it is more interesting to note that there was no income gradient in the utilisation of outpatient and inpatient care services. While outpatient and inpatient utilisation were the same across income quintiles, there was a distinct pro-rich distribution for the use of private health care services and, conversely, a pro-poor distribution for public care (Health Policy Research Associates et al., 2013, pp. 55–6).

To increase the accessibility of private care, the government has repeatedly announced its intention to reform the country's health care financing system to provide 'consumers with a wider choice in the purchase of health services from both the public and private sectors' (Malaysia, 2001, p. 495). The financing mechanism that has garnered the most attention thus far has been that of social health insurance (Tangcharoensathien et al., 2011).

Social health insurance is seen as an appropriate replacement for general taxation-financed health care, as both public funding sources, with their pre-payment and fund pooling features, can provide financial risk protection to the public. This remains an important policy

Box 9.5 Systems observations: interactions between modes of health financing and delivery

The separate financing and health care delivery systems in Malaysia do not just shape equity of health and financial outcomes. As described within this chapter and elsewhere in this book, this structure has shaped how the health system functions as a whole. Because of the movement of patients and health workforce between the public and private health systems in Malaysia, decisions on financing policies should take impacts on both into account even though the policy may, on the surface, only target one or the other

consideration in the welfare-conscious governance of the country. To date, there have been no major reforms to the country's financing system. However, various agencies, including the MoH, have made preparations for the yet-to-happen change, in the absence of which, some of these changes have been diverted to other uses. Changing the way health care is financed in Malaysia from general taxation to social health insurance is a major endeavour that would require a major change in the mindset of health managers. As shown in Case Study 9.1, resistance to change within the public sector can impede the adoption of newer and more efficient accounting systems.

9.4 Conclusions

This short review of the trends in health financing in Malaysia outlines the rise in private funding of health care, especially private household OOPPs, since the 1980s. This trend is related to the expansion of the private provision of care. With few minor exceptions, there is a clear division between public funding for public care and private funding for private care. With this dichotomy in place, the government has found it increasingly difficult to commit sufficient public funds to meet the growing health care needs of the population. Cost sharing, which describes the partial transfer of the health financing burden from public funding to private pockets, entered the government policy lexicon in the 1980s. To enable cost sharing, the government has put in place policies to enhance the growth of the private health sector to encourage the consumption of private care by the segments of the population that can afford to pay, while at the same time, public funds have been committed to support public provision of care.

In 2018, the government announced that it would explore a health care scheme that aims to create a national health financing scheme 'to provide assistance for primary care treatment for the B40[13] households to ensure comprehensive health coverage' (Malaysia, 2018, pp. 11–20). Under this scheme, referred to as PeKa B40, which has since been rolled out in April 2019, public funding from general taxation would be used to pay for private care for the poor.[14] This new development may herald the tearing down of the wall dividing public funding from private provision, leading to more efficient use of health care resources for the benefit of all in Malaysia.

9.5 Key Messages from Malaysia's Experience

9.5.1 What Went Well and Not So Well?

- For the first 45 years, with a relatively young population, it was possible to achieve relatively good outcomes with relatively low health care expenditure.
- However, the system needs to adapt to new challenges to continue reaping such benefits (relatively affordable health care).
- With a hybrid public–private financing and delivery system:
  - The public sector, which is welfare-oriented, uses pooled tax funds to provide:
    - access and financial protection to the poor, and
    - protection from catastrophic health expenditure for households – a safety net for all sectors of the population.
  - The private sector initially complemented the public sector by catering for those who could afford it, *but* it now has an increasing share of OOPP expenditure due to:
    - low private health insurance uptake, and
    - fee-for-service provider payment mechanisms.
  - This threatens social efficiency in the provision of health care.

9.5.2 *Trends and Challenges*

- Health expenditure is likely to rise (due to an ageing population, epidemiology and technology).
  - With the current system, this is likely to result in rising OOPPs.
  - If pooled funding is used to address OOPPs in the private sector, there is likely to be increased utilisation of the private sector with higher health expenditure unless prices are controlled effectively.

References

Arrow, K. (1963). Uncertainty and the welfare economics of medical care. *American Economic Review*, LIII, 941–73.

Barraclough, S. (1999). Constraints on the retreat from a welfare-orientated approach to public health care in Malaysia. *Health Policy*, 47, 53–67.

Central Bank of Malaysia. (2005). *Insurance Annual Report 2005*. Kuala Lumpur: Central Bank of Malaysia.

Chan, C. K. (2014). The Malaysian health system in transition: the ambiguity of public and private. Municipal Services Project. Occasional Paper No. 26. Kingston.

Chee, H. L. (2007). *Medical Tourism in Malaysia: International Movement of Health Care Consumers and the Commodification of Healthcare*. ARI Working Paper Series No. 83. Singapore: Asia Research Institute, National University of Singapore.

Chee, H. L. (2008). Ownership, control, and contention: challenges for the future of health care in Malaysia. *Social Science & Medicine*, 66, 2145–56.

Chee, H. L. and Barraclough, S. (2007). The growth of corporate health care in Malaysia. In H. L. Chee and S. Barraclough, eds., *Health Care in Malaysia: The Dynamics of Provision, Financing and Access*. New York: Routledge, pp. 19–39.

Department of Statistics Malaysia. (2013). *Report of the 2012 Household Income and Basic Amenities Survey*. Putrajaya: Department of Statistics Malaysia.

Government of Malaysia. (1982). *Fees (Medical) Order 1982 [P.U. (A) 358/1982]*. Kuala Lumpur: National Printers Malaysia Bhd.

Government of Malaysia. (1998). *Private Healthcare Facilities and Services Act 1998 (Act 586)*. Kuala Lumpur: National Printers Malaysia Bhd.

Government of Malaysia. (2006). *Private Healthcare Facilities and Services (Private Hospitals and Other Private Healthcare Facilities) Regulations 2006 [P.U. (A) 138/2006]*. Kuala Lumpur: National Printers Malaysia Bhd.

Government of Malaysia. (2013). *Private Healthcare Facilities and Services (Private Hospitals and Other Private Healthcare Facilities) [P. U. (A)358/ 2013]* Kuala Lumpur: National Printers Malaysia Bhd.

Health Policy Research Associates, Institute for Health Systems Research and Institute for Health Policy. (2013). *Malaysia Health Care Demand Analysis: Inequalities in Healthcare Demand and Simulation of Trends and Impact of Potential Changes in Healthcare Spending*. Kuala Lumpur: Institute for Health Systems Research.

Institute for Health Systems Research. (2013). *Cost Analysis of Delivering Outpatient Services in a Public Hospital*. Putrajaya: Ministry of Health Malaysia.

Institute for Public Health. (2015). *National Health Morbidity Survey 2015. Volume 2: Non-communicable Diseases, Risk Factors and Other Health Problems*. Kuala Lumpur: Ministry of Health Malaysia.

Institut Tadbiran Awam Negara Malaysia. (1994). *Dasar-dasar Pembangunan Malaysia*. Kuala Lumpur: Institut Tadbiran Awam Negara Malaysia.

Malaysia. (1966). *First Malaysia Plan 1966–1970*. Kuala Lumpur: Government of Malaysia.

Malaysia. (1970). *Second Malaysia Plan 1970–1975*. Kuala Lumpur: Government of Malaysia.

Malaysia. (1976). *Third Malaysia Plan 1976–1980*. Kuala Lumpur: Government of Malaysia.

Malaysia. (1981). *Fourth Malaysia Plan 1981–1985*. Kuala Lumpur: Government of Malaysia.

Malaysia. (1986). *Fifth Malaysia Plan 1986–1990*. Kuala Lumpur: Government of Malaysia.

Malaysia. (1990). *Sixth Malaysia Plan 1990–1995*. Kuala Lumpur: Government of Malaysia.

Malaysia. (1996). *Seventh Malaysia Plan 1996–2000*. Kuala Lumpur: Government of Malaysia.

Malaysia. (2001). *Eighth Malaysia Plan 2001–2005*. Kuala Lumpur: Government of Malaysia.

Malaysia. (2018). *Mid-term Review of the Eleventh Malaysia Plan 2016–2020*. Putrajaya: Government of Malaysia.

Malaysian Productivity Corporation. (2016). *Reducing Unnecessary Regulatory Burdens on Business: Medical Professional*. Petaling Jaya: Malaysian Productivity Corporation.

Ministry of Health Malaysia. (2006). *Malaysia National Health Accounts Project: Report on the MNHA Classification System (MNHA Framework)*. Putrajaya: Ministry of Health Malaysia.

Ministry of Health Malaysia. (2007). *Health Facts 2007*. Putrajaya: Ministry of Health Malaysia.

Ministry of Health Malaysia. (2008). *Malaysia National Health Accounts Project: Health Expenditure Report 1997–2006*. Putrajaya: Ministry of Health Malaysia.

Ministry of Health Malaysia. (2010). *Health Facts 2010*. Putrajaya: Ministry of Health Malaysia.

Ministry of Health Malaysia. (2015). *Annual Report 2014*. Putrajaya: Ministry of Health Malaysia.

Ministry of Health Malaysia. (2018a). *Health Facts 2018*. Putrajaya: Ministry of Health Malaysia.

Ministry of Health Malaysia. (2018b). *Malaysia National Health Accounts: Health Expenditure Report (1997–2016)*. Putrajaya: Ministry of Health Malaysia.

Ministry of Health Malaysia. (2019). *Malaysia National Health Accounts: Health Expenditure Report 1997–2017*. Putrajaya: Ministry of Health Malaysia.

Ministry of Health Malaysia and Harvard T. H. Chan School of Public Health. (2016). *Malaysian Health Systems Research Volume 1: Contextual Analysis of the Malaysian Health System March 2016*. Putrajaya: Ministry of Health Malaysia.

Mustapha, F. I., Omar, Z. A., Mihat, O., Noh, K. M., Hassan, N., Bakar, R. A. et al. (2014). Addressing non-communicable diseases in Malaysia: an integrative process of systems and community. *BMC Public Health*, 14. Online article. https://bmcpublichealth.biomedcentral.com/articles/10.1186/1471-2458-14-S2-S4

Ng, C. W. (2005). Contributions of the Employee Provident Fund and the Social Security Organisation towards affordable health care. Masters thesis, Public Health (Health Services Management), University of Malaya.

Ng, C. W. (2019). Price setting and price regulation in health care: case study of Malaysia. In S. L. Barber, L. Lorenzoni and P. Ong, eds., *Price Setting and Price Regulation in Health Care: Lessons in Advancing Universal Health Coverage*. Geneva: World Health Organization, Organisation for Economic Co-operation and Development, pp. 165–96.

Ng, C. W., Mohd Hairi, N. N., Ng, C. J. and Adeeba, K. (2016). Universal health coverage in Malaysia: issues and challenges. In N. P. Tey, K. C. Cheong and R. Rajah, eds., *Revisiting Malaysia's Population-Development Nexus*. Kuala Lumpur: University of Malaya Press, pp. 175–96.

Phua, K. H. (1989). The development of health services in the colonies: a study of British Malaya and Singapore. *Asia-Pacific Journal of Public Health*, 3, 315–23.

Rasiah, R., Wan Abdullah, N. R. and Tumin, M. (2011). Markets and healthcare services in Malaysia: critical issues. *International Journal of Institutions and Economics*, 3, 467–86.

Roemer, M. I. (1991). *National Health Systems of the World*. New York: Oxford University Press.

Rohaizat, Y. (2004). Financing health care in Malaysia: safety net for the disadvantaged groups including pensioners, elderly people, the poor and the disabled. *NCD Malaysia*, 3, 43–6.

Rozita, H. H. (2000). Financing health care through general taxation in Malaysia. In S. Sararaks, ed., *International Conference on Evidence-Based Practice: Towards Evidence-Based Policymaking in Health Sector Development*, 4–6 September 2000. Kuala Lumpur: Ministry of Health Malaysia, pp. 243–54.

Tangcharoensathien, V., Patcharanarumol, W., Ir, P., Aljunid, S. M., Mukti, A. G., Akkhavong, K. et al. (2011). Health-financing reforms in southeast Asia: challenges in achieving universal coverage. *The Lancet*, 377, 863–73.

van Doorslaer, E., O'Donnell, O., Rannan-Eliya, R. P., Somanathan, A., Adhikari, S. R., Garg, C. C. et al. (2007). Catastrophic payments for health care in Asia. *Health Economics*, 16, 1159–84.

Varghese, C., Nongkynrih, B., Onakpoya, I., McCall, M., Barkley, S. and Collins, T. E. (2019). Better health and wellbeing for billion more people: integrating non-communicable diseases in primary care. *British Medical Journal*, 364, 1327. DOI: http://10.1136/bmj.1327

Wagstaff, A., Flores, G., Hsu, J., Smitz, M.-F., Chepynoga, K., Busmam, L. R. et al. (2018a). Progress on catastrophic health spending in 133 countries: a retrospective observational study. *Lancet Global Health*, 6, e169–79.

Wagstaff, A., Flores, G., Hsu, J., Smitz, M. F., Chepynoga, K., Busmam, L. R. et al. (2018b). Progress on impoverishing health spending in 122 countries: a retrospective observational study. *Lancet Global Health*, 6, e180–92.

Westinghouse Health Systems. (1985). *Malaysia. Health Services Financing Study. Final Report Kuala Lumpur*. Kuala Lumpur: Westinghouse Health Systems.

World Health Organization. (2010). *World Health Report 2010: Financing for Universal Coverage*. Geneva: World Health Organization.

Xu, K., Saksena, P., Jowett, M., Indikadahena, C., Kutzin, J. and Evans, D. B. (2010). *Exploring the Thresholds of Health Expenditures for Protection against Financial Risk: World Health Report 2010. Background paper No. 19*. Geneva: World Health Organization.

Yu, C. P., Whynes, D. K. and Sach, T. H. (2008). Equity in health care financing: the case of Malaysia. *International Journal for Equity in Health*, 7, 15.

System Analysis Case Study 9.1: Development of a Case-Mix System for Improving Efficiency in Ministry of Health Hospitals

Chiu-Wan Ng, Tharani Loganathan, Kuan-Joo Lim and David T. Tan

Case-mix systems are patient classification tools that describe the mix of cases being treated in a health care facility. The diagnosis-related group (DRG) system is one of the most common case-mix systems used in acute care hospitals. This system allows hospital managers to use a consistent method to classify patients by diagnostic groups, the medical procedures they undergo and the cost of treatment received. The information generated can be used to improve hospital performance in terms of efficiency and quality of care. In addition, DRGs can be used as the basis for hospital payment systems aimed at increasing technical efficiencies within individual hospitals and promoting equity in funding shares between hospitals (Reid, 2005). DRG-based hospital payment systems have been implemented in several countries in the Association of Southeast Asian Nations (ASEAN) region, including Singapore, Indonesia and Thailand (Lim, 2004; Mathauer & Wittenbecher, 2013).

Efforts to develop a case-mix system for Malaysian public hospitals started during the period in which there was policy interest to establish social health insurance as the country's main health financing mechanism (Rohaizat, 2005). Within the context of the proposed nationwide reform, a case-mix-based hospital payment system was viewed as a tool that could provide the data necessary for comparing case performance across hospitals to enhance quality, equity and efficiency of health care services (Figure 9-A). What began as a research effort in 1996 with participation from local academics and MoH officers led to the adoption of DRG systems in two public academic teaching hospitals in 2002 (Hospital Universiti Kebangsaan Malaysia) and 2013 (Hospital Universiti Sains Malaysia).[15] Within the MoH hospital network, the aptly named Malaysian DRG system was rolled out gradually from 2010, and by October 2017, the system had been implemented in 50 hospitals.[16]

To date, major health financing reforms have yet to materialise and MoH hospitals are still being funded predominantly from general taxation. The Malaysian DRG system has not been used for hospital reimbursement purposes. Instead, the focus has been on the use of the

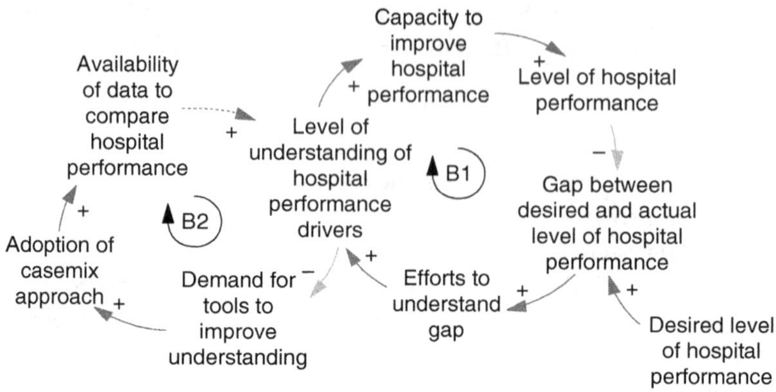

Figure 9-A Concerns over sustainable health care financing and quality of care are creating an impetus to improve hospital performance. In response, efforts are being made to understand performance shortfalls to increase capacity for improving hospital performance, creating a balancing loop that should reduce the performance gap (B1). However, limited levels of understanding of hospital performance drivers hinder this and have created a demand for further tools to improve understanding. One potential tool is adopting a case-mix approach to accounting, which would generate the necessary data to facilitate comparisons of treatment performance across hospitals, improving understanding (B2 loop). Case-mix accounting achieves this by tracking costs per medical case instead of aggregating costs into line items.

information collected to improve the efficiency and quality of care, especially with respect to services provided by cluster hospitals. Cluster hospitals are groups of specialist and non-specialist MoH hospitals providing different levels of services located within a defined geographical area. These groups are formed to maximise resource use by sharing clinical leadership, usually provided by the lead specialist hospital, and by facilitating patient care at the most appropriate level according to individual clinical needs. Patient referral protocols have been developed to ease patient transfer from a higher level of care at one hospital to a lower level of care at another, or vice versa. The MoH monitors the quality of patient care within and between hospitals using information mined from the Malaysian DRG system. The cluster hospital initiative was started in 2014, and by 2018, there were 13 clusters, involving 18 specialist and 28 non-specialist hospitals, throughout the country (The Star Online, 2018). In addition to vast amounts of clinical information, the Malaysian DRG system also captures information on the cost of care. This is a treasure trove of information that has yet to be fully utilised.

Hospital expenditure makes up the largest share of public funding for health each year. In 2016, this amounted to 62.5% of public expenditure (Ministry of Health Malaysia, 2018, p. 40). Clinical and cost data from DRG systems can be used not just to control individual hospital costs but also to compare performance across hospital networks (Reid, 2005). To fully utilise DRGs as a tool for controlling costs, hospital budgets need to be DRG-based. However, this is not currently being done for hospitals implementing the Malaysian DRG system. Public MoH hospitals are funded through global budgets. The accounting system used at MoH hospitals is known as the Modified Budgeting System (MBS), where hospital funding is partially based on historical spending and performance targets to be achieved in the year. Hospital managers do not need to examine detailed hospital costs by the number of different cases treated; they only need to ensure that they do not exceed the annual allocations for different hospital programmes.

Thus the potential for the Malaysian DRG system to be used as a tool for improving hospital efficiency has yet to be fully realised. That said, the existing system has only been developed for inpatient services at hospitals and lacks a framework for addressing other major hospital services provided in day-care, outpatient and specialist clinics and emergency departments. Until the system expands to cover these services, case-mix budgeting cannot fully replace the existing methods. However, the major hurdle to the adoption of a DRG-based hospital payment system may be the institutional mindset, which is resistant to changing from the line item hospital payment system that the MoF, the functional payor of public services funded by the federal government, has established across all government agencies (Figure 9-B). Although the existing practice does not generate useful data for evaluating hospital performance, internal familiarity, MoF dictates and the lack of mechanisms by which case-mix can contribute to decision-making create strong resistance to changing existing accounting practices. The situation is complicated by ownership issues over the Malaysian DRG system. The technical programmes within the MoH lead the work to develop and maintain the system, with input from health care professionals. However, administrators within the non-technical programmes manage the ministry's annual hospital budgets using a line

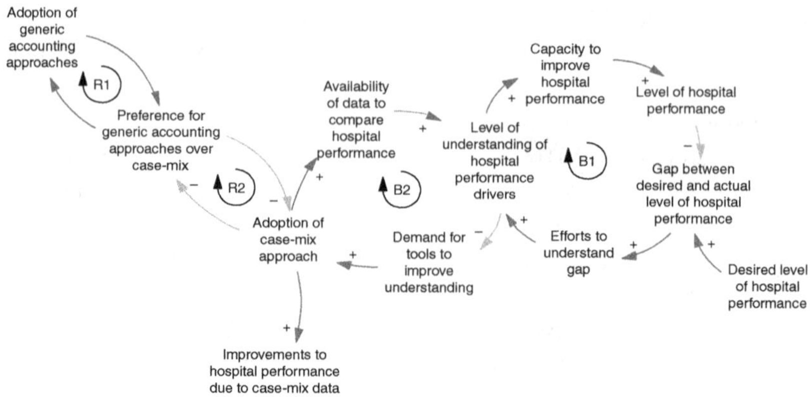

Figure 9-B Institutional pressures keep generic accounting approaches in place over the adoption of the case-mix approach. The pre-existing adoption of generic accounting approaches has created ways of thinking and acting among administrative personnel that would be disrupted by the adoption of case-mix accounting. This creates a dominant reinforcing loop (R1) that competes against another reinforcing loop (R2) that would support case-mix accounting. Even when parallel case-mix accounting systems are created and maintained, improvements in hospital performance are limited, as the data are not used at national level to allocate resources and evaluate hospital-level performance.

item format. As the two accounting systems are incompatible, the hospitals that utilise case-mix are forced to run two parallel accounting systems, increasing the administrative workload. Further work is needed to reconcile the line item accounting format to the bundling of costs based on DRGs produced by the Malaysian DRG system. Until then, the full potential of DRGs for improving hospital performance will not be realised.

Systems Lessons

Systems analysis in this case study demonstrates the dynamics through which long-established institutional procedures create pressures that mitigate against the ability of the system to introduce initiatives to modernise management. This is especially true when the costs of changing procedures directly impact the party responsible for decision-making but the benefits do not.

References

Lim, E. K. (2004). Case mix in Singapore – 5 years on. *Annals of the Academy of Medicine of Singapore*, 33, 660–1.

Mathauer, I. and Wittenbecher, F. (2013). Hospital payment systems based on diagnosis-related groups: experiences in low- and middle-income countries. *Bulletin of the World Health Organization*, 91, 746–56a.

Ministry of Health Malaysia. (2018). *Malaysia National Health Accounts: Health Expenditure Report (1997–2016)*. Putrajaya: Ministry of Health, Malaysia.

Reid, B. (2005). Case-mix and the control of hospital costs. *Malaysian Journal of Public Health*, 5(Supplement 2), 125–30.

Rohaizat, Y. (2005). Proposed national health care financing mechanism for Malaysia: the role for case-mix. *Malaysian Journal of Public Health*, 5(Supplement 2), 91–8.

The Star Online. (8 January 2018). *Subra: Cluster Hospital Concept Is Cost-Effective*. Online article. https://www.thestar.com.my/metro/metro-news/2018/01/09/subra-cluster-hospital-concept-is-costeffective-he-says-aim-to-deliver-high-quality-services-to-the

Notes

1. Examples of public funding for health are taxation and social health insurance. For both, state involvement is crucial. Political commitment from the state is required for adequate allocation of taxes to fund health care. For social health insurance, the state must maintain the governance structures (and often the agency) to implement the insurance system.
2. Private household OOPPs for health refer to payments made by individuals and households for health care that are not reimbursed by any third-party payers such as employers or health insurers. These are payments that come mainly from savings. However, if the OOPPs needed are very large and if savings are insufficient, households may be forced to source funds from the sales of assets or even from loans. The implications of such actions on the welfare of affected households, especially the poorer ones, will be elaborated on later in the chapter.
3. The HSFS was conducted by a consulting company, Westinghouse Public Applied Systems, and was funded by the Asia Development Bank.
4. The HSFS reported all expenditure estimates in Malaysian ringgit, where one Malaysian ringgit was equivalent to US$0.42 in 1983.
5. The HSFS gathered information from private hospitals and private health care practitioners. The private health expenditures were then categorised into hospitals (3.8% of total expenditures), mines and

estates (0.2%), voluntary bodies (0.1%), insurance (0.6%) and 'direct payments' (18.8%).

6. Unless otherwise indicated, all expenditure figures obtained from the MNHA quoted in this chapter (in text, tables and graphs) are in 2017 prices using GDP deflators available from https://databank.worldbank.org/source/world-development-indicators#, accessed on 1 November 2019.
7. The Malaysian Productivity Corporation (MPC) is an entity under the Ministry of International Trade and Industry created to enhance Malaysia's global competitiveness. Information on the MPC can be obtained from www.mpc.gov.my/background.
8. Comprising funding from government agencies, social security organisations, private insurers and private corporations.
9. User fees, in the context of health care, are fees for health care services charged by health care providers. User fees are applicable for both public and private providers in Malaysia. In the case of public providers, the policy to maintain low user fees was intentional to ensure that care remains affordable to facilitate access to care. Funds from general taxation make up the resultant shortfall in cost recovery. In contrast, fees in the private sector are set at cost plus profits to ensure the financial viability of the private providers.
10. In December 2019, the government announced that it would stop regulating the consultation fees of private medical doctors and dentists. As of March 2020, when a new government took over administration of the country, the relevant sections of the laws have not yet been revised.
11. GLCs are defined as companies with a primary commercial objective and in which the Malaysian government has a direct controlling stake and not just percentage ownership.
12. Information obtained from the Council's website (www.mhtc.org.my/about-us/), accessed on 5 July 2019.
13. Generally referring to households earning below RM 4,000 a month.
14. Information obtained from the PeKa B40 website (www.pekab40.com.my/manfaat.html), accessed on 5 July 2019.
15. Information obtained from https://news.usm.my/index.php/english-news/2215-usm-launches-husm-tariff-using-case-mix-system, accessed on 19 November 2019.
16. Information obtained from http://medicaldev.moh.gov.my/casemix/about-us/malaysiandrg/, accessed on 19 November 2019.

10 Health Information

NURAIDAH M. MARZUKI, FAZILAH S. ALLAUDIN, SUPATHIRATHEAVY RASIAH AND JO. M. MARTINS

10.1 Introduction

Earlier chapters discussed how health development in Malaysia has been part of a systematic approach to socio-economic development since independence. This chapter elaborates on how information has supported this process. Like most developing countries, Malaysia faced challenges in generating adequate, accurate and timely information to support health development. This chapter illustrates the strategies Malaysia adopted to address those challenges. The chapter also illustrates how components of the health system such as governance and healthcare services stimulated the incremental development of the health information system.

10.2 Nature of Information and Main Sources

The information Malaysia used in supporting health development included health information collected primarily for the health sector and information collected for more general purposes such as population censuses and vital statistics. In this context, the World Health Organization (WHO) has suggested that health information involves the production, analysis and dissemination of information on three major dimensions of health (World Health Organization, 2007):

- Determinants of health
- Performance of the health system
- Health status

The main sources of information are:

- Censuses of the population
- Household surveys

- Civil registration of vital events
- Public health surveillance
- Medical records
- Data on health services
- Data on health systems resources in the nature of human resources, health infrastructure and financing

Additionally, there are data on materials such as vaccines and drugs, as well as findings from health systems research. Over time, although in a generic sense the dimensions of the health system and the methods of collection have remained substantially those mentioned above, the instruments used have advanced with the evolution of information technology (IT) and the evolution of health concerns as the country has experienced socio-economic and epidemiological transitions.

10.3 The Era of Rapid Development (1960s–1970s): Health Information Helped Address Health Concerns

During this phase of development, data collection and compilation were mostly manual, resulting in slow, sometimes incomplete data and limited analysis. Data flowed from health facilities to district health offices, where it was compiled and transmitted to state health departments, which in turn did further compilation before transmitting it to the Ministry of Health (MoH) at national level. Each MoH programme had its own data collection system, occasionally resulting in conflicting information. Systems for checking data comprehensiveness were limited. Additionally, there was no central compilation and analysis of information from other agencies such as local authorities, the Ministry of Defence and the Ministry of Education (MoE), as well as private sector health services. Annual reports, such as those of the MoH and the Department of Statistics (DoS), were the most readily available sources of information.

10.3.1 People and Their Health

During the immediate post-independence years, the MoH used a range of information that was already available to develop health priorities and to monitor the implementation of health interventions. For example, empowered by the relevant legislation, the DoS conducted population censuses through household surveys that provided basic information on the number, location and characteristics of the people in the country. The DoS also collected data on births and deaths; police throughout the country, together with hospitals, were responsible for registering and reporting births and deaths. Thus the 1957 census showed that three-quarters of Malaysian people lived in rural areas (Department of Statistics, 1960), and the DoS provided annual population estimates between censuses using data from the existing system of registering births and deaths. Additionally, registering births and deaths provided annual information on fertility and infant mortality. For example, fertility was about three times the replacement level, and infant mortality was high and the associated life expectancy was relatively low (Fernandez et al., 1975).

The MoH also collected and compiled data from hospitals on causes of admission and of death. Deaths registered by the police were not usually medically certified. However, the limited available information indicated that most mortality was related to infectious diseases such as malaria and tuberculosis (Roemer, 1976). Surveys of education status showed that about three-quarters of the adult population (≥15 years of age) were illiterate (Ministry of Education Malaysia, 1967). Similarly, household budget surveys showed that most people in rural areas lived below the poverty line (Roslan, 2001). Concerns about toddler mortality rates (1–4 years of age), known to be associated with malnutrition, led to a joint applied nutrition programme by the MoH and other ministries (education, information and agriculture). An evaluation study performed in 1979 showed enhanced child nutrition practices and weight gains (Ministry of Health Malaysia, 1982; Chapter 4).

Legislation required the reporting of dangerous and infectious diseases to the MoH, and such information provided the basis for the disease control measures described in Chapter 6. Once the various disease control programmes had been developed, each established its own information system, including the monitoring of disease and deaths and programme activities (Chapter 6).

Household surveys, such as those for 1957–1958 and 1973–1974 (Young et al., 1980), also yielded an assessment of household use of health services and their distribution among different income groups.

10.3.2 Health Workforce

Legislation required the registration of nurses, midwives, doctors, dentists and pharmacists in both the public and private sectors (Chapter 8; Federation of Malaya, 1957), providing annual estimates of the distribution of health professionals. For example, the number of nurses and doctors per head of population was relatively low. Also, while health-related information showed that the major determinants of health were related to the poor living conditions in rural areas, information from the registration of health professionals indicated that most nurses worked in public hospitals, while more than half of the doctors were in the private sector (Department of Statistics, 1964; Chapter 3; Chapter 8). Such information guided the formulation of policies related to human resources (Chapter 8). Annual registration data enabled monitoring of the progress made to increase low numbers in relation to the growing population. In addition, an annual census of doctors and dentists in the private sector carried out since the 1970s (e.g. Department of Statistics, 1975) enabled assessment of the public–private distribution of the health workforce and guided the mobilisation of scarce health professionals, especially for rural areas.

10.3.3 Health Facilities and Services

The MoH routinely collected information on public sector health facilities and their basic activities, such as number of admissions and ambulatory patient encounters. This information indicated that most hospitals and clinics were located in urban centres and that most hospitals in the private sector were relatively small and most were concerned with maternity services. Such information guided planning for expanding the rural health service and strengthening the public hospital network (Chapters 4 and 5). For example, there were an average of two public sector beds per 1,000 people (excluding special institutions) (Federation of Malaya, 1959). This would be considered a relatively high ratio for a young population, although some beds were reserved for patients with tuberculosis and other infectious diseases. At that time, data collected from hospitals were rudimentary, such as number of admissions and patient encounters. It did not permit the evaluation of functions. About 20 years after independence, a purpose-designed survey of hospitals showed low occupancy rates in small hospitals but very high occupancy in larger hospitals in the greater urban centres (Chapter 5; Institute for Public Health, 1983), triggering several initiatives for improving services in smaller hospitals.

In rural areas in 1960, there was only one main health centre per 600,000 people, one sub-centre per 320,000 people and one midwife clinic per 120,000 people (Ismail, 1971). Data were also collected on the number of visits to health centres for maternity and child health and on public hospital outpatient services. Such information mainly supported decisions related to staff deployment and the supply of medical products, including vaccines, to public sector facilities. After 17 years of rigorous expansion of the rural health service, the MoH conducted a household survey: a high proportion of villages were 'underserved', and this finding triggered the re-vamping of the rural health service (Chapter 4) to rapidly increase access to front-line staff through revised staffing patterns and mobile clinic services. In 1968, an environmental sanitation survey in selected rural areas indicated that only 4% of the population was served with piped water, and the remainder obtained water from either unprotected wells or untreated surface water (Ministry of Health Malaysia, 1982), and this triggered a re-vamped approach to rural sanitation (Chapter 7). Annual data compiled and analysed by the MoH enabled the government to monitor progress in comparison to the targets, as discussed in Chapters 4–8.

10.3.4 Health Financing

During this phase of development, information available on health financing was mostly from the government's financing of health services and their administration in the public sector. At about the time of independence, public sector expenditure on health amounted to about 1.4% of the gross domestic product (GDP) (Federation of Malaya, 1957; 1959; 1961; Department of Statistics, 1999; Chapter 9). Since the 1970s, the annual census of private doctors, dentists, maternity homes and hospitals also reported revenues of, and expenditures incurred in, related private practice (Department of Statistics, 1975). Central government agencies used this annual census mostly to monitor growth in private health sector employment and economic activity. Household expenditure surveys such as that for 1957–1958 yielded an estimate of households' health-related expenditures (Roemer, 1976; Chapter 9).

10.3.5 Information Supported the Assessment of Progress

10.3.5.1 Effectiveness

Household surveys indicated that although still high, poverty, closely associated with health status in Malaysia, had declined by 1980 to 37% of the population (46% in rural areas) (Chapter 3). Registers of communicable diseases indicated that substantial progress had been achieved in the incidence of diseases usually associated with childhood, such as mumps and whooping cough (Chapter 6; Ministry of Health Malaysia, 1982). This progress was reflected in the fall in communicable diseases as a cause of death in mortality statistics compiled by the DoS and in infant and maternal mortality during the period (Department of Statistics Malaysia, 1991; Chapters 3–7).

10.3.5.2 Costliness

Information on the annual expenditure on health service delivery and administration was available only for the public sector. The government used such information as part of the annual review process, and the evaluations were associated with the preparation of the Malaysia Plans and their mid-term reviews. Also, although the DoS collected some limited information on the private practices of doctors, dentists, hospitals and maternity homes, this was not aggregated to obtain an overall picture nor used in planning. Estimates indicate that overall annual expenditure was under 2% of the GDP for the substantial health improvements recorded during the 1960s and 1970s.

10.3.5.3 Equity

Malaysia used a variety of instruments and data sources to produce a useful assessment of equity in the distribution and access to health services, outcomes and financial burden. Disaggregation and analysis of the various types of data for demonstrating trends in differences between urban and rural areas and between population groups provided evidence on progress towards the goal of reducing inequity illustrated in Chapters 3–7. Physical access to healthcare improved in rural areas. Household surveys indicated that spending on public healthcare benefited mostly those living in poverty and with lower household incomes (Young et al., 1980).

10.4 The Era of Transition and Consolidation (1980s–1990s)

In the two decades of the 1980s and 1990s, Malaysia experienced a major socio-economic transition, with most people becoming urban-based, a lower proportion of dependent children and a larger proportion of young adults. The success in the prevention and management of communicable diseases also led to an epidemiological transition. These changes drove the need for better health-related information. International development in IT and the growing capacity and competence in the MoH for managing healthcare services (Chapters 4, 5 and 8) facilitated and supported the further development of health-related information.

10.4.1 People and Their Health

The population censuses, vital statistics, disease registers and surveys of internal migration continued to provide information on population growth and characteristics as well as disease occurrence. The MoH used this information to assess the population covered by services such as immunisation and to assess the progress made in reducing mortality and disease incidence. Household living condition surveys indicated that poverty was substantially reduced during the 1980s and 1990s (Chapter 3). Nevertheless, continuing concerns regarding possible lags in reaching the poor and their health led to health assessments of the very poor to ascertain the appropriate support to be provided (Ministry of Health Malaysia, 1992).

However, changing disease patterns drove the need for better information. For example, non-communicable diseases were not notifiable, and the only available data were those collected from admissions and deaths in public sector hospitals. Similarly, dental health data were limited to the provision of dental service. The need for community-wide information led the MoH to initiate large-scale population-based surveys that were to become a regular feature in the future. An example is the first National Health and Morbidity Survey in 1986–1987, a comprehensive household survey on access and use of health services, health-related behaviour and morbidity from non-communicable diseases such as hypertension and diabetes mellitus (Institute for Public Health, 1988). The survey was repeated in 1996 (Institute for Public Health, 1999) and more frequently in subsequent decades. Other examples include oral health surveys of six-year-old school children (Dental Division, 1972a) and of adults (Dental Division, 1972b), which provided data on oral health and the need for services. Such surveys subsequently formed a regular surveillance system on oral health.

Another aspect of health information was health systems research (HSR). The driver motivating the development of HSR was the thrust to improve management within the MoH to respond better to the national policy of improved effectiveness and efficiency (Chapters 4 and 5). Beginning with a small unit within the Institute for Public Health, which at the time was mainly a training institution, HSR proved its value to the MoH and was soon developed into a major programme with international credentials, subsequently meriting its own institution.

10.4.2 Health Workforce

During this phase of development, new legislation commenced requiring the registration of additional categories of personnel – assistant medical officers, opticians and optometrists – thereby increasing the human resources information database. However, as the numbers of health professionals increased, the system's capacity for updating the database regularly was limited (World Health Organization, 2014). Therefore, the registers maintained by the respective boards became less valuable as a source of information for planning and policies regarding the health workforce. Mainly, the boards used the information to regulate professionals (Chapter 12). Meanwhile, information required for health workforce planning was deficient, contributing to gaps in planning. For example, the progressive transfer of health personnel education from the MoH to the MoE resulted in information lags between the two ministries, creating a barrier to forward planning by the MoH, the main user of health personnel. Furthermore, the MoE did not obtain data from all sources that produced health personnel, namely private sector institutions and foreign institutions. The time lag and incomplete data later resulted in serious problems of employment, as discussed in Chapter 8 and Case Study 8.1.

Box 10.1 illustrates the initial development of HSR in Malaysia.

Box 10.1 Health systems research provided information for managerial decision-making

Prior to 1980, the general perception was that research was the prerogative of researchers in research institutes who published results in journals, and health system managers had little interest in or access to such information. The Fourth Malaysia Development Plan (1981–1985) adopted health systems research as a tool to provide appropriate focused information to address the problems experienced in implementing programmes (Pathmanathan, 1988). Few researchers were available or had the competence to perform such research.

A small group of staff at the Public Health Institute developed short training programmes specifically designed for multi-disciplinary teams of staff who managed health districts, hospitals and state-level health programmes. This training programme eventually gained international recognition and was replicated in several countries (Varkevisser et al., 2003). The programme aimed at providing basic research competence to a wide array of health staff and at encouraging the use of information in decision-making at every level in the health system. Examples of the programme's outputs included measles immunisation coverage in a local area improving from 44% to 66%, reduced instances of non-availability of prescribed medication at dispensing counters through improved local record-keeping of medicine stocks, and reduced waiting times at hospital outpatient clinics by re-deployment of staff and re-scheduling of their work programmes.

Lessons arising from the experience included the need to discourage beginner teams from selecting complex problems. For example, an attempt to compare the cost-effectiveness of the 'flying doctor' services versus static clinics for remote population groups resulted in frustrating and inconclusive findings. Conversely, successful projects such as the measles immunisation spurred state-level managers to expand the initiative state-wide and seek means of ensuring that every client contact with the health system, whether in a hospital or a private clinic, would be an opportunity to encourage immunisation.

Thirty years after its initiation, the programme continues to flourish, largely because healthcare managers at every level of the system appreciate its usefulness and have adapted it in various forms to suit their particular needs and constraints.

10.4.3 Health Facilities and Services

Information from the sources described earlier in this chapter continued to provide data that showed, for example, that although the number of total hospital beds increased, the beds-to-population ratio in the public sector declined, partly compensated by the substantial rise in private sector beds (Chapter 5). Data showing the rising prevalence of small private hospitals was a factor in triggering the formulation of new legislation to regulate private hospitals. Similarly, data showing the increased utilisation of health centres in the public sector for ambulatory care contributed to the transfer of outpatient services from hospitals to health centres (Chapter 4). The introduction of the quality assurance programme (QAP) in several MoH programmes contributed to better data quality, such as in the accuracy in International Classification of Diseases (ICD) coding of deaths or discharges from hospitals. It also resulted in better use of information, as the QAP required evidence of remedial measures by institutions, whose performance on selected indicators suggested the need for immediate improvement (Chapter 5).

10.4.4 Health Financing

As described earlier, information on health expenditure was limited to that in the public sector, and there was uncollated and limited information on the private sector. Rising concerns about the sustainability of the healthcare financing system prompted the need for more comprehensive information on health expenditure. The first major assessment of healthcare financing was carried out in the 1980s by external consultants (Westinghouse Health Systems, 1985) in conjunction with the study of the possible introduction of social health insurance in Malaysia (Chapters 3 and 9). The study provided sufficient information for a policy decision not to implement social health insurance. A household health expenditure survey provided information on out-of-pocket expenditure on health for 1996 (University Malaya, 1999). This led to awareness of the need to gain better understanding of the financial implications of the structural changes taking place to households and the financing of public and private health services. The MoH has undertaken recent estimates on health financing of both the public and private sectors for the late 1990s and consequent years (Malaysian

National Health Accounts Unit, 2017). These studies indicate that health financing as a proportion of the GDP rose from 1983 to 2000, with an increasing proportion from the private sector (Chapter 9). This information shows that the government policy of placing greater emphasis on the provision of private health services has a price, and there is a need to provide public sector services as part of the social safety net.

10.4.5 Information Technology Development

Struggling with the increasing amount and varied quality of data generated by the different programmes, the MoH took a significant step towards improving the accuracy and comprehensiveness of health information. It established a central information documentation unit responsible for routinely collating information on all programme activities; checking comprehensiveness and accuracy; and analysing and publishing information on health status, human resources and health service delivery, using DoS information as the denominator. These publications became the source of official information, replacing the several different reports published by individual programmes (i.e. Information and Documentation System) (Ministry of Health Malaysia, 2001; Selvaraju, 2006). The rising availability of computerisation supported the implementation and effectiveness of this initiative to centralise and standardise data generated by the MoH. Progress was incremental, dictated by the cost of new technology and the capacity for training staff at district and state levels to acquire computer literacy.

Another important development was the proposal to establish a telehealth programme, beginning with a Telehealth Pilot Project (Ministry of Health Malaysia, 1997; Suleiman, 2001) to increase IT use to promote the integration of the collection of health information from a variety of sources. Three major modes were envisaged:

- Lifetime health plans
- Teleconsultation
- Information and education

The first was to provide a lifelong personal health record linked to an electronic medical record. The second was to consist of a multimedia network for face-to-face consultation of individuals and health professionals or among healthcare providers to enhance clinical support. The third was to establish knowledge databases and interactive training programmes and make health information available to the public and to health professionals. By 2000, several projects had been initiated, such as the Medical Care Information System for collecting patient information in MoH hospitals, the Communicable Disease Control Information System for collecting information for the surveillance and management of communicable diseases, and the Maternal and Child Health System for collecting and analysing information from MoH services (Ministry of Health Malaysia, 2002).

As one of the pioneering efforts in telehealth globally, the Telehealth Pilot Project encountered numerous implementation challenges and was stopped for re-evaluation in 2000. Subsequently, the scope and financing of telehealth implementation was scaled back. The Information Management Division remains responsible for telehealth as a whole; however, in practice, the various projects emerging from the original initiative have been taken over by the relevant MoH divisions, which determine the pace, scope and objectives in their implementation.

As discussed in detail in Case Study 10.1, systems interoperability was a key obstacle to implementing and scaling up the telehealth project. This continues to be a challenge, with no overall interoperability standard defined yet. At present, interoperability issues are being addressed on a case-by-case basis based on the needs of a particular application or system. The Health Informatics Centre (HIC) has been working to develop and promote the adoption of standards and terminology for the healthcare industry in Malaysia and to audit documentation to ensure data quality. While adherence to standards set by the HIC has been good, data quality remains a work in progress.

10.4.6 Assessment of Progress in Health Outcomes

10.4.6.1 Effectiveness

Household surveys indicated that poverty, a major factor associated with health, declined from about 37% in 1980 to 9% in 1999 (Chapter 3). The registration of births and deaths provided evidence that health service interventions were most successful in reducing infant, maternal and adult deaths. When death rates reached low levels, concerns about data accuracy and comprehensiveness began to surface. For example, as less than half of the deaths were medically certified,[1] there was insufficient information on the causes of death. The MoH established a system of confidential enquiry into maternal deaths to provide sufficient information to institute preventive measures for the future. These enquiries also led to the recognition that misclassifications of the cause of death were distorting the disease profiles constructed from this data source. Registers of notifiable diseases showed a continuing decline in the incidence and mortality of the major communicable diseases, while hospital statistics suggested increased morbidity and deaths from non-communicable diseases (Chapters 3 and 6). Household health surveys (Institute for Public Health, 1988; 1999) provided evidence of the growing importance of non-communicable diseases and related behaviour and led the MoH to establish Healthy Lifestyle programmes (Chapter 6).

10.4.6.2 Costliness

Concerns about healthcare financing continued during this phase of development. Studies indicated that Malaysia's total expenditure on health was relatively low compared to its GDP. Recognising the need for more comprehensive information on healthcare expenditure, the MoH developed the National Health Accounts (NHA) programme. The NHA uses standardised international NHA methodology to provide annual information on health expenditure. The data cover public and private sectors, are adjusted for inflation to support trends analysis, and include aggregated and sufficiently disaggregated information on the sources of funds and expenditure to support policy and planning decisions (Malaysian National Health Accounts Unit, 2015). The data provided by the NHA continued to support efforts to re-organise the country's healthcare financing system.

10.4.6.3 Equity

The information available for both service coverage and health outcomes of the population in different states indicated that access and use of services continued to improve in those states with the greatest need. Differences continued to prevail, but they became smaller (Chapters 3–7). Household surveys also showed that exempting the poor from fees for public health services lessened the financial burden for the poorer people (Chapter 9).

Box 10.2 System observations: closing the feedback loop to improve data collection

Health information systems are crucial to creating learning feedback loops that enable health system strengthening. However, the actors who collect the data may not recognise its value, resulting in poor data quality. In developing this volume, we came across several accounts in which data collection and entry were low priorities for both hospital administrators and ground-level medical personnel, who were motivated by tasks that had direct impacts on patient outcomes. When data were used to evaluate and improve hospital performance, however, hospital administrators responded by making proper data entry a high priority and communicated that to the hospital workforce (Figure 10.1).

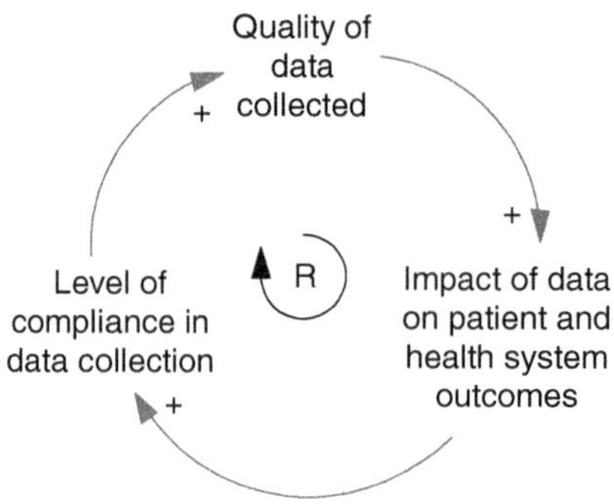

Figure 10.1 Reinforcing loop showing how compliance with data collection improves the quality of data, enabling positive impacts on health outcomes. When health system personnel are able to observe these impacts, the intrinsic motivation improves the level of compliance in data collection. Conversely, when this connection is not made, data collection can be perceived as a box-ticking exercise, compromising the quality of data collected.

10.5 Health Information in the 2000s

10.5.1 People and Their Health

The decennial census of population and inter-census estimates continued, and they showed that the majority of people lived in urban

Box 10.3 System observations: use of health information for single- and double-loop learning

Health information can be used to improve the implementation of health strategies towards existing goals (single-loop learning). Such learning seeks to improve the performance of the health system within existing paradigms and is important for health system strengthening. The role of household health surveys in the establishment of 'Healthy Lifestyle' programmes provides a different example in which health information catalysed a paradigm shift. Here, health information was used to determine whether the existing goals of the health system were appropriate and adequate (double-loop learning)

areas, with the possible exception of Kelantan (Department of Statistics, 2011). The proportion of registered deaths that were medically certified increased from 39% in 2000 to 51% in 2014. However, the quality of data on the cause of death remained inadequate for policy and planning. For example, in 2013, the cause of death classification for 30% of deaths was unacceptable. Among the medically certified deaths, 12.5% were assigned to 'symptoms, signs and ill-defined conditions'; among the non-medically certified deaths, 60% were assigned to 'old age' (Omar et al., 2019). The continued use of household health surveys provided more abundant information on health-related behaviour and the characteristics of the users of services, while some surveys focused on specific health aspects such as adult nutrition (Institute for Public Health, 2014), non-communicable diseases (Institute for Public Health, 2015), maternal and child health (Institute for Public Health, 2016), and adolescent (Institute for Public Health 2018) and elderly health (Institute for Public Health, 2019). This information supported the refinement of health strategies and programmes in specific areas discussed in Chapters 4–6.

10.5.2 Health Workforce

Institutional re-organisation transferred responsibility for the pre-service education of most categories of health personnel to the MoE (Chapter 8). As a result, within the MoH, all aspects of human resource management became the purview of the civil service arm of the MoH. As discussed in Chapter 12, the consequence was policies and management focused on MoH staff but not on the health workforce of the country. Information aspects of the health workforce that were essential for policy and planning were dispersed between various ministries and between departments within the MoH. Examples of such information include entry and output from training programmes, entry and exit from the workforce, geographic- and discipline-specific deployment and ratios between various categories. No single agency is responsible for collating, aggregating and analysing nationwide information. Spurred by a WHO effort to construct the health workforce profiles of member countries, the MoH initiated a major study (World Health Organization, 2014) to compile nationwide information that provided sufficient information for identifying key gaps in policies and impending problems in the workforce, some of which are illustrated in Chapter 8. Efforts are ongoing to institutionalise the routine collation and analysis of such information and to strengthen policy and planning by using it to make estimated projections for workforce requirements and supplies for the future.

10.5.3 Health Facilities and Services

The MoH maintains an inventory of health facilities in the public and private sector that enables it to monitor trends in the number of and the capacity of public and private facilities per head of population. This information supports policies and planning, for example, for expanding hospitals or clinic networks (Chapters 3–5). However, information on services availability in health facilities is limited to the public sector. The MoH conducted facility surveys through its Clinical Research Unit (Clinical Research Centre, 2014) in the private and public sector for a few years, creating a comprehensive picture that enabled the analysis of gaps and utilisation patterns, particularly of specialised services in hospitals and clinics. However, in subsequent years, although the private sector provided much of the information required by new legislation, the MoH did not institutionalise mechanisms for collating and analysing such information. The quality of services provided by health facilities in the public and private sectors became available from the quality accreditation programme (Malaysian Society for Quality in Health, 2018; Chapter 12).

Growing management competence in the MoH and international emphasis on evidence-based decision-making in healthcare produced a thirst for a wide variety of information. For example, several clinical specialist groups established disease registers for their specialities to provide evidence of the effectiveness of clinical interventions. In response to requests from MoH programmes, the National Institutes of Health (NIH) conducted an increasing number of studies to evaluate interventions or analyse problems. Examples include evaluation of the cluster hospital concept (Institute of Health Management, 2016), analysis of healthcare demand (Health Policy Research Associates et al., 2013) and attitudes towards tobacco smoking (Tee et al., 2012). Similarly, local universities produced increasing numbers of studies related to the Malaysian health system and its programmes. There is a growing challenge in keeping track of such outputs and providing convenient access to researchers and managers.

10.5.4 Health Financing

The NHA programme started by the MoH in 2001 (Ministry of Health Malaysia, 2018) made a major difference to the information available and the periodic assessment of health financing in both the public and the private sector and their relative evolution since 1997 (e.g. Malaysian National Health Accounts Unit, 2017). NHA data are quoted widely in reports and discussions, demonstrating that it has raised wide awareness of the issues related to health financing. Analysis of health expenditure showed substantial growth in health expenditure as a proportion of the GDP, from 3.3% in 2000 to 4.6% in 2015, and the relative importance of private health expenditure, which amounted to almost half (48.5%) of the total (Chapter 9).

10.5.5 Medical Products

In addition to information related to the regulation of pharmaceutical products in Malaysia and the use of pharmaceutical products and medical devices, the MoH has conducted surveys since 2004 on the use and prices of medicines (e.g. Ministry of Health Malaysia, 2006) and also later on medical devices (e.g. Ministry of Health Malaysia, 2009). Price negotiations for the procurement of medicines for the MoH use some of this information (Chapter 11).

10.5.6 *Information Technology Development*

The initial proposals for the greater use of IT in MoH information systems (Ministry of Health Malaysia, 1997) were further developed in proposals for a Malaysian Health Data Warehouse (MyHDW) (Ministry of Health Malaysia, 2013). This continues to be under development, with all the constraints usually encountered with IT systems development of a very comprehensive nature. By 2016, progress had been achieved in the collection, storage and processing of information on each hospital inpatient and in the production of related reports (Ministry of Health Malaysia, 2018).

The growing interest in producing and using information from research led the MoH to take the lead in establishing a national process to identify research priorities that guide public sector funding for research in Malaysian academic institutions as well as the NIH under the MoH (Suleiman & Merican, 2000). The rapid escalation in the volume of information from different systems created the need to create and maintain websites providing convenient access. It also required discussion forums to disseminate information. The NIH took the lead in collaborating with local and international academic institutions to provide regular forums for disseminating information and encouraging discussion. While this is evidence of progress, many institutions continue to struggle with issues of systematic cataloguing of research and providing access to research products. Another aspect of access to information is that while the MoH has a wealth of data from various sources, researchers outside the MoH system experience difficulty accessing it. Processes for making the data more accessible without compromising integrity are in the developmental stages.

10.5.7 *Health Outcomes*

10.5.7.1 Effectiveness

Chapters 3–7 demonstrated the substantial gains in health status but also the more recent plateau in infant and maternal mortality and in diseases such as dengue and tuberculosis, and the rapid increase in ill health due to non-communicable disease. Recent studies also indicate potential lacunae in the health information system. For example, a recent multi-dimensional study on urban child poverty shed light on childhood undernutrition, with high levels of stunting and maternal anaemia in the urban poor, which exists side by side with the problem of obesity among children nationwide (UNICEF, 2018). Another study indicated higher levels of avoidable mortality than in comparator countries of the Organisation for Economic Co-operation and Development (OECD) (Ministry of Health Malaysia & Harvard T. H. Chan School of Public Health, 2016). The output of studies such as these served to stimulate the Malaysian health system into making course corrections (Chapter 12).

10.5.7.2 Costliness

Information from the NHA programme (Malaysian National Health Accounts Unit, 2017) provided significant insights into the cost of health services in the public and private sectors, which increased by 1.3% of the GDP during the 15-year period of 2000–2015. This information also gave an indication of the service specialisation of the private sector in medical services and its costliness and increasing share of health expenditure (about 49% in 2015) (Chapters 3 and 9).

A major feature of the health system is technological change in medical care. While the MoH produces studies assessing new technologies and their cost-effectiveness, the use of such information is limited to MoH facilities and insurance agencies (Chapter 5).

10.5.7.3 Equity

Surveillance of poverty levels in Malaysia has shown a continuing fall in poverty levels in all states. However, although the gap has narrowed, there continues to be a higher proportion of people living below the poverty line in states with a higher proportion of people in rural areas (Chapter 3). Some concerns have been raised about the use of the current poverty line and the assessment of poverty in Malaysia (Ravallion, 2019), and suggestions have been made for alternative assessment methods that would better reflect current conditions. Information on estimated life expectancy at birth reflects the continuing difference among states in most cases (Department of Statistics Malaysia, 2017). As far as equity in access is concerned, household surveys show that health services in the public sector provide a degree of access to people in rural areas for most essential services, but the usual disadvantage of distance and travel remains. Although there is a financial burden associated with high out-of-pocket disbursements by those who use medical services in the private sector (Ministry of Health

Malaysia & Harvard T. H. Chan School of Public Health, 2016), services supplied almost free by the public sector tend to diminish the financial burden and improve financial access for those most in need.

10.6 Lessons from the Malaysian Experience

Health information systems developed in incremental stages, spurred by growing demands from policymakers and managers from different levels in the healthcare system. The growing managerial competence and increasing complexity of healthcare services contributed to the growing demand for information. Conversely, information provided by the health information systems contributed substantially to the development of the healthcare system and provided evidence for making corrections in the direction of development. User demand contributed to improving the quality and timeliness of information. Digitalisation contributed immensely to the development of the health information system but also presented serious challenges related to governance and human and financial capacity.

During the development process, several information sub-systems grew in response to specific needs. A continuing challenge for the health information system is to co-ordinate and harmonise information generated by different sub-systems. Another continuing challenge is to provide adequate and timely access to information without jeopardising the integrity of various healthcare services.

10.7 Key Messages from Malaysia's Experience

10.7.1 What Went Well?

- Spurred by demands from increasingly competent managers and clinicians, the health information system, in incremental steps:
  - used information from health and non-health sources (census, income),
  - steadily improved the timeliness and quality of data, and
  - embraced initiatives that added analytic and evaluative information (health systems research, quality improvement, disease registries, technology assessment, NHA).

- The utilisation of data and information spurred improvement in data quality.
- Continuing efforts are needed to harmonise and standardise data generated by different information sub-systems that evolve with growing healthcare systems.

10.7.2 What Did Not Go So Well?

- Inadequate infrastructure, managerial capacity and demands on financial and human resources hampered ambitious digitalisation plans.
- In the interests of safeguarding confidentiality, academicians and researchers outside the MoH have inadequate access to health information.
- There is inadequate collated, analysed information on private sector healthcare and on occupational and environmental health.

10.7.3 Trends and Future Challenges

Increasing digitalisation is expected to bring great benefits if the system is able to address the difficult challenges of platform interoperability and concerns about confidentiality in relation to legal requirements, personal privacy and commercial interests.

References

Clinical Research Centre. (2014). *National Medical Care Survey*. Kuala Lumpur: Ministry of Health Malaysia.

Dental Division. (1972a). *Dental Epidemiological Survey of School Children in West Malaysia 1970–71*. Kuala Lumpur: Ministry of Health Malaysia.

Dental Division. (1972b). *Dental Epidemiological Survey of Adults in Peninsular Malaysia 1970–1971*. Kuala Lumpur: Ministry of Health Malaysia.

Department of Statistics. (1960). *1957 Population Census of the Federation of Malaya*. Kuala Lumpur: Department of Statistics.

Department of Statistics. (1964). *Malaysia Official Yearbook 1964*. Kuala Lumpur: Department of Statistics.

Department of Statistics. (1975). *Census of Professional and Institutional Establishments: Private Sector 1973*. Kuala Lumpur: Department of Statistics.

Department of Statistics. (1999). *Malaysia Economic Statistics: Time Series*. Kuala Lumpur: Department of Statistics.

Department of Statistics. (2011). *Population Distribution and Basic Demographic Characteristics Report 2010*. Kuala Lumpur: Department of Statistics.

Department of Statistics Malaysia. (1991). *Vital Statistics Time Series: Peninsular Malaysia 1911–1985*. Kuala Lumpur: Department of Statistics.

Department of Statistics Malaysia. (2017). *Abridged Life Tables, Malaysia, 2015–2017*. Kuala Lumpur: Department of Statistics.

Federation of Malaya. (1957). *Report of the Medical Department for the Year 1956*.

Federation of Malaya. (1959). *Report of the Medical Department for the Year 1958*.

Federation of Malaya. (1961). *Report of the Medical Department 1960*.

Fernandez, D. Z., Hawley, A. H. and Predaza, S. (1975). *The Population of Malaysia*. Paris: Committee for International Cooperation in National Research in Demography.

Health Policy Research Associates, Institute for Health Systems Research and Institute for Health Policy. (2013). *Malaysia Health Care Demand Analysis: Inequalities in Healthcare Demand and Simulation of Trends and Impact of Potential Changes in Healthcare Spending*. Kuala Lumpur: Institute for Health Systems Research.

Institute for Public Health. (1983). *Study of Hospital Utilization in Peninsular Malaysia*. Kuala Lumpur: Ministry of Health, Malaysia.

Institute for Public Health. (1988). *National Health and Morbidity Survey 1986–1987*. Kuala Lumpur: Ministry of Health Malaysia.

Institute for Public Health. (1999). *National Health and Morbidity Survey 1996*. Kuala Lumpur: Ministry of Health Malaysia.

Institute for Public Health. (2014). *National Health and Morbidity Survey 2014*. Kuala Lumpur: Ministry of Health Malaysia.

Institute for Public Health. (2015). *National Health and Morbidity Survey 2015*. Kuala Lumpur: Ministry of Health Malaysia.

Institute for Public Health. (2016). *National Health and Morbidity Survey 2016*. Kuala Lumpur: Ministry of Health Malaysia.

Institute for Public Health. (2018). *National Health and Morbidity Survey 2017*. Kuala Lumpur: Ministry of Health Malaysia.

Institute for Public Health. (2019). *National Health and Morbidity Survey 2018*. Kuala Lumpur: Ministry of Health Malaysia.

Institute of Health Management. (2016). *Cost Effectiveness Analysis of Cluster Hospital Pilot Projects on Transforming Healthcare Services in Malaysia*. Kuala Lumpur:Ministry of Health Malaysia.

Ismail, A. M. (1971). *Rural Health*. Kuala Lumpur: Ministry of Health Malaysia.

Malaysian National Health Accounts Unit. (2015). *Malaysia National Health Accounts: Health Expenditure Report 1997–2013*. Putrajaya: Ministry of Health Malaysia.

Malaysian National Health Accounts Unit. (2017). *Malaysia National Health Accounts: Health Expenditure Report 1997–2015*. Putrajaya: Ministry of Health Malaysia.

Malaysian Society for Quality in Health. (2018). *Annual Report, 2018*. Kuala Lumpur: Malaysian Society for Quality in Health.

Ministry of Education Malaysia. (1967). *Educational Statistics of Malaysia 1938 to 1967*. Kuala Lumpur: Ministry of Education Malaysia.

Ministry of Health Malaysia. (1982). *Annual Report Ministry of Health Malaysia 1980*. Kuala Lumpur: Ministry of Health Malaysia.

Ministry of Health Malaysia. (1992). *Annual Report Ministry of Health Malaysia 1990*. Kuala Lumpur: Ministry of Health Malaysia.

Ministry of Health Malaysia. (1997). *Malaysia's Telemedicine Blueprint: Leading Healthcare into the Information Age*. Kuala Lumpur: Ministry of Health Malaysia.

Ministry of Health Malaysia. (2001). *Indicators for Monitoring and Evaluation of Strategy for Health for All*. Kuala Lumpur: Ministry of Health Malaysia.

Ministry of Health Malaysia. (2002). *Annual Report Ministry of Health Malaysia 2000*. Kuala Lumpur: Ministry of Health Malaysia.

Ministry of Health Malaysia. (2006). *Malaysian Statistics on Medicine 2004*. Putrajaya: Ministry of Health Malaysia.

Ministry of Health Malaysia. (2009). *Malaysian Statistics on Medical Devices 2007*. Putrajaya: Ministry of Health Malaysia.

Ministry of Health Malaysia. (2013). *Malaysian Health Data Warehouse (MyHDW) 2011–2013*. Putrajaya: Ministry of Health Malaysia.

Ministry of Health Malaysia. (2018). *Annual Report Ministry of Health 2016*. Putrajaya:Ministry of Health Malaysia.

Ministry of Health Malaysia and Harvard T. H. Chan School of Public Health. (2016). *Malaysian Health Systems Research Volume 1: Contextual Analysis of the Malaysian Health System March 2016*. Putrajaya: Ministry of Health Malaysia.

Omar, A., Ganapathy S. S., Annuar, M. F. M., Khoo, Y. Y., Jeenanathan, C., Awaduddin, S. M., Yn, J. L. M. and Roo, C. (2019). Cause-specific mortality estimates for Malaysia in 2013: results from a national sample verification study using medical record review and verbal autopsy. *BMC Public Health*, 19(1), 110. DOI: http://10.1186/s12889-018-6384-7

Pathmanathan, I. (1988). Health systems research as a management tool in Malaysia. In World Health Organization, *Health Systems Research in Action: Case Studies from Botswana, Columbia, Egypt, Indonesia, Malaysia, the Netherlands, Norway and the United States of America*. Geneva: World Health Organization. Online report. http://apps.who.int/iris/handle/10665/59074

Ravallion, M. (2019). *Has Malaysia Virtually Eliminated Poverty?* Economics & Poverty. Online article. www.economicsandpoverty.com/2019/01/21/has_malaysia_virtually_eliminated_poverty

Roemer, M. I. (1976). *Health Care Systems in World Perspective*. Chicago, IL: Health Administration Press.

Roslan, A. H. (2001). *Income Inequality, Poverty and Development Policy in Malaysia*. Paris: UNESCO.

Selvaraju, S. (2006). *Health Information Management: Malaysian Experience*. Health Informatics Center, Ministry of Health Malaysia, pp. S32–38.

Suleiman, A. B. (2001). The untapped potential of telehealth. *International Journal of Medical Informatics*, 61(2–3), 103–12.

Suleiman, A. B. and Merican, I. (2000). Research priorities: future challenges. *Medical Journal of Malaysia*, 55(1), 1–6.

Tee, G. H., Hairi, N. N. and Hairi, F. (2012). Attitudes towards smoking and tobacco control among pre-clinical medical students in Malaysia (short communication). *International Journal of Tuberculosis and Lung Disease*, 16(8), 1126–8. DOI: http://10.5588/ijtld.11.0254

UNICEF. (2018). *Children Without: A Study of Urban Child Poverty and Deprivation in Low-Cost Flats in Kuala Lumpur*. Putrajaya: UNICEF Malaysia.

University Malaya. (1999). *National Household Health Expenditure Survey 1996: Final Report*. Kuala Lumpur: University of Malaysia.

Varkevisser, C. M., Pathmanathan, I. and Brownlee A. (2003). *Designing and Coordinating Health System Research Projects*. Amsterdam: KIT and International Development Centre.

Westinghouse Health Systems. (1985). *Malaysia Health Services Financing Study*. Kuala Lumpur.

World Health Organization. (2007). *Strengthening Health Systems to Improve Outcomes: WHO Framework for Action*. Geneva: World Health Organization.

World Health Organization. (2014). *Human Resources for Health Country Profiles: Malaysia*. Manila: WHO Regional Office for the Western Pacific.

Young, K., Bussink, W. C. F. and Hasan, P. (1980). *Malaysia, Growth and Equity in a Multiracial Society*. Washington, DC: World Bank.

System Analysis Case Study 10.1: Challenges in Introducing Telehealth

Nuraidah M. Marzuki and David T. Tan

Introduction

Telehealth uses ICT for a wide range of applications in healthcare, ranging from information management to remote care. Many benefits from ICT use are scale-dependent. For example, integrated electronic patient records for a patient are only dependable if all the health providers for that patient are part of a common information system. When a telehealth standard is in common use, the benefit of adopting that standard is high, reinforcing interoperability (Figure 10-A, R1 loop). However, when there is no prevailing standard in practice or in policy, incompatible practices can proliferate (Figure 10-A, R2 loop).

Background to Telehealth in Malaysia

The push for telehealth in Malaysia was part of a national strategy, known as the Multimedia Super Corridor programme, for accelerating ICT use and moving toward a knowledge-based economy. Telehealth implementation was meant to follow a roadmap from 1997, beginning with a five-year Telehealth Pilot Project with four components: Teleconsultation, Mass Customised and Personalised Health Information and Education, Lifetime Health Plan, and Continuing Medical Education. A total of RM 100 million was allocated for this phase of telehealth implementation (Economic Planning Unit, 1996; 2001).

The move towards telehealth was widely welcomed in the healthcare sector, as it was perceived to address many health system needs by improving the coverage and quality of service delivery, including the equitable distribution of specialised care. It would also improve the health information system, thus providing the data necessary for better use of medical products, health financing and policymaking (Suleiman, 2001).

Telehealth was implemented in a top-down manner. This push from the top was necessary to create co-ordinated action across the MoH for the systemic changes needed to implement telehealth. Unfortunately, the knowledge and exposure regarding the need for health

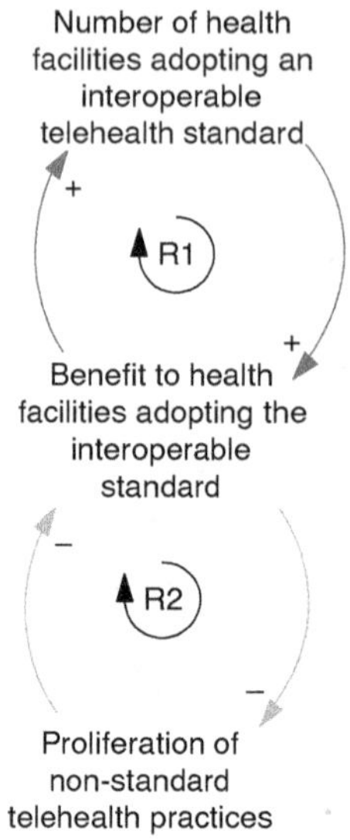

Figure 10-A For telehealth functions that cut across health facilities, the more health facilities adopt and operate within a particular interoperable telehealth standard, the greater the benefit for other facilities to adopt that standard, creating a reinforcing cycle (R1 loop). However, when there is not a critical mass of health facilities operating to a single standard, the proliferation of incompatible telehealth standards can occur, as facilities seek to set the definitive standard or simply meet locally relevant needs with locally available resources.

interoperability was rather scarce in the 1990s, resulting in the insufficient establishment of standards that would ensure interoperability. This problem was exacerbated by varying levels of IT infrastructure and perceived needs across health facilities. As a result, the push for telehealth adoption did not create a critical mass of health facilities operating to the same standards. Instead, a range of telehealth systems proliferated without strict conformance to standards, undermining interoperability (Figure 10-B).

Persistence of Incompatible Standards

Malaysia's attempt to adopt telehealth was one of the earliest efforts globally. As such, a range of unforeseen challenges emerged and the

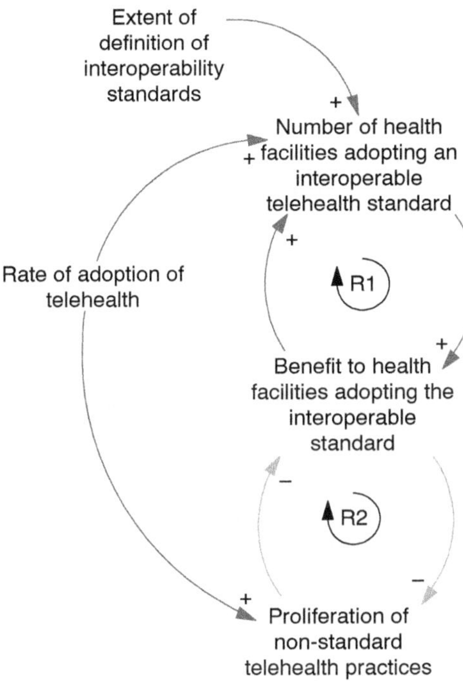

Figure 10-B The push for the adoption of telehealth could increase the number of facilities adopting an interoperable telehealth standard or lead to the proliferation of incompatible standards. Due to the lack of technical guidance and enforcement, a proliferation of incompatible standards occurred.

targets intended for the Telehealth Pilot Project were not achieved. The national push for telehealth was revised pending re-evaluation and new directions. Although unsuccessful, the pilot project provided valuable lessons and experience and increased expertise that could be built upon.

One of the key obstacles was the fragmentation of telehealth systems and practices that emerged in the Telehealth Pilot Project. With a variety of disparate systems in operation, enabling system interoperability would have incurred additional costs, as facilities that had already launched telehealth would have to be upgraded to new ICT systems and infrastructures (Figure 10-C, R3 loop). This would be both costly and disruptive. For health facilities that had not yet strongly

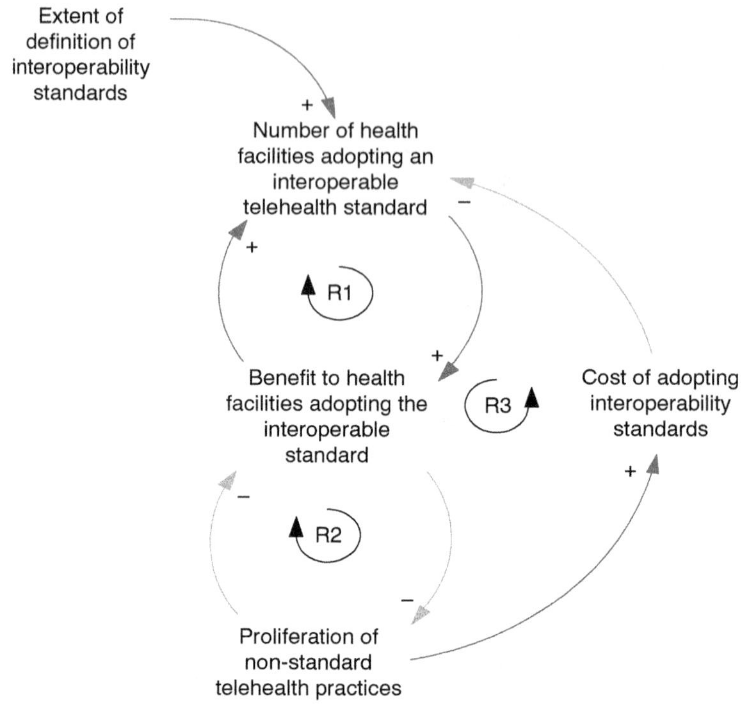

Figure 10-C The proliferation of incompatible telehealth standards actually increases the cost of adopting interoperable standards (R3 loop) due to health facility operations and structures coming to rely on incompatible telehealth software.

invested in telehealth, the limited number of facilities with which they could achieve interoperability limited benefits, while uncertainties regarding the future of interoperability standards increased risks (Figure 10-D, R4 loop).

Systems Lessons

Systems analysis of the experience of telehealth in Malaysia illustrates the importance of path dependence **and** lock-in in the development of information and communication technology (ICT) in healthcare. Malaysia's pioneer efforts with telehealth were timely and foresighted, even though they did not yield the desired results. However, the proliferation of telehealth practices has created a

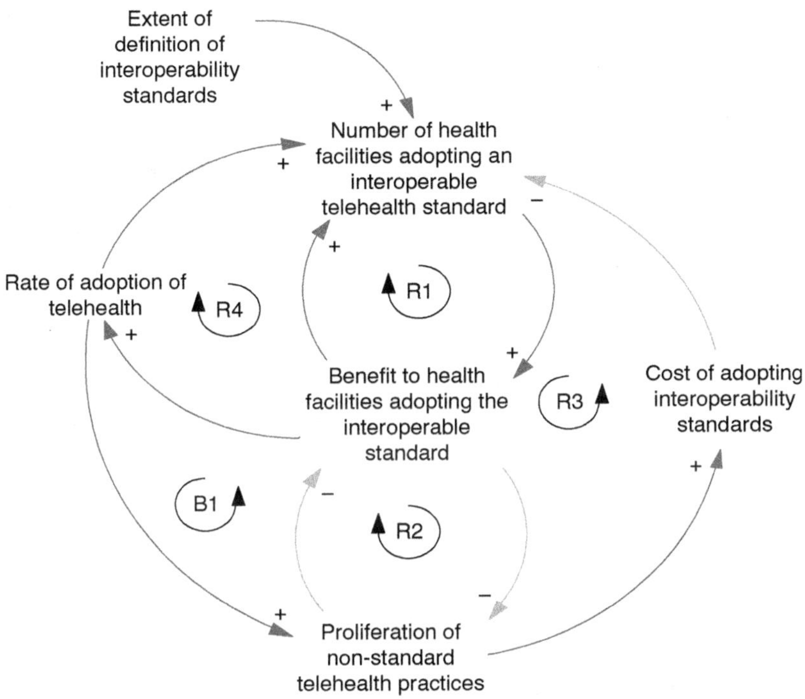

Figure 10-D The lack of a critical mass of health facilities operating on the same telehealth standard reduces benefits for certain functions, such as health information exchange. The lack of immediate benefits to health facilities discourages the adoption of telehealth, which in turn makes it difficult to achieve a critical mass (R4 loop).

persistent problem for interoperability. It is important to design health system experiments to 'fail forward' when lock-in is a real possibility. In such cases, it may be more important to avoid unacceptable outcomes than to aim for full-scale success in implementation.

References

Economic Planning Unit. (1996). *Seventh Malaysia Plan 1996–2000*. Kuala Lumpur: Economic Planning Unit.

Economic Planning Unit. (2001). *Eighth Malaysia Plan 2001–2005*. Kuala Lumpur: Economic Planning Unit.

Suleiman, A. B. (2001). The untapped potential of telehealth. *International Journal of Medical Informatics*, 61(2–3), 103–12.

Note

1. Medically certified deaths are those that are certified by physicians and include cause of death. Other deaths are certified by local police, who provide a 'lay' opinion on the cause of death reported by relatives.

11 *Medical Products*

THOMAS PARAIDATHATHU
AND CHEE HAN LIM

11.1 Introduction

Medical products and devices make up one of the 'building blocks' of the World Health Organization (WHO) framework for analysing health systems. Safe and effective medicines, vaccines and medical devices are fundamental to a functioning health system. However, health systems deal with many challenges in trying to ensure that such products are available, affordable, effective and safe and used appropriately (World Health Organization, 2018). This chapter analyses the role of medical products in the development of the Malaysian healthcare system since independence 60 years ago. Medical products as discussed in this chapter include modern (allopathic) pharmaceuticals (both prescription and non-prescription), vaccines, health supplements and traditional medicines but do not cover medical devices. Medical products confer enormous benefits to health. However, they also have potential harmful effects, either through their inherent properties or through misuse and abuse. Therefore, this chapter addresses concerns about medical products' access and affordability, alongside the aspects of safety and quality.

11.2 The Scene at Independence

Malaysia inherited a system in which traditional medicines were used side by side with modern (allopathic) medicines. Traditional medicines mostly originated from medicinal plants and had their roots in Malay, Chinese or Indian traditional medicine practices (Harun, 2006; Heggenhougen, 1980; Tate et al., 2005). The largely rural population, who had very limited access to modern medical care, depended heavily on traditional medicines. Almost all allopathic medicines were imported from Britain through the British Crown Agents and delivered

Box 11.1 Legislation to safeguard the people vis-à-vis medical products

- Registration of Pharmacists Act 1952
- Poisons Act 1952 and Regulations
- Sale of Drugs Act 1952
- Dangerous Drugs Act 1952
- Medicines (Advertisement and Sale) Act 1956

to the public either through the public sector health service or private sector doctors (general practitioners) or sold in private pharmacies (Harun, 2017). As described in earlier chapters, these health services were largely urban-based. Although there was legislation to regulate practitioners of allopathic medicine, there was no legislation or system to oversee traditional medical practitioners and traditional medical products. During the years immediately before independence, there was little awareness among the public regarding the safety and efficacy of pharmaceuticals.

Furthermore, opium addiction was a serious problem. Therefore, the government enacted several laws (Box 11.1) that sought to:

- ensure that potentially toxic medicines and substances were adequately controlled and handled only by adequately trained healthcare professionals;
- protect society from adulterated or unwholesome drugs, drugs deleterious to health and counterfeit drugs; and
- prevent the public from being misled, resulting in the wrong use of medicines, ignorance of toxicity or ineffective treatment for life-threatening illnesses.

11.3 The First Phase of Evolution (1960–1970s): Focus on Increasing Access

11.3.1 The Driving Forces

Earlier chapters discussed how the first couple of decades following independence focused on increasing access to healthcare for the rural population through integrated development of the health sector within the broader socio-economic development of the country. A key component of the healthcare system was the supply of medicines free of charge to patients who attended public sector facilities. The budget of the Ministry of Health (MoH) bore the cost of these drugs. The number of health facilities, particularly in rural areas, increased rapidly (Chapters 3 and 4), and national programmes for controlling communicable disease spread throughout the country (see Chapter 6). All of these required a reliable supply of medicines and vaccines. Therefore, the initial focus was on the import, storage, distribution and dispensing of medicines (Pharmaceutical Services Programme, 2013).

11.3.2 Import, Production and Purchase of Medicines

For the first 15 years, most medicines were imported, and the Crown Agents had a near monopoly on the import of medicines and vaccines for public sector facilities (Federation of Malaya, 1962; British Resident Selangor, 1903). Subsequently, local agents took over this role. However, parallel import of a patented product from an alternative source was allowed, and this provided a less costly alternative source for a patented product. A few multinational pharmaceutical companies also imported and distributed medicines to the few private pharmacies and wholesalers, which in turn supplied them to private medical practitioners and public sector facilities.

The public pharmaceutical sector initially focused on developing logistics to ensure supply to the rapidly expanding network of healthcare facilities. The MoH constructed a large central Government Medical Store (GMS) that became responsible for acquiring supplies from agents and in turn supplying medicines to all MoH facilities through a transport network. Hospitals and state stores submitted invoices and obtained most of their medicines from the GMS (Box 11.2).

Meanwhile, the GMS progressively developed the capacity for manufacturing medicines, and by 1970, it manufactured more than 150 types of pharmaceutical products, including tablets, large-volume intravenous fluids, injections in ampoules (including morphine and pethidine) and galenicals.[1] A few large hospitals supplemented the GMS production capacity by manufacturing intravenous solutions and galenicals for their own use. There were only a few private pharmaceuticals manufacturers, such as Glaxo and Sterling Drugs, which

Box 11.2 Management of the flow of medicines in the MoH system to ensure uninterrupted supply at the front line

- The GMS operated on a trust account of RM 40 million, with which it bought its initial stock.
- State stores and hospitals received funds through their budget and used it to purchase supplies from the GMS.
- If the GMS was unable to meet a request for supply, facilities could purchase a limited amount from the private sector.

were foreign companies with manufacturing plants in Malaysia (B. Yeap, recollections of early pharmacy services in Malaysia, personal communication to Thomas Paraidathathu, 2016). Moreover, the Institute of Medical Research (IMR) also produced a range of vaccines for a time (Ramanathan et al., 1976). The first Malaysian private pharmaceutical manufacturing company was the Malayan Pharmaceutical Factory (MPF) in Petaling Jaya. By the 1970s, more pharmaceutical manufacturers were set up in Melaka, Sungai Petani, Port Klang and Bangi (Malaysia Competition Commission, 2017). Thus, while hospitals and the GMS catered to the government hospitals, the private pharmaceutical manufacturers catered mainly to the private hospitals and clinics and sometimes, through tenders, also supplied the MoH.

11.3.3 Quality and Safety

During this phase of development, the system relied on the legislation that was already in place. However, from time to time, the MoH also issued circulars to ban the import and use of certain drugs or chemicals, such as phenformin, or re-classified them in the Poisons List to restrict their use. There was hardly any enforcement capacity; therefore, the MoH gradually built up the capacity for oversight. Box 11.3 shows the key landmarks in this process.

Prior to 1985, Malaysia did not require local registration of a medicine. Unless the MoH banned a product, importers or manufacturers could sell it in the country. Additionally, some manufacturers in the country used premises that were unsuitable for manufacturing and

Box 11.3 Landmarks in developing institutional capacity for oversight of pharmacy and pharmaceutical trade

1969: Government Medical Store (GMS).
1969: Pharmaceutical Chemistry Department in the MoH to cater for rising needs.
1970: National Pharmaceutical Control Laboratory (NPCL) for quality assurance of pharmaceuticals.
1976: Pharmacy Enforcement Unit in MoH to enforce legislation related to pharmacy and pharmaceutical trade.
1978: NPCL converted into National Pharmaceutical Control Bureau (NPC) to perform regulatory functions.
1984: Control of Drugs and Cosmetics Regulations in June 1984 'marked the dawn of the regulatory era'.
1985: Drug Control Authority under the chairmanship of the Director General of Health for 'ensuring quality, safety and efficacy of pharmaceutical products prior to marketing'. The NPCB became its secretariat.

(*Source*: Pharmaceutical Services Programme, 2013)

preparing medicines (e.g. garages and shophouses). They had a very poor understanding of the concept of good manufacturing practice (GMP). The quality of medicines and their compliance with pharmacopoeia standards were unknown (S. Selvaraja, experiences as a pharmacy regulator, personal communication to Thomas Paraidathathu, 2018). Furthermore, there were no inspections of manufacturing premises or licensing requirements from the MoH.

Also, as local registration of a product was not required, the Malaysian government suspected that some multinational pharmaceutical companies were 'dumping' their products in the country. For example, an analgesic product containing the drug dipyrone, which the US FDA[2] had banned, was available in Malaysia.

However, this period also witnessed the first baby steps for improving the quality of medicines dispensed at public sector facilities. Patients used to bring their own containers to public sector hospitals and clinics for oral solutions, lotions and eye drops.[3] Such containers had inconsistent levels of cleanliness and sizes. Therefore, in 1979, the

MoH decided to supply medicines in plastic containers, enabling standardised and hygienic packing. Moreover, pre-packing speeded up the dispensing process. In the private sector, quality and safety depended on the professional integrity of the medical profession and private pharmacies and their adherence to professional and legal requirements to prevent wrongful use of prescription medication. In 1983, inspired by the WHO initiative on essential drug lists, the MoH produced its own Blue Book, listing essential drugs for MoH facilities. This formed the basis for standardising the availability of medicines at each level of the facility in MoH services.

11.3.4 Prescription, Dispensing and Human Resources

During the first decade after independence, the very few Malaysian pharmacists trained mainly in Singapore, Australia or the United Kingdom. At the start of the second decade after independence, a local university established a training programme, but its output was limited. As population growth was relatively rapid, the ratio of pharmacists to population remained low. Dispensing medication was the responsibility of medical assistants[4] in the public sector facilities and of clinic assistants under the supervision of doctors in private sector clinics. To address the need for personnel, particularly for hospital pharmacies, an allied health profession of dispensers was introduced, with one year's training in a newly established Dispensers Training School followed by on-the-job training at hospitals. Gradually, the dispensers replaced medical assistants for dispensing in the public sector facilities (Pharmacy and Supplies Programme, 1996; G. Singh, experiences as a dispenser in the early years, personal communication to Thomas Paraidathathu, 2012).

11.3.5 Outcomes

Although there is no direct information on the availability of and access to medicines and vaccines, the success in reducing vaccine-preventable deaths (see Chapter 4) and malaria (see Chapter 6) and the rapid increase in the utilisation of hospitals and clinics (see Chapters 4 and 5) suggest adequate access to and use of basic medicines and vaccines. As discussed in Chapters 4–6, the availability and use of effective vaccines and medicines contributed to the changing profile of hospital bed utilisation.

11.4 The Second Phase (the 1980s–1990s): Strengthening Quality and Safety

11.4.1 The Driving Forces

During the next two decades after independence, Malaysia experienced stable politics, continued economic growth with a few downturns, rapid urbanisation due to rural-to-urban migration, and a demographic and epidemiologic transition (see Chapter 3). The incidence of communicable diseases declined while the prevalence of non-communicable diseases increased. (see Chapters 3–6). Meanwhile, the advent of newer pharmaceutical products and international research on effectiveness and risks changed medical care practices. One example is the management of eclampsia of pregnancy, where the use of magnesium sulfate enabled nurses in more remote settings to initiate effective management without awaiting the availability of a doctor.

11.4.1.1 International Influences

The generic drug industry flourished around the world, and in response, multinationals differentiated their products as better quality and supported by strong research. At the same time, the issue of the increasing presence of counterfeit medicines on the market, especially in some African countries, highlighted the need for stricter regulatory controls and enforcement. While countries like the US, the United Kingdom, Germany and Australia had well-established drug regulatory agencies such as the United States FDA and the Australian Therapeutic Goods Administration (TGA), many developing countries did not have good regulatory control of medicines. The WHO encouraged developing countries to establish regulatory systems for medicines and to participate in international collaboration for sharing of information of reports of adverse drug reactions (ADR) and adulterated and counterfeit medicines (Raranawijitrasin & Wondermagegnehu, 2002).

11.4.2 Import, Production and Sale: Quality and Safety

11.4.2.1 Strengthened Governance Capacity: Legislation and Regulatory Requirements

Concerns about drug efficacy, quality and safety made it imperative that the government take steps to strengthen the governance process.

This included the enactment of legislation (Box 11.1), building laboratory capacity and human resource competence for pharmaceutical analysis and for educating manufacturers, monitoring compliance with regulations, and enforcement of regulations. The Control of Drugs and Cosmetics Regulations (CDCR) 1984 under the Sale of Drugs Act established the Drug Control Authority (DCA) and gave it powers. The legislation included two key requirements for pharmaceutical products prior to sale in Malaysia: first, the registration of pharmaceutical products, and second, the licensing of manufacturers and wholesalers and of products for clinical trials. The CDCR established criteria for manufacturing facility location and required suitably qualified personnel, such as pharmacists, chemists and biochemists, and proper quality control procedures, both during manufacturing and for the finished product.

Empowered by the CDCR 1984, the DCA assumed responsibility for ensuring that medicines were safe, efficacious and of suitable quality prior to sale in Malaysia. The DCA implemented three initiatives: first, prior to registration and subsequent sale, the DCA instituted a process that included laboratory testing according to established pharmacopoeias or other standards and the evaluation of a dossier submitted by the manufacturer or applicant (on behalf of the manufacturer). Applications for the registration of imported medicines had to be accompanied by a Certificate of Free Sale (CFS), Certificate of Pharmaceutical Product (CPP) or an equivalent certificate from a competent authority in the country of manufacture, thus addressing the issue of the dumping of products not sold in the country of manufacture. All registered medicines were identified by a unique registration number intended to increase consumer confidence in the product's safety and efficacy.

11.4.2.2 Stronger Monitoring Complemented by Education and Information

Second, the DCA inspected manufacturers to ensure compliance with GMP guidelines published by the WHO (World Health Organization, 2011). In conjunction, the MoH provided education regarding GMP and established a system to provide reliable information to the public and healthcare providers regarding medical products.

Third, the DCA initiated a pharmacovigilance system through a voluntary reporting system, whereby healthcare professionals and members of the public were encouraged to report suspected ADR. Initially, the number of reports to the Malaysian Adverse Drug Reactions Advisory Committee (MADRAC) was not encouraging. Subsequently, the National Pharmaceutical Control Bureau introduced a number of initiatives such as letters of appreciation to encourage people, especially healthcare personnel, to submit suspected reports. Malaysia has been a participant of the WHO Adverse Drug Reactions Monitoring Programme since 1987 (Raranawijitrasin & Wondermagegnehu, 2002), and reports of ADR are sent to the WHO Collaborating Centre for International Drug Monitoring in Uppsala, Sweden.

The introduction and enforcement of the CDCR is believed to have increased consumer confidence regarding the quality, safety and efficacy of medicines in Malaysia. A number of popular combination products that were available prior to 1985 are no longer available in Malaysia. They included products for which there was no good scientific rationale, such as Franol, which was a combination product for asthma that contained theophylline, ephedrine and phenobarbitone.[5] Products without proven efficacy or with unacceptable risk-to-benefit considerations and low-quality, cheap generics became almost nonexistent in the Malaysian market.

11.4.2.3 Production Evolved

As a result of the regulatory changes, in the 1990s, government hospitals ceased the bulk manufacturing of pharmaceutical products such as intravenous fluids, eye drops, mixtures and creams because of difficulty complying with GMP requirements.

Simultaneously, the national policy to privatise selected public sector activities reached the pharmaceutical sector. During the 1980s, the GMS had continued to manufacture and supply medicines to government institutions, and the annual turnover increased from RM 100 million in 1984 to RM 150 million by 1994 (R. Kumarasingham, recollections of early pharmacy services in Malaysia, personal communication to Thomas Paraidathathu, 2016). In 1994, the GMS was privatised, and soon, under the name of Pharmaniaga,[6] it acquired other manufacturing plants, became a large, fully integrated healthcare company and took on manufacturing, logistics, distribution, sales, marketing and supply of equipment. Pharmaniaga received an initial 15-year concession (up to 2009) for supplying to MoH institutions 700 items on the Approved Products Purchase List (APPL) and set up an integrated information system for the MoH institutions to order and monitor their supply of medicines. Initially, there were complaints of steep increases in prices, but these issues appear to have diminished over time. Stock-outs or low stocks of medicines at public healthcare facilities occurred occasionally, and patients received smaller amounts of medicines and had to refill more frequently.

Meanwhile, the local pharmaceutical industry grew. By the 1990s, the number of pharmaceutical manufacturers increased to more than 50, and all complied with international GMP standards. They also began exporting to other countries. In 1990, Malaysia exported a total of about RM 70 million worth of medicinal and pharmaceutical products (SITC[7] 541) and medicaments (including veterinary medicaments) (SITC 542), which was equivalent to about 5% of the total chemicals export of the year (Pharmaceutical Society, 2002).

11.4.3 Purchase: Effectiveness and Cost of Medicines

In the face of the growing choice of available medicines, the need for rational choice became a priority, particularly considering the national policy of providing highly subsidised medicines almost free to clients in public sector healthcare facilities. In 1983, the MoH established a system for selecting medicine eligible for purchase by the MoH through the Ministry of Health Medicines Formulary (MOHMF). An MoH review panel comprising representatives from different clinical disciplines uses criteria such as efficacy, safety, budget impact and ethical considerations for selecting items from the MOHMF. Other methods of selection include multi-criteria decision analysis (MCDA). The review panel aims to ensure that selection is transparent, predictable and considers the value to the community of patients and the cost of a drug. For example, if the cost of a drug were so prohibitive that only a fraction of the patients who need it would receive it, it would not qualify for inclusion in the MOHMF. The MOHMF is updated regularly, and in 2017, there were 1,676 drugs in the list. Other healthcare providers in the public sector, such as teaching hospitals and the Ministry of Defence, have their own formularies.

11.4.4 Prescription, Dispensing and Human Resources

For the first 25 years of independence, there was only one pharmacy school in Malaysia, with a small output that was augmented by a trickle of pharmacists trained abroad. In 1990, there were only 1,239 registered pharmacists (less than 1 per 10,000 population) (Ministry of Health Malaysia, 2000). The rapid expansion of the pharmaceutical sector was accompanied by the concentration of the available pharmacists in the private sector. In 1996, 77% of pharmacists were in the private sector (Ministry of Health Malaysia, 2000).

Due to the limited availability of pharmacists, their traditional role in the MoH during the 1950s to 1980s was in functions related to improving medicine quality and safety, enforcing standards for medicines and in the procurement and supply of medicines for patients. In the public sector, dispensing remained in the hands of assistant pharmacists, and in the private sector, largely in the hands of clinic assistants and their supervisory doctors. With the gradually increasing availability of human resources, pharmacists in MoH hospitals began to advise on individualised drug therapy, re-constituting cytotoxic drugs, providing medication counselling and developed drug information systems in hospitals (Ministry of Health Malaysia, 2002). By 1995, three other pharmacy programmes had begun in Malaysia, thereby boosting production output. The first graduates from these programmes began coming into the market by the end of the 1990s.

11.5 The Third Phase (2000s–2010s): Growing Concerns about Affordability

11.5.1 Import, Production and Sale: A Stable Regimen for Quality and Safety

The National Pharmaceutical Regulatory Agency (NPRA)[8] succeeded in constructing a good regulatory framework for pharmaceuticals, and it gained international recognition. Co-ordination with customs authorities was strengthened to monitor consignments of products such as saccharin, beta-agonists, precursor and essential chemicals liable to be misused, for example in illegal traffic in narcotic drugs (Ministry of Health Malaysia, 2002). Additionally, the scope of monitoring extended to traditional products adulterated with poisons such as fenfluramine. In 2002, the NPRA became a member of the Pharmaceutical Inspection Co-operation Scheme (PIC/S), an international non-binding, informal co-operative arrangement between regulatory authorities in the field of GMP of medicinal products. This indicated that the NPRA adhered to internationally acceptable GMP inspection standards. Indirectly, it also validated the standard of the local pharmaceutical industry. The NPRA is also an active member of the ASEAN (Association of Southeast Asian Nations) harmonisation initiatives for the regulatory control of pharmaceuticals. In addition, Malaysia was accepted in 2013 into the Organisation of Economic Co-operation and Development (OECD) system for Mutual Acceptance of Data (MAD) in the assessment of pharmaceuticals. New medicines that are needed in Malaysia but that require more evidence of safety and efficacy are sometimes given conditional registration. Recently, a vaccine for dengue was given a two-year conditional registration. Phase IV clinical trials are still to be conducted, and therefore it has not been given full marketing authorisation.

After an initial slow start during the 1990s, the reporting of ADR to MADRAC improved, accompanied by appropriate regulatory action by the DCA. Figure 11.1 shows the rise in the number of received reports from 2010 (7,079) to 2017 (15,936). The MoH conducted post-marketing surveillance of pharmaceutical products to ensure that registered products continued to adhere to stipulated standards of quality and conditions of use.

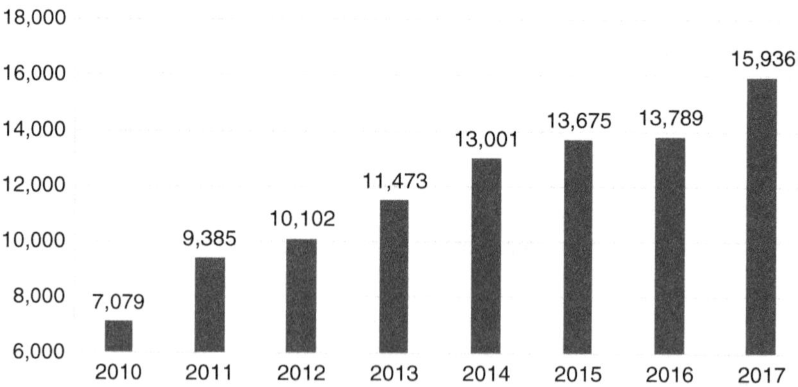

Figure 11.1 Number of received reports of ADR.
Sources: Ministry of Health Malaysia, 2010; 2011; 2012a; 2013; 2014; 2015; 2016; 2017.

Counterfeit medicines amounted to less than 5% of all marketed pharmaceutical products. A significant contributor to this healthy scenario is the access to good-quality medicines at low or no cost at government healthcare facilities. The instances where counterfeit medicines were discovered involved medicines with high consumer demand such as Panadol and Viagra. Since 2005, a product-specific hologram was introduced as an additional safety feature for all registered drugs.

Advertisements. In the 2000s, Malaysia adopted a national policy of promoting medical tourism. In response, the Medicine Advertisements Board (MAB) relaxed the conditions related to advertisements for medicines, provided improved guidelines and simplified the approval process for over-the-counter (OTC) drugs, functional medicines and health supplements. However, the industry is pushing for similar relaxations to the direct-to-consumer advertisement of controlled medicines, but this is not allowed. Simultaneously, the MoH strengthened efforts to provide reliable information to the public and healthcare providers through its centralised information centre and programmes such as Know your Medicines and Ask your Pharmacist. Meanwhile, the private sector took the initiative to produce the MIMS (Monthly Index of Medical Specialities), a reference publication for Malaysian medical professionals providing updated prescribing information and drug availability.

11.5.2 Supply Logistics, Prescription, Dispensing: Availability of Medicines

In the MoH system, logistics improved with the increased use of information technology that facilitated modernised inventory management and enhanced storage facilities. The volume of prescriptions in MoH facilities increased rapidly. For example, there was a 12% increase in one year during 2016–2017 (Ministry of Health Malaysia, 2017). Approximately 30–40% of these are repeat prescriptions for patients with chronic illnesses such as diabetes and hypertension who had prescriptions for 3–6 months' duration. However, dispensing was monthly to monitor for any side/adverse effects, efficiently manage resources, avoid extensive stock holding and reduce medicine wastage resulting from improper storage or expiration. This dispensing practice caused inconvenience and travel costs to patients, congestion, and longer waiting times at pharmacy counters, particularly in the larger healthcare facilities. Several initiatives addressed this challenge. A digitalised Integrated Drug Dispensing System (*Sistem Pendispensan Ubat Bersepadu*, or SPUB) has enabled patients to obtain their prescriptions at any MoH facility and to do so through an appointment system that enables prior preparation of the prescription, thus drastically reducing waiting times. Other innovations have increased access and convenience. The drive-through pharmacy is a concept borrowed from the fast food and banking industries. The Medicines by Post scheme sends medicines to the patient's home by a courier company for a fee of RM 6. The Locker4u scheme provides designated lockers, secured by a key/personal identification number (PIN), where patients can collect their medicines from hospitals at their own convenience. Patients who use these initiatives are very satisfied (98% satisfaction) with these services (Pharmaceutical Services Programme, MoH Malaysia, 2016).

As the availability of pharmacists increased, the scope of their service expanded, with more MoH hospitals providing pharmaceutical services such as parenteral nutrition, therapeutic drug monitoring, cytotoxic drug reconstitution, clinical and ward pharmacy services, and medication therapy adherence clinics and promoting quality use of medicine.

11.5.2.1 Human Resources

The production of pharmacists increased rapidly. The number of local pharmacy degree programmes increased rapidly to 22. The expansion was largely due to 17 institutions in the private sector; Chapter 8 discusses this phenomenon. The number of pharmacists per 10,000 population increased 4-fold within 14 years, namely from 1.02 in 2000 to 4.08 in 2014. The profile of the pharmacy workforce evolved rapidly (Figure 11.2). Two factors contributed to a rapid increase in the public sector workforce of pharmacists. First, in 2004, the government introduced a two-year period of compulsory service in the public sector for new graduates. Initially, there were concerns that this move would result in a shortage in the private sector, but it was expected that such a shortage would be short-lived, as market forces would continue to entice them to the private sector.

However, a second factor intervened. The government amended its civil service conditions, resulting in pharmacists receiving higher starting salaries and better opportunities for career advancement. As a

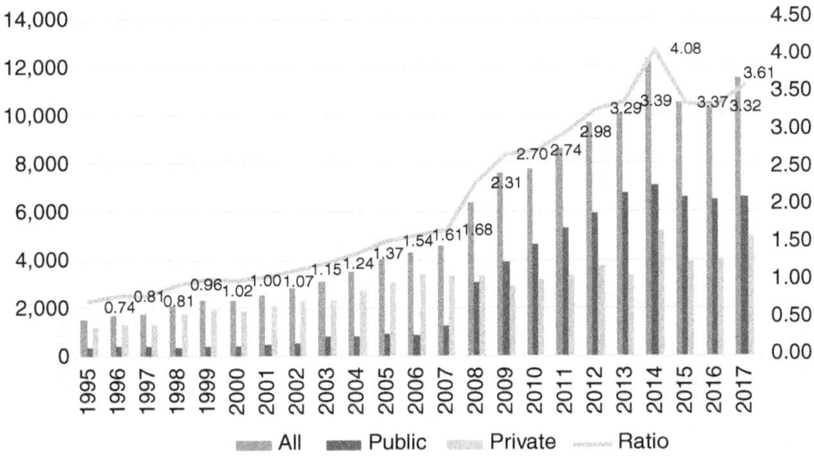

Figure 11.2 Number and ratio of pharmacists per 10,000 population.
Sources: Ministry of Health Malaysia, 1995; 1996; 1997; 1998; 1999; 2001; 2019a; Suleiman & Jegathesan, n.d.

result, more pharmacists chose to remain in the public sector, and by 2009, the numbers in the public sector overtook those in the private sector. The sudden influx of new graduates was similar to that experienced in the medical workforce, discussed in Chapter 8. Its consequences for the public sector were similar – several administrative adjustments were required to accommodate the new graduates, who required supervision and monitoring during the first years of their service prior to full registration.

Meanwhile, the number of pharmacy assistants continued to increase, rising from 1.01 per 10,000 population in 2002 to 1.87 in 2017 (Figure 11.3). Until 2012, they were almost exclusively in the public sector, when the numbers in the private sector began to increase gradually. By 2005, the number of pharmacists had overtaken that of assistant pharmacists.

The increased availability of pharmacists produced other changes. First, their role in the public sector started to expand gradually to cover direct services to clients. Second, the simultaneous influx of large numbers of new graduates, both medical and pharmacy, stretched the capacity of the public sector to absorb them to the limit. This resulted in a push from the public sector into the private sector, in contrast to earlier years, when the attraction of the private sector had caused

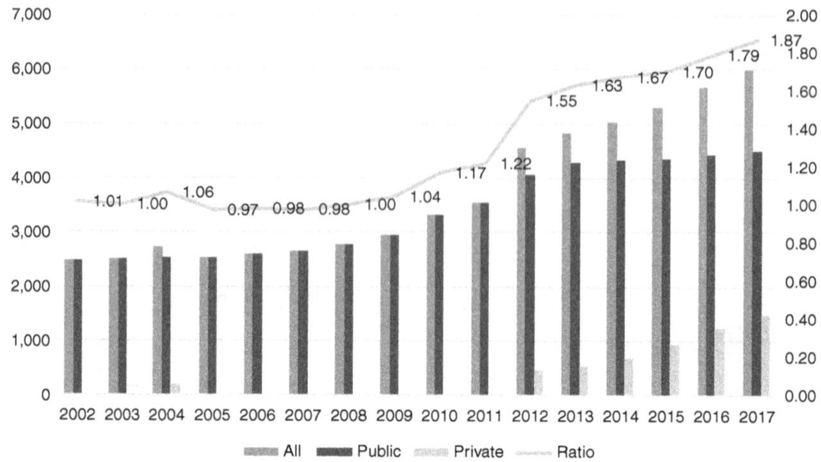

Figure 11.3 Number and ratio of assistant pharmacists per 10,000 population. *Source:* Ministry of Health Malaysia, 2019a.

movement of both professions out of the public sector. Some indication of the stress to the private sector is the ongoing controversy between the pharmacy and medical professions regarding the separation of prescription and dispensing functions in the private sector. Pharmacists argue that this would be in the best interests of patients in order for them to obtain cost-effective medicines and avoid unnecessary use of medications and their side effects. The counter-arguments from the medical profession include: (a) that the relative scarcity of private pharmacies in rural areas would limit access to medicines, and (b) that 'patients go to pharmacies to buy medicines after consulting the doctor once, and then continue buying prescription-only medicines without a prescription'. General practitioners (GPs) further acknowledge that in the face of multiple challenges, including a fee schedule that has been unrevised for 27 years, 'most GPs survive because the sale of medicines provides a small margin of profit' (Philip, 2019). The economic factors underlying the controversy are evident.

11.5.3 Affordability and Pharmaceutical Pricing

In October 2006, in line with WHO recommendations, the Malaysian National Medicine Policy (NMP) (*Dasar Ubat Nasional*, or DUNas)

Box 11.4 System observations: path dependency in dispensing practices

The parallel development of dispensing practices in public healthcare facilities and private clinics provides a good illustration of path dependency in health systems. The lack of pharmacists in the early years of the health system (Section 11.3.4) resulted in other health personnel taking on the dispensing role. In public healthcare facilities, economies of scale kept the dispensing role specialised such that assistant pharmacists (Section 11.4.4) and then pharmacists were later able to take on this role. In private clinics, however, prescription and dispensing remained closely linked in the absence of policy or systemic incentives to separate these functions.

came into force. It covers all aspects of medicines. The objectives of DUNas are to improve the health outcomes of Malaysians through:

1. Promoting equitable access to essential medicines.
2. Ensuring the availability of safe, effective and affordable medicines of good quality.
3. Promoting quality use of medicines by healthcare providers and consumers.

Affordability is an important component of DUNas to ensure that cost does not become a barrier to equitable healthcare. To this end, DUNas encourages 'Efforts … to promote healthy competition towards fair, transparent and sustainable cost-effective treatments' (Ministry of Health Malaysia, 2012b).

Rising healthcare cost is a global phenomenon, albeit the rates grow differently by country. Malaysia's medical inflation rates for 2019 were forecast to be about 5.7 times higher than that of general inflation (Aon, 2019). While there are many contributing factors to rising healthcare costs, higher drug costs is a significant factor. Drug affordability is a legitimate concern for patients with critical illnesses and those who require chronic therapy. Estimated conservatively, the health expenditure on medical goods in 2017 was 8%, or RM 4.55 billion of the national total health expenditure (Ministry of Health Malaysia, 2019b).

11.5.3.1 Public Sector

The public sector provides care for the majority of patients in Malaysia. For example, 70% of hospital admissions in 2017 were in public healthcare facilities. Hence the government budget allocation for medicine procurement is a concern. The total amount allocated for medicine procurement has remained about the same since 2014 (Figure 11.4) despite a yearly increase in public demand for drug treatment (Figure 11.5). In 2017, the allocation for medicine procurement for the MoH was about 10% (RM 2.38 billion) of the MoH operating expenditure.

The government has to balance budget limitations against factors such as drug accessibility, value and (opportunity) cost and the rising demand for effective, quality and safe drug treatment. It does this through careful planning and procurement strategies.

The MoH practices an open tender policy for pharmaceutical products listed in the APPL (about 700 items determined by the MoH, which includes many items from the National Essential Medicines List) and the MoH National Tender (about 300 items). The MoH uses international best practices, for example, the WHO procurement process and workflows, for medicine procurement. Thus the process uses the indicative drug price based on market survey when calling for the open tender. This ensures that government central purchase obtains products that offer the best value. The MoH Procurement Board selects successful bidders after bids pass through the Technical and Financial Evaluation Committees.

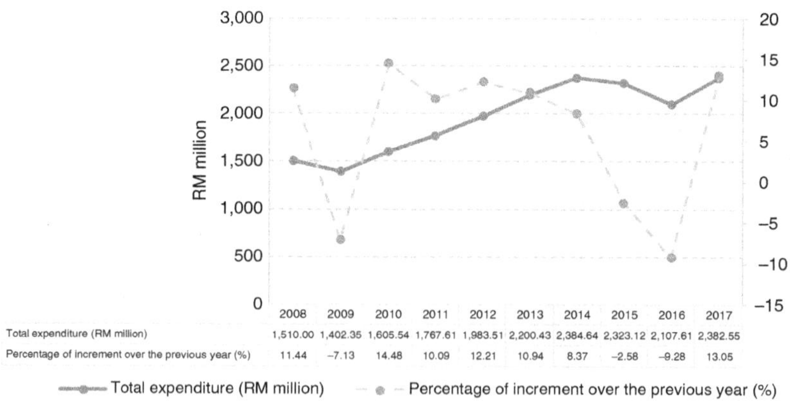

Figure 11.4 MoH medicine expenditure, 2008–2017.
Source: Pharmaceutical Services Programme, Ministry of Health Malaysia, 2018.

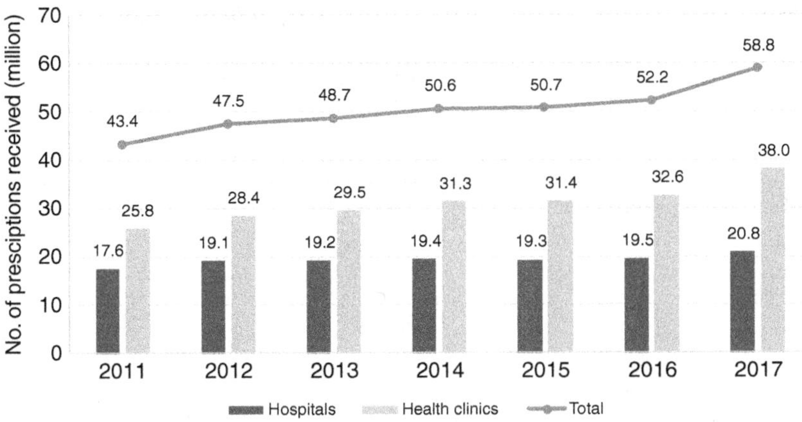

Figure 11.5 Number of outpatient prescriptions received, 2011–2017.
Source: Pharmaceutical Services Programme, Ministry of Health Malaysia, 2018.

Only local purchase orders with a total value of less than RM 500,000 are exempted from open tender. Generally, generic medicines provide value while meeting budget constraints and public demand. Thus, in 2017, about 60% of drugs procured and dispensed were generics (30% local manufacture, 70% imported) (Pharmaceutical Services Programme, Ministry of Health Malaysia, 2018).

In its attempts to meet the increased demand for drug treatment, the government seems to have tried to keep the price it pays for drugs low to curb the escalation of its expenditure on drugs. However, the price the government pays for generic and originator drugs, although substantially lower than that charged in the private sector, has remained above the international reference median price (Table 11.1). Figure 11.5 shows that, from 2014 to 2017, despite no significant increase in its budget for medicine procurement, the MoH managed to provide an additional 8.2 million outpatient prescriptions. MoH management of budget disbursement in three-month staggered periods instead of annual disbursement to individual hospitals and clinics promotes prudent planning and more accurate forecast of local demand, thereby reducing the risk of drug shortage or wastage.

As described, in the development since the 1990s, Pharmaniaga, although a private entity and concessionaire, continues to play an important role in logistics and storage service provision to MoH health

Table 11.1 *Price comparisons in private sector outlets*

	Generics		Originators	
	Public sector	Private sector	Public sector	Private sector
Median price compared to international reference price (MPR)	1.2	2.5	1.6	8.6
	Generics		**Originators**	
	Hospitals	Pharmacies	Hospitals	Pharmacies
Mark-up in the private sector	51%	22.4%	167%	94.7%

Source: Pharmaceutical Services Programme, Ministry of Health Malaysia, 2018.

facilities nationwide, even if the request is made by a health facility in a remote area. In addition, it handles the open tender processes on behalf of the MoH and the Ministry of Finance (MoF). As a local generic drugs manufacturer, Pharmaniaga may also bid for government procurement tenders. As Pharmaniaga is responsible for handling the bids, the issue of potential disadvantage to other competitors has been considered. The response to this was that bids by Pharmaniaga must be submitted at least two weeks before the close of tenders.

11.5.3.2 Private Sector

Much expenditure on medical products is in the private sector. For example, the private sector spent RM 3.55 billion or 77% of the total medical goods expenditure[9] in 2016, and there is a wide range of prices for medical products. Higher procurement prices due to the lack of economies of scale and high mark-ups by service providers or retailers[10] are the principal contributory factors (Table 11.1).

As about 30% of inpatients use private hospitals, they pay a substantial price for medicines. The mark-up in private hospital prices is not transparent for patients or their insurance companies, and this asymmetry of information is a contributor to market failure. For certain life-saving and critical-care prescription drugs that are under patent protection, the implications are significant. For example, gefitinib, a cancer drug, cost 190.8 days of minimum wage per treatment in 2017, while trastuzumab, a breast cancer drug, cost 551.7 days of minimum wage, that is, more than 1 year of minimum wage (Pharmaceutical Services Programme, Ministry of Health Malaysia, 2018).

The cost of patented drugs is a barrier to access, and their generic competitors allow more patients to afford the drugs, hence resulting in increased sales. The government policy of favouring the lowest-priced generic drug procurement and the timely entry of generic drugs into the market has had strong effects in terms of drug affordability for patients. An illustrative example in Malaysia is that the originator pharmaceutical company was willing to reduce the price of trastuzumab[11] by about 52% to win an MoH tender to compete with a local drug company that had also bid to supply a biosimilar drug.

In view of the potentially significant positive impact of generics on public expenditure on medicine, the Malaysian intellectual property patent law (Patents Act 1983) could be reviewed to expedite generic entry, for example, by reviewing patent criteria and the mechanism for allowing pre-grant and post-grant opposition. Furthermore, the introduction of Bolar-type[12] provisions in regulatory approval would protect local manufacturers from harassment through threats of legal action. Under the government drug procurement public tender process, local generic drug manufacturers have a slight preference of a 10–15% higher price margin advantage, given the experience that local producers can provide a more consistent and reliable drug supply.

Although Malaysia has price controls on a number of food items and petrol, it has thus far not imposed price controls on medicines. By and large, medicines are affordable, especially since the government provides high-quality, safe and effective medicines primarily through the MoH at almost no cost to the patient. The presence of a competitive local generic manufacturing industry certainly helps in ensuring that generic products remain affordable. However, the challenge is in ensuring that imported patented innovator products are also affordable. If costs become prohibitive for the government to purchase patented drugs for a large number of patients, it can use provisions under the agreement on Trade-Related Aspects of Intellectual Property Rights (TRIPS) to make such medicines available at a cheaper price for public non-commercial use.

In addition, Malaysia is one of the initial six co-sponsoring nations that proposed a resolution at the 72nd World Health Assembly that makes the pricing of medical products more transparent, and the resolution was adopted on 28 May 2019. The price information inputs are the cornerstone for the effectiveness of any future policies on drug price monitoring and control.

11.5.4 The Case of Right to Government Use

In early 2000, the costs of certain antiretroviral (ARV) drugs that were imported and under patent were so high that it limited the country's ability to provide treatment to HIV-infected patients requiring it. In spite of negotiations, a suitable price could not be agreed upon. In 2003, the Malaysian government exerted rarely used powers to acquire the drugs through a tender to a local pharmaceutical company to import and supply selected generic versions of patented ARV drugs manufactured by the Indian company Cipla. This was possible by using a provision provided under the TRIPS agreement in line with the Doha Declaration 2001 by members of the World Trade Organization (WTO) and the provision of the Rights of Government under the Patents Act 1983 (World Trade Organization, 2001). The medication would be solely for the use of patients managed by MoH facilities. On completion of the 'government use' licensing period, the MoH was able to negotiate with the multinational companies for better prices and therefore no longer required the use of special provisions. A similar situation arose in 2017 for medication for hepatitis C; it is the subject of Case Study 12.1 in Chapter 12.

The government has indicated that it will not hesitate to use this mechanism in public health emergency situations where a large number of patients do not have access to affordable treatment. Malaysia is the first and one of only a few countries in the world to exercise this right to provide access to a patented product as part of its public health policy.

11.5.5 Pharmaceutical Trade Sector in Malaysia

Pharmaceutical products are important trade items for Malaysia. In 2017, their trade amounted to RM 6.45 billion or 0.36% of total trade. However, the import of pharmaceutical products was about six times larger than the total export value (Figure 11.6). This

Box 11.5 System observations: the need for an equitable international system for drug development and public good

The cost of medication and other medical technologies is a limiting factor in the advancement of universal healthcare (UHC). Managing the tension between public goods and private incentives to develop and produce medical technologies is an ongoing challenge that transcends national boundaries, as seen here and in Case Study 12.1. There are significant provisions for low-income countries under international law, though obstacles to exercising these provisions exist and need to be addressed. An equitable framework for cost sharing between middle-income and high-income countries remains absent. The current approach of case-by-case resolution is opaque, drains resources and favours countries with political or economic leverage, thus creating inequitable outcomes.

created a trade deficit of RM 4.6 billion in 2017. In accordance with the government's Economic Transformation Programme, a project was implemented in 2010 to provide incentives for the local production of generics for export. Subsequently, the sales of generic and patented medicines as a percentage of prescription drugs have seen a reversal, with generics overtaking patented drugs in 2013 (Malaysia Competition Commission, 2017). The local pharmaceutical manufacturing sector started to pick up and saw a 63.7% increase in the export value from 2013 to 2017 compared to a 31.3% increase in the value of imported medicines (Figure 11.6). The increased export value for formulated products (medical products) for human use (Table 11.2) contributed 81.0% of all pharmaceutical products export in 2017.

11.6 Key Messages from Malaysia's Experience

11.6.1 What Went Well?

- The medical products subsystem at various times in development:

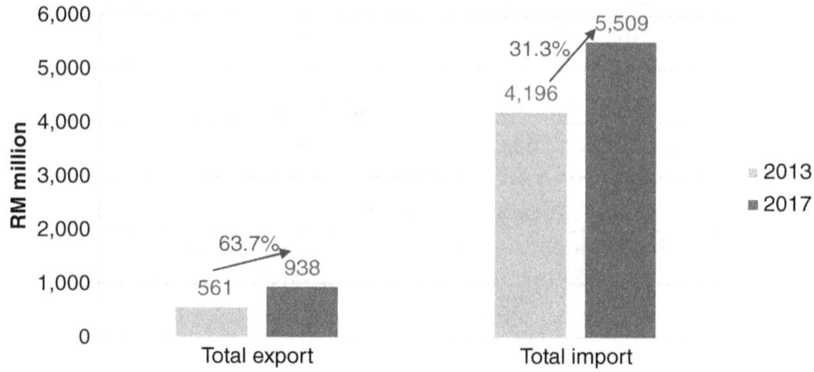

Figure 11.6 Export and import value of pharmaceutical products to Malaysia, 2013 and 2017.
Source: Department of Statistics Malaysia, 2018.

 - ○ Responded to demands from rapidly expanding health services and more variety and higher costs of internationally available medical products.
 - ○ Dealt with hazards and stresses such as trade in illicit and dangerous drugs, dumping of poor-quality and unsafe medicines, misuse and abuse of allopathic and traditional medical products, internationally rising costs of pharmaceuticals, and patent protection.
 - ○ Served its purpose despite facing constraints, including human resources and budgetary limitations.
- The health system successfully improved access, safety and quality of imported and local products, quality of local production, and cost control through incremental steps in strengthening:
  - ○ logistics and production capacity,
  - ○ legislation, monitoring and enforcement,
  - ○ education and negotiation.

11.6.2 What Did Not Go So Well?

- The inability to moderate the high and increasing cost of medical products in the private sector.

Table 11.2 *Export and import value of pharmaceutical products to Malaysia by product category, 2013–2017*

		2013				2017			
		Export		Import		Export		Import	
No.	Product category	Value (RM million)	%	Value (RM million)	%	Value (RM million)	%	Value (RM million)	%
1	A1: Formulated products for human use	453.1	80.8	3,548.9	84.6	760.5	81.0	4,551.1	82.6
2	A2: Formulated products for veterinary use	6.1	1.1	80.0	1.9	25.2	2.7	66.1	1.2
3	A3: Vaccine products for human and veterinary use	6.1	1.1	231.8	5.5	11.6	1.2	415.3	7.5
4	B1: Vitamins	34.0	6.1	162.7	3.9	86.3	9.2	262.7	4.8
5	B2: Antibiotics	61.8	11.0	173.0	4.1	54.9	5.8	214.1	3.9
Total		561.0	100.0	4,196.4	100.0	938.5	100.0	5,509.2	100.0

Source: Department of Statistics Malaysia, 2018.

11.6.3 Trends and Challenges

- Challenges in traditional medicines and health supplements:
  - Adulteration
  - Inappropriate marketing and use
  - Sale as health foods to bypass regulation of medical products
- Pressure from the pharmaceutical industry for patent protection.
- Implementation of price control tools.
- National formulary for all public sector health facilities to enable them to have economies of scale in purchasing and to have uniform policies such as antibiotic policies.

References

Aon. (2019). *2019 Global Medical Trend Rates Report – Global Benefits*. Online report. www.willistowerswatson.com/en-MY/Insights/2018/11/2019-global-medical-trends-survey-report

British Resident Selangor. (1903). *Indent for Supplies: Letter to the Crown Agents*. Selangor.

Department of Statistics Malaysia. (2018). *Nilai Import Produk Farmaseutikal ke Malaysia*. Online report. www.data.gov.my/data/en_US/dataset/nilai-import-produk-farmaseutikal-ke-malaysia

Federation of Malaya. (1962). *Parliamentary Debates (House of Representatives): Official Report*. Government of Malaysia.

Harun, H. (2017). *Medicine and Imperialism II: A History of Colonial Health Policy in British Malaya*. Harudin Harun.

Harun, M. P. (2006). *Kitab tib: Ilmu perubatan Melayu*. Perpustakaan Negara Malaysia: Kementerian Kebudayaan, Kesenian, dan Warisan Malaysia.

Heggenhougen, H. K. (1980). Bomohs, doctors and sinsehs: medical pluralism in Malaysia. *Social Science and Medicine*, 4, 235–44.

Malaysia Competition Commission (MyCC). (2017). *Market Review on Priority Sector under Competition Act 2010: Pharmaceutical Sector*. Kuala Lumpur: Malaysia Competition Commission.

Malaysian Medical Association. (1980). *The Future of the Health Services in Malaysia*. Kuala Lumpur: Malaysian Medical Association.

Ministry of Health Malaysia (MoH). (1995). *Health Facts*. Kuala Lumpur: Ministry of Health Malaysia.

Ministry of Health Malaysia (MoH). (1996). *Health Facts*. Kuala Lumpur: Ministry of Health Malaysia.

Ministry of Health Malaysia (MoH). (1997). *Health Facts*. Kuala Lumpur: Ministry of Health Malaysia.
Ministry of Health Malaysia (MoH). (1998). *Health Facts*. Kuala Lumpur: Ministry of Health Malaysia.
Ministry of Health Malaysia (MoH). (1999). *Health Facts*. Kuala Lumpur: Ministry of Health Malaysia.
Ministry of Health Malaysia (MoH). (2000). *Health Facts*. Kuala Lumpur: Ministry of Health Malaysia.
Ministry of Health Malaysia (MoH). (2001). *Health Facts*. Kuala Lumpur: Ministry of Health Malaysia.
Ministry of Health Malaysia (MoH). (2002). *Annual Report*. Kuala Lumpur: Ministry of Health Malaysia.
Ministry of Health Malaysia (MoH). (2010). *Annual Report*. Putrajaya: Ministry of Health Malaysia.
Ministry of Health Malaysia (MoH). (2011). *Annual Report*. Putrajaya: Ministry of Health Malaysia.
Ministry of Health Malaysia (MoH). (2012a). *Annual Report*. Putrajaya: Ministry of Health Malaysia.
Ministry of Health Malaysia (MoH). (2012b). *Malaysian National Medicines Policy [Dasar Ubat Nasional (DUNas)]*, 2nd ed. Putrajaya: Ministry of Health Malaysia.
Ministry of Health Malaysia (MoH). (2013). *Annual Report*. Putrajaya: Ministry of Health Malaysia.
Ministry of Health Malaysia (MoH). (2014). *Annual Report*. Putrajaya: Ministry of Health Malaysia.
Ministry of Health Malaysia (MoH). (2015). *Annual Report*. Putrajaya: Ministry of Health Malaysia.
Ministry of Health Malaysia (MoH). (2016). *Annual Report*. Putrajaya: Ministry of Health Malaysia.
Ministry of Health Malaysia (MoH). (2017). *Annual Report*. Putrajaya: Ministry of Health Malaysia.
Ministry of Health Malaysia (MoH). (2019a). *Human Resource for Health (HRH) Database*. Putrajaya: Ministry of Health Malaysia.
Ministry of Health Malaysia (MoH). (2019b). *Malaysia National Health Accounts: Health Expenditure Report 1997–2017*. Putrajaya: Ministry of Health Malaysia.
Mortimer, A. (1946). Medical or mobile dispensary vital. Letter to the State Medical and Health Officer, Selangor.
National Pharmaceutical Regulatory Agency. (2019). *Drug Registration Guidance Document (DRGD)*, 2nd ed. Putrajaya: Ministry of Health Malaysia.

Paraidathathu, T. (2019). *Pharmacy in Malaysia: History and Development*. Kuala Lumpur: University of Malaya Press.

Pharmaceutical Services Programme. (2013). *Our History*. Online webpage. www.pharmacy.gov.my/v2/en/content/our-history.html

Pharmaceutical Services Programme. (2016). *Kajian Kepuasan Pelanggan Perkhidmatan Tambah Nilai Farmasi* (Pharmacy Value Added Services Patient Satisfaction Survey). Ministry of Health Malaysia, unpublished.

Pharmaceutical Services Programme. (2018). *Medicine Price Monitoring in Malaysia: Survey Report 2017*. Putrajaya: Ministry of Health Malaysia.

Pharmaceutical Society. (2002). *Malaysia Export, Import and Deficit in Pharmaceuticals: Annual Report*. Online report. www.mps.org.my/news master.cfm?&menuid=38&action=view&retrieveid=2436

Pharmacy and Supplies Programme. (1996). *Annual Report*. Kuala Lumpur: Ministry of Health Malaysia.

Philip, A. (2019). The GP: an endangered species. Online letter. www.thes tar.com.my/opinion/letters/2019/05/06/the-gp–an-endangered-species

Ramanathan, K., Cheah, W. C. and Dondero, T. J. (1976). *75 Years of Medical Research in Malaysia: 1901–1976*. Kuala Lumpur: Institute for Medical Research.

Raranawijitrasin, S. and Wondermagegnehu, E. (2002). *Effective Drug Regulation: A Multicountry Study*. Geneva: World Health Organization.

Suleiman, A. B. and Jegathesan, M. (eds.). (n.d.). *Health in Malaysia: Achievements and Challenges*. Kuala Lumpur: Ministry of Health Malaysia.

Tate, M., Khoo, K. K. and Selvamany, G. (2005). *History of Medicine in Malaysia: The Foundation Years*. Kuala Lumpur: Academy of Medicine of Malaysia.

Tong, S., Tilakavati, K. and Pt, T. (2009). 1st CORFIS Report 2007–2008: Community-based cardiovascular risk factor intervention strategies (CORFIS): inaugural CORFIS phase I report 2009.

World Health Organization (WHO). (2018). *Annual Report: Promoting Access to Safe, Effective, Quality and Affordable Essential Medical Products for All*. Geneva: World Health Organization, Medicines, Vaccines and Pharmaceuticals.

World Health Organization (WHO). (2011). *WHO Expert Committee on Specifications for Pharmaceutical Preparations*. Geneva: World Health Organization.

World Trade Organization (WTO). (2001). *Declaration on the TRIPS Agreement and Public Health*. World Trade Organization. Online publication. www.wto.org/english/thewto_e/minist_e/min01_e/mindecl_ trips_e.htm

System Analysis Case Study 11.1: Challenges in Regulating Traditional Medical Products

Thomas Paraidathathu, Chee Han Lim and David T. Tan

Malaysia is one of the few countries that has taken on the task of registering traditional medicines. Normally, medicines are registered based on safety, efficacy and quality through evidence obtained from clinical trials and laboratory testing. Unlike typical drug registration, traditional medicines in Malaysia are not subjected to clinical trials for efficacy, with claims based instead on their use by indigenous populations over hundreds or thousands of years (Box 11-A). Thus they are evaluated for registration by the DCA based primarily on safety and quality. Although most traditional medicines contain ingredients from natural sources, mainly plants and mineral sources, it is dangerous to take their safety for granted (National Pharmaceutical Regulatory Agency, 2019). Safety is evaluated through the absence of ingredients from plants with a known history of toxicity and adverse effects and through only allowing plant and mineral ingredients with a historical record of safety. The DCA recognises the lack of stringent clinical evidence and thus only allows indications/claims for traditional medicines to be of a general nature.

When the registration of traditional medicines was first started, the concern was about the presence of heavy metals such as lead and mercury and the high microbial content in such products. Lead and mercury were sometimes deliberately added to the products in accordance with traditional practice or inadvertently through plant uptake in contaminated soils. High microbial content resulted from poor manufacturing practices. Adverse consequences from the improper manufacture and use of traditional medicines prompted the registration process, in which a heavy metals or microbial burden above permissible levels will not be registered by the DCA (National Pharmaceutical Regulatory Agency, 2019).

This in turn increased manufacturer awareness and compliance with quality and safety requirements (Figure 11-A, B1 loop).

The NPRA has taken a mentoring approach with manufacturers of traditional medicines and conducted training for them on aspects of GMP and about working together so that they could collectively

Box 11-A Usage and popularity of traditional and complementary medicines (T&CM)

The belief in T&CM and its associated modalities such as acupuncture, massage, *tui na*, etc. is much more prevalent in the Chinese community than in the Malay and Indian communities. Chinese patients often switch between T&CM and modern medicine according to the system they believe is more effective. An estimated 69% of the Malaysian population uses T&CM in their whole life and 55% use T&CM each year (Maihebureti et al., 2011).

Unfortunately, there are also cases of patients with incurable diseases like cancer who stop the chemotherapy prescribed by their oncologist and switch to T&CM and succumb to the disease. The MoH has attempted to integrate some traditional medicine practices in its healthcare facilities since 2007. More than 18 MoH hospitals now provide T&CM services such as acupuncture and Malay massage for chronic pain and post-stroke management, herbal therapy as adjunct therapy for patients with cancer, Malay postnatal treatment, and shirodhara (ayurvedic treatment) for insomnia, stress and mild anxiety (Traditional and Complementary Medicine Division, 2017). Some private hospitals that provide T&CM services are the Tung Shin Hospital in Kuala Lumpur and Lam Wah Ee Hospital in Penang.

The Traditional and Complementary Medicines Act 2016 provides for the regulation of T&CM services, registration of practitioners and accreditation of T&CM qualifications by a Traditional and Complementary Medicine Council. There are approximately 16,050 T&CM practitioners in Malaysia (Traditional and Complementary Medicine Division, 2017). As the majority of T&CM service providers are in the private sector, most patients will probably pay out of pocket (OOP) for the treatment. OOP health expenditure[13] for T&CM in 2017 was RM 541 million, tripling since 2006 (RM 180 million) (Malaysian National Health Accounts Unit, 2019).

manufacture in good facilities. Most traditional medicine manufacturers are not as well-resourced, financially and physically, as the large pharmaceutical manufacturers, and so the NPRA has encouraged them

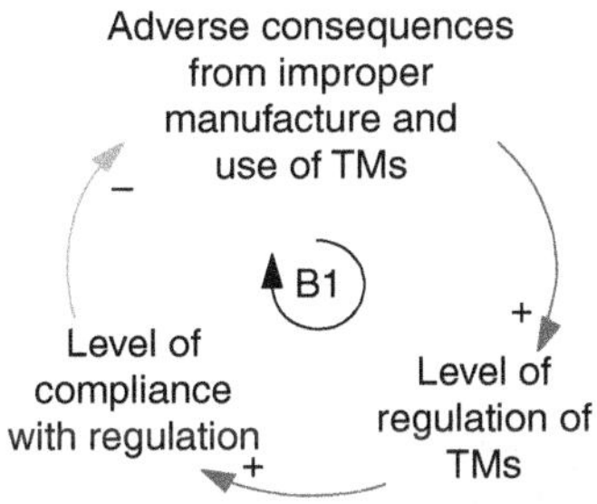

Figure 11-A The registration and regulation of traditional medicines was in response to the adverse health impacts from the improper manufacture and use of traditional medicines and has successfully reduced poor practice and consequent outcomes.

to improve gradually and where possible to work co-operatively. Some of these efforts have borne fruit and a number of traditional medicine manufacturers have facilities that comply with GMP standards equivalent to those of modern medicine manufacturers.

These regulations have not harmed the traditional medicine market, with the market value projected to reach RM 32 billion in 2020 (The Malaysian Reserve, 2019). However, the regulations have created costs, whether directly through upgrading facilities and manufacturing processes or indirectly by stopping practices that make traditional medicines more marketable. An example of the latter is the adulteration of traditional medicines with chemical substances to generate physiological responses that convince the user of its effectiveness. Common adulterants are chemicals that include corticosteroids, substances for treating erectile dysfunction, appetite suppressants and antihistamines. Many of these chemical compounds are controlled substances with the potential to cause serious adverse effects. Such practices have created an escalating arms race between regulators and unscrupulous traditional medicine manufacturers and suppliers (Figure 11-B, R1 and B2 loops), with regulation and enforcement continually having to play catch-up with new strategies and practices aimed at bypassing existing regulations. Some of these experiences are detailed below.

In response to the adulteration problem, traditional medicine products in the marketplace are randomly sampled, along with follow-up investigations of reports of ADR or reports from consumers

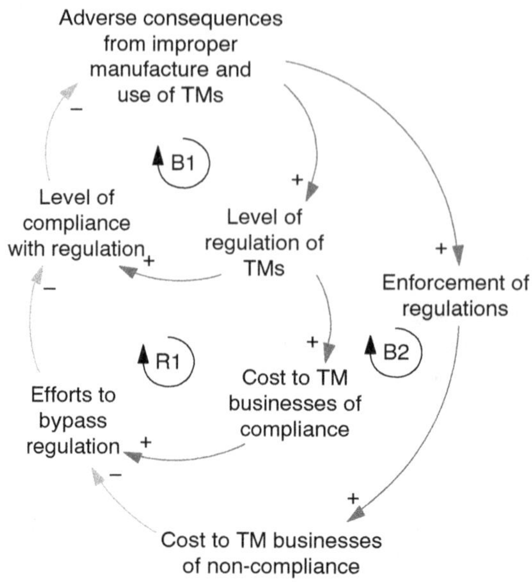

Figure 11-B Regulation of traditional medicines creates costs to traditional medicine businesses, which some actors attempt to bypass (R1), creating a race to close regulation loopholes (B1) and enforce existing regulations (B2).

(Paraidathathu, 2019). Proof of adulteration will lead to the revocation of product registration and withdrawal from the market, along with prosecution of the suspected parties. In 2018, there were 629 confiscations of suspected adulterated products, which resulted in 167 prosecutions in court (Ministry of Health Malaysia, 2019).

One challenge to prosecution is the difficulty in pinpointing the stage at which product adulteration takes place: manufacturing, re-packing or even distribution. It was common practice in traditional medicine manufacturing to use premixes of the herbal ingredients (which contained the different herbal ingredients, fillers, diluents, etc.) and manufacture the finished product in Malaysia. When an adulterated product was detected, the manufacturer would often claim ignorance and blame the supplier of the premix for adding the adulterant. To address the problem, the DCA no longer allows the use of premixes in the manufacture of traditional medicines (National Pharmaceutical Regulatory Agency, 2019).

With the crackdown on the adulteration of registered traditional medicines, sales of unregistered traditional medicines have risen. In recent years, the availability of unregistered traditional medicines sold as sex stimulants and adulterated with corticosteroids and drugs for erectile dysfunction has increased. These products do not enter the Malaysian market through legitimate entry points but are smuggled into the country instead. This has led to increased enforcement action against smuggling. Approximately 88 hotspots have been identified throughout the country, and through constant surveillance and raids, about 60% are now considered 'clean' (Paraidathathu, 2019). In response to the increased surveillance and frequent raids, the suppliers of these unregistered products have now resorted to marketing them not as traditional medicines but as 'health foods', which are less strictly regulated. Greater collaboration between the Food Division of the MoH and the NPRA is needed to address this.

In addition to addressing the problem of improper manufacture of traditional medicines from the supply side, it is also possible and important to address demand-side issues, changing consumer preferences to provide competitive advantages for compliance (Figure 11-C). For example, the MoH has taken various initiatives to warn the public about consuming unregistered products, such as the Kenali Ubat Anda (Know Your Medicines) campaign that educates the public about medicines. Other measures, such as better publicity of certification or voluntary quality standards that go above and beyond minimum requirements, may provide further incentives for good manufacturing and marketing practice.

Systems Lessons

Systems analysis illustrates the dynamics of interactions when health system regulations to protect the public are in conflict with commercial interests. These regulatory measures can and do produce positive public health outcomes but, with sufficient financial incentive, actors will find ways to bypass and evade regulations. The health system needs to recognise and monitor these responses and deal with the challenges innovatively. Where feasible, finding ways to align commercial interests with public protection may alleviate the regulatory arms race.

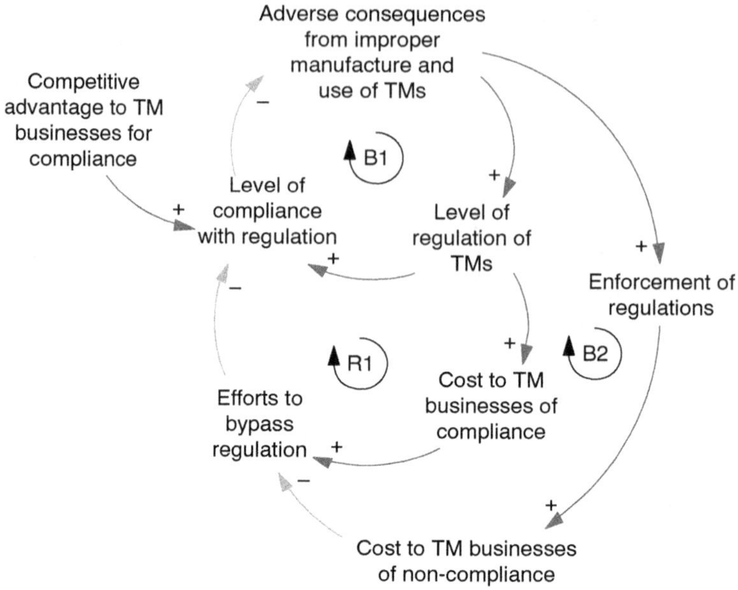

Figure 11-C Creating benefits for traditional medicine businesses for compliance with regulation can reward good actors and reduce attempts to bypass regulation.

References

Maihebureti, A., Sharifa Ezat, W. P. and Syed, M. A. (2011). Role of traditional and complementary medicine in universal coverage. *Malaysian Journal of Public Health Medicine*, 11, 1–5.

Malaysian National Health Accounts Unit. (2019). *Malaysia National Health Accounts: Health Expenditure Report 1997–2017*. Putrajaya: Ministry of Health Malaysia.

The Malaysian Reserve. (2019). *Local Herbal Industry Poised to Hit RM32b Market Value in 2020*. Online article. https://themalaysianreserve.com/2019/10/29/local-herbal-industry-poised-to-hit-rm32b-market-value-in-2020/

Ministry of Health Malaysia. (2019). *Interview with Officers of Enforcement Division*. Putrajaya: Ministry of Health Malaysia.

National Pharmaceutical Regulatory Agency. (2019). *Drug Registration Guidance Document (DRGD)*, 2nd ed. Putrajaya: Ministry of Health Malaysia.

Paraidathathu, T. (2019). *Pharmacy in Malaysia: History and Development*. Kuala Lumpur: University of Malaya Press.

Traditional and Complementary Medicine Division. (2017). *Traditional Complementary Medicine Blueprint 2018–2027 Health Care*. Putrajaya: Ministry of Health Malaysia.

Notes

1. Galenicals are creams, ointments and lotions.
2. US Food and Drug Administration.
3. Patients were given eye drops in a bottle and provided with a straw to instil the drops (G. Singh, personal communication to Thomas Paraidathathu, 2012).
4. Allied health personnel had a key role in delivering healthcare. In hospitals, a key category currently known as medical assistants were previously known as dressers and later as hospital assistants. Upgraded training programmes preceded each change in terminology and were accompanied by upgraded remuneration.
5. Phenobarbitone is a respiratory depressant, hence unsuitable for asthma.
6. Initially known as Southern Task, the privatised entity changed its name a few times and became known as Pharmaniaga Logistics Sdn Bhd.
7. Standard International Trade Classification, the code used for 2,970 commodity categories.
8. Previously known as the National Pharmaceutical Control Bureau.
9. This covers only medical products dispensed to outpatients. The expenditure item is categorised by functions of healthcare. Other medical goods expenditure goes to 'services of curative care'.
10. Medicine Prices Monitoring 2017 Report, Pharmacy Programme, Ministry of Health.
11. A breast cancer drug for HER2- (erb-b2 receptor tyrosine kinase 2)-positive patients.
12. Legal exemptions (or research exemptions) from infringement for certain patent acts concerning the development and submission of testing data to a regulatory agency.
13. By function of healthcare. Source: Malaysian National Health Accounts Unit, 2019.

12 *Leadership and Governance*

JO. M. MARTINS AND INDRA PATHMANATHAN

12.1 Introduction

This chapter explores the influence of leadership and governance on the development of the health system in Malaysia during the 60 years since independence. Governance refers to 'a wide range of steering and rule-making related functions carried out by governments/decisions makers as they seek to achieve national health policy objectives' (World Health Organization, 2019). It includes the policies and systems structures that facilitate the regular operation of a health system. Leadership has been defined as 'the art of motivating a group of people to act towards achieving a common goal' and includes elements of inspiring and directing (Ward, 2019). This concept has been extended to apply to institutions as leaders (Washington et al., 2008). Leadership occurs at many levels of the system, and its characteristics, development and impact on the health system have been analysed variously (Hartley, 2008; West et al., 2015).

Leadership and governance are strategic elements in a health system (West et al., 2015). Their performance has an impact on:

- the direction and priorities of the system,
- the development and bonding of the various inputs into a coherent set of activities and services, and
- collaboration with relevant public entities and the formation of coalitions with other organisations and civil society in the pursuit of public interest and social welfare.

Leadership and governance are key to planning and implementing activities, evaluating outcomes, and the shifts and corrections needed. By their very nature, they operate in a political and socio-economic context, and outcomes depend on political and social acceptance of objectives and their operational forms. This, in turn, enhances the mobilisation of resources and their application to achieve set goals. They are of greater importance in multi-ethnic societies, such as Malaysia, to minimise tensions arising from differences in perspectives and actual conditions, as well as to create a political framework that can manage the development process in spite of constraints. The development process could either address one set of constraints at a time or follow a more holistic path by addressing a number of related ones simultaneously and benefiting from the synergy of complementary thrusts that enhance outcomes across the system (Pourbohloul & Kieny, 2011).

12.2 The Ministry of Health: Context and Structure

12.2.1 National Governance Context

The Malaysian Constitution provides a federal type of government, with division of powers between the federal and state governments. At the federal level, the legislature consists of a lower House of Representatives, elected through nationwide elections, and a partially appointed Senate. Each state has its own State Assembly elected by statewide elections. The parliamentary type of government has an executive (Cabinet), headed by a prime minister who is a member of the lower house and a number of ministers. The hereditary Malay heads (Sultans) of some states elect from among themselves a monarch (Supreme Ruler) who serves for a fixed term. The monarch has limited powers and follows the advice of the prime minister of the day. The rulers, on the advice of their governments, appoint the members of the independent judiciary, both at federal and state level. While some powers are exclusive to either the federal or the state governments, there are some overlapping areas where powers are conjoint. The federal government has powers concerned with health and the provision of health services and others relevant to health such as the environment, labour and education (Commissioner of Law Revision, 2014), whereas states have powers over land.

Malaysia adopts a holistic approach wherein health policies are formulated and developed within the context of wider major national development policies set by the Prime Minister's Department (PMD) and Cabinet and articulated in various Malaysia Plans. Health professionals in the Ministry of Health (MoH) have the primary responsibility of advising the government on health priorities and formulating health programmes and interventions according to these priorities. Achieving balanced development with greater equity and poverty alleviation has been a national aim, with the reduction of differences between groups of people and regional areas a key priority. Another aspect of priority-setting has been the need to balance health service development with human resources availability and fiscal constraints (Economic Planning Unit, 1991; 2015; Chapters 3–9). National priorities and health needs have evolved as economic and social development took hold with growing urbanisation (Chapter 3). For example, the Eleventh Malaysia Plan (2016–2020) moved priorities from eradicating poverty to improving the living conditions of the 40% of all households that have the lowest income (Economic Planning Unit, 2015). The MoH policies responded accordingly.

12.2.2 MoH Organisational Structure

At federal level, the MoH, headed by a Cabinet-level minister, has two arms. The administrative arm, headed by the Secretary General and staffed by civil servants from the country's general public civil service, is responsible for public service personnel administration, finance and procurement. The health professional arm, headed by the Director General (DG) and staffed by healthcare professionals, focuses on planning, implementing and evaluating service delivery and the wider concerns that affect the health of the community. It appears that areas under the DG's responsibility tend to be concerned with the whole system beyond the health services provided by the MoH, while those under the more direct administration of the Secretary General tend to relate to the provision of services by the MoH and public service administration.

The organisational structure of the MoH follows the conventional separation of public health and community-based services from medical and hospital services, with separate areas of responsibility for research and technical support, including planning, engineering services, the National Institutes of Health, dental care, and pharmaceutical goods and supplies. Each state has a state-level health department responsible for administration and delivering services, and its organisation reflects the conventional separation of public health and community-based services from medical and hospital services (Ministry of

Health Malaysia, 1975; 2018). There are smaller administrative entities at district and hospital levels. As described in Chapters 4, 5, 6 and 8, the evolution over the past 60-year period has seen growing professional and managerial competence, beginning at the federal level and gradually trickling down to the district and hospital levels.

12.3 The MoH as an Intersectoral Leader

The MoH is expected to exercise institutional leadership and governance for health. It sets the health agenda and ensures its place in the broader national agenda, sets policies that shape how public and private health sectors operate and interact, creates regulations for health and safety and collaborates internationally for health.

12.3.1 Inter-ministerial Leadership

The MoH is the major source of technical expertise for health. It formulates and administrates health-related legislation and regulations, provides training for nursing and other allied health professional personnel and is the major provider of health services in Malaysia. However, health is dependent not merely on health services but also on what people do and their work and living conditions. Consequently, the MoH often lacks both the direct authority and supervision of substantial areas of relevance to health risks management and their impact on health that fall under the responsibility of other ministries or agencies such as environment, transport or food services. This diversity of authority and responsibilities requires the MoH to provide, at times, leadership and technical support in collaborative approaches with other federal and state agencies and civil society in the pursuit of policies and practices that enhance the health status of Malaysians.

Historically, several other ministries have played influential roles in health development. The PMD plays a major role in developing national policy that guides health policies and translating it into five-year plans with mid-term reviews and longer-term outline perspective plans. This process enables performance evaluation and corrections. The Ministry of Finance addresses fiscal needs from development and operational demands. As MoH revenue amounts to only a small fraction (3% in 2016) of its operational expenditure, it is dependent on the fiscal resources of the federal government through the Ministry of

Finance (Ministry of Health Malaysia, 2018; Chapter 9). The role of the Ministry of Education (MoE) has expanded from training medical students to include the training other health professionals. The MoE also administrates a number of university teaching hospitals and has partnered with the MoH in providing health-enhancing services and promoting healthy practices in school-age children. Finally, co-ordination across different levels of government has also been important, with federal, state and local governments sharing responsibilities in areas such as the promotion and maintenance of healthy conditions at a local level, such as the preparation and sale of food in urban areas.

New and emerging challenges to public health have triggered changes in the roles and inter-relationships between ministries. For example, as health concerns related to environmental, occupational or lifestyle issues rise in importance, the corresponding ministries have an increasing responsibility for health. However, there are examples where professional specialisation in the relevant ministries has created gaps in their ability to respond. The MoH has stepped in to address these gaps or ensure proper ownership by other ministries. For example, the professional strength of the agencies concerned with the environment (e.g. the Department of Chemistry) led to a focus on chemistry rather than on bacteriology. In the case of labour, safety concerns focused on risks from mechanical devices and not on exposure to and contamination by biological agents. The MoH supported the relevant ministries in developing the needed expertise.

Although the MoH is the acknowledged leader for issues related to health, in practice, leadership has taken on different forms and has been manifested by different institutions. For example, Chapter 7 provides an example where the MoH provided leadership by facilitating other agencies that had the primary responsibility of providing safe water and sanitation to develop the professional competence required to perform their function adequately. Similar examples are evident in the management of other environmental and occupational health risks (Chapters 4, 6 and 7). As other ministries and agencies acquired greater capacity to address the changing environmental, labour and social scene, the role of the MoH evolved and became a supportive one.

Sometimes leadership is a shared role. For example, universities under the MoE are responsible for the academic training of medical practitioners. However, the MoH, as the leading provider of healthcare, takes the lead in defining the competencies required in the medical workforce, while the universities take the lead in designing and implementing the curriculum. However, the MoH provides much of the practical training and internship of doctors in its public hospitals and is therefore the final authority to decide whether the new doctor is competent to practice without supervision (Chapter 8). Civil society has also demonstrated leadership in health. Chapter 6 provides examples of situations where non-governmental organisations (NGOs) provided leadership for successful advocacy for national policies and programmes to tackle tuberculosis and HIV/AIDS.

12.3.2 Leading and Governing Service Delivery in the Public and Private Sectors

The private sector has a significant role in the delivery of healthcare in Malaysia. An important governance question is whether the provision of health services is a public or a private matter and the role of government in its provision and financing. The nature of health services does not make market mechanisms effective to ensure efficiency and social, or even private, satisfaction in meeting health needs. Much of healthcare has the characteristics of what have been termed *public goods*,[1] which makes market competition an inadequate means of achieving efficiency or ensuring equity in their distribution in view of income inequalities and poverty. Further, health services, like education, have attributes that can give them social merit that society needs to determine independently of preferences determined by price and consequently the living standards of more than one generation. Further, the health service 'market' is characterised by commonly designated 'market failures' that preclude assumptions regarding the maximising of consumer utility (or welfare) and efficiency in the allocation of resources and their use. Among other attributes, the health 'market' is characterised by few providers, especially in the case of hospitals, with restrictions to entry due to licensing and other constraints; prices that are sometimes determined by providers or insurers; asymmetry of information between consumers and providers, as the consumer is dependent on the supplier to determine services received; and, as previously mentioned, considerable externalities, especially in the case of infectious diseases. These characteristics of the health services 'market', especially in the case of services provided by the private sector, do not allow the efficient performance of social objectives of consumer sovereignty and efficiency (Martins, 2004).

Thus governance of the health system in Malaysia has to address the balance between public and private provision of services, their relative costs and equity in their distribution. First, the relative scarcity of medical personnel and their concentration in urban centres led to the provision of public sector primary healthcare in rural areas, where most people lived, by allied health personnel. This was a low-cost but effective delivery of basic healthcare. Complemented by environmental services, it contributed to improved equity in access to health services (Chapters 3, 4 and 8).

As medical personnel became more abundant and people more urbanised, with easier geographical access to both public and private health services, the provision of lower-cost public services still played the important function of benchmarking the price of private services, keeping private fees in check. However, to retain medical personnel, the governance of public services had to keep the remuneration of medical personnel in the public sector at an acceptable level (Chapters 8 and 9). These balancing efforts have kept total health expenditure in Malaysia at the middle level of 4.0% of the gross domestic product (GDP) in 2014, compared with its neighbouring countries – 6.5% in Thailand, 4.9% in Singapore and 2.8% in Indonesia (Ministry of Health Malaysia, 2017) – and added about 15 years to the life expectancy of Malaysians (Chapters 3 and 9).

The governance of health services raises some potential conflicts of interest for the MoH. An obvious one is that the MoH is both a regulator and a provider of services. This governance issue is only partly addressed by the establishment of state administrations of public sector health services that are accountable and subjected to oversight by the central administration of the MoH. However, the MoH is, in turn, subjected to oversight by agencies in the PMD and the Ministry of Finance.

In addition, a number of governance issues arise from the government-stated interest in the promotion of the private sector in general and private health services in particular. The government has nominated health as one of the National Key Economic Areas. Although a number of economic activities are included, such as the production of pharmaceutical and medical devices, with some emphasis on their economic and export value, an area more directly related to health services is medical tourism (Prime Minister's Department, 2017). The Malaysian government has promoted medical tourism since the late 1990s (Ormond et al., 2014; Chandran et al., 2017). It is fostered by the Malaysia Healthcare Travel Council (MHTC), an initiative of the Ministry of Finance. The council's membership also includes the ministries of relevance to tourism, the MoH, and other agencies such as the Association of Private Hospitals of Malaysia (Malaysia Healthcare Travel Council, 2020). There is no obvious evidence of the direct relevance of medical tourism to the health of Malaysians, as its objective is an economic one. This is reflected in the absence of any apparent reference to medical tourism in the annual reports of the MoH (e.g. Ministry of Health Malaysia, 2018). There is not much specific information on the value of medical tourism and its contribution to economic activity. An estimate by the MHTC for 2017 of the value of medical tourism was that it represented the equivalent of about 0.1% of the value of Malaysia's exports in that year (Malaysia Healthcare Travel Council, 2017; Malaysia External Trade Development Corporation, 2018).

However, this economic interest has led to pressure on the MoH to reduce the regulatory burden on private health services in its administration of the Private Healthcare Facilities and Services Act. In this context, a study mandated under the Tenth Malaysia Plan to modernise business regulations conducted a regulatory review with the aim of reducing unnecessary regulatory burdens on private hospitals (Malaysia Productivity Corporation, 2014a). The review focused on the private hospital sector, as this is deemed a high-value-added, high-knowledge-based and growing sector. It found that regulations covering private hospitals were excessively prescriptive and made several recommendations for reducing the regulatory burden. It is noteworthy that the annual report of the same agency – related to the Ministry of International Trade and Industry – for 2013–2014 mentions rising costs and innovation as the major issues to be addressed by private hospitals and makes no mention of the burden of regulations (Malaysia Productivity Corporation, 2014b).

The regulation of medical personnel has been an important point of consistency across the public and private health sectors. Health services are dependent on the competence of medical, nursing and other professional personnel. Malaysia uses the mechanism of licensing via statutory bodies to manage these standards of practice, and this process has evolved and became more comprehensive over time (Chapter 8). For example, the Nurses Act 1950 provided for a Nursing Board to supervise the training and registration of nurses and oversight of their practice (Chong et al., 2011). The Medical Act 1973 gave the Malaysian Medical Council the authority to evaluate the qualifications of medical practitioners and their registration (Malaysian Medical Council, 2018). This was important because of the past shortages and recruitment from countries with varied training and degrees of competence. The licensing and/or registration of other health professions has continued over the years to ensure appropriate and safe professional practice (e.g. Allied Health Professions Act 2016) (Lim, 2016).

12.3.3 Regulations for Health and Safety

In the health sector, Malaysia uses regulation and licensing for two major purposes. The first is to manage threats to community health arising from the spread of disease or deleterious elements in the environment in which people live. The second is to protect the community from fraudulent or potentially harmful practices by healthcare providers or through the sale of medical and food products. The regulations give legal authority to various agencies for their enforcement, with sanctions for their infringement.

Initial regulatory activity by the MoH addressed infectious disease (Chapter 6), medical personnel (Section 12.3.2) and medical products (Chapter 12). In later years, however, as urbanisation and industrialisation increased the health risks of water supply contamination, changes to the Constitution allowed the federal government and the MoH to play a greater role in water supplies and sewerage and their regulation (Water Services Industry Act 2006) (Wahab, 2011; Pidgeon, 2012). The MoH plays an active role in the National Drinking Water Quality Surveillance Programme (Ministry of Health Malaysia, 1998). The growth in the commercialisation of food supplies, including international trade, has added to health risks in food supply and consumption, leading to the strengthening of the Food Act 1983 and its regulations.

Most Malaysians are of working age and are employed in a wide range of activities with varied degrees of health risk and disability risk. Consequently, occupational safety is a major factor in the maintenance of health. The Occupational Safety and Health Act 1994 aims at maintaining safe working conditions and applies sanctions for adverse practices. Although the administration of related regulations and surveillance lies with the Ministry of Labour, the MoH remains concerned about the surveillance of occupational diseases in order to identify the causes and sources that can direct remedial action, in addition to the promotion of the health of the large labour force in health services (Ministry of Health Malaysia, 2018).

Malaysia has used health legislation and regulation sparingly, perhaps in part due to limitations in institutional bandwidth and capacity. The lead time for enacting and enforcing new legislation is lengthy, taking five or more years for food legislation, for example. This indicates the complexity of the processes, which include stakeholder engagement, legal expertise and availability to draft the legislation, and developing the enforcement capacity and mechanisms for implementation. Such capacity might require financial resources, digital monitoring, laboratory services, the establishment of procedures and guidelines, and the training of enforcement and prosecution staff. In addition, the nature of the imperatives for legislation influenced political will and support, which in turn influenced the priority of enacting and implementing legislation effectively and the system capacity to do so.

Table 12.1 illustrates this through contrasting examples of the development of legislation to safeguard against hazards in food, where strong foreign trade imperatives proved much stronger than domestic imperatives that involved balancing health concerns against the growth of local food services.

While it is important to allow sufficient time to garner stakeholder support and build system capacity, long lead times in developing legislation and regulation can be detrimental. A problem may develop in the intervening period, resulting in the need for repeated re-drafting of legislation. It weakens governance capacity and engenders frustration among groups experiencing negative impact and among enforcement authorities. An example from Case Study 5.1 in Chapter 5 is the long delay in enacting legislation to govern the behaviour of third-party agencies that serve as intermediaries between employers and healthcare providers for their employees.

12.3.4 *International Collaboration*

As with most developing countries, the development of Malaysia's health system has had some external support, specifically from the

Table 12.1 *Differing imperatives influenced the system behaviour in formulating health legislation*

	Characteristics of the imperatives for legislation	Lead time for formulation of legislation and preparatory activities
Example No. 1: **Legislation to safeguard the public against health hazards and fraud and to ensure hygiene and sanitary practices in the preparation and sale of food** • Food Act 1983 • Food Regulations 1985 • Food Hygiene Regulations 2009	The domestic market was the target, with public health as the imperative, i.e.: • Malaysian public exposed to health hazards • Malaysian stakeholder support was required • Malaysian enforcement capacity had to be strengthened	**Lead time: 5 years** During the interval: • Support garnered through the gradual enforcement of a code of practice • Staff numbers and competence developed for monitoring and enforcement • Laboratory services strengthened
Example No. 2: **Legislation to ensure that the quality of fish and fishery products exported to the European Union (EU) meet EU requirements and certifications** • Food Regulations 2009 *(Issuance of Health Certificate for Export of Fish and Fish Product to the European Union)*	The EU was the target market, with trade as the imperative, i.e.: In June 2008, the European Commission de-listed all Malaysian fish and fishery processing establishments at Malaysia's request to avoid an EU ban on imports of Malaysian fish and fishery products valued at RM 600 million per year	**Lead time: 2 years** During the interval, Malaysia: • Enacted legislation equivalent to EU requirement • Strengthened the capacity of competent authorities through organisational re-structuring and recruiting additional staff • Increased the financial allocation

• Fisheries Regulations 2009 *(Quality Control of Fish for Export to the European Union)* • Fish Marketing Regulations 2010 • Fisheries Development Authority of Malaysia Regulations 2010 *(Recognition of Fish Landing Site for Fish Export to European Union)*	*Outcomes:* May 2009: Malaysia resumed exports to the EU of fish and fishery products processed from local aquaculture and imported raw materials September 2010: Malaysia resumed exports of fishery products processed from local capture fishery raw materials	• Provided official guarantees of the control of exports of fishery products along the supply chain to meet EU requirements

multilaterals. The World Health Organization (WHO) has been a source of technical advice on the management and prevention of both communicable and non-communicable diseases as well as health personnel training and the organisation of community- and hospital-based services. Malaysia has also collaborated with international financial institutions such as the Asian Development Bank and the World Bank. International support for the Malaysian health system has been predominantly technical in nature, with limited financial support, to cover some infrastructure development rather than for the delivery of programmes. As discussed in Chapter 6, the limited reliance on international financial support contributed to the ability of the MoH to design programmes based on national priorities and directions, integrating new initiatives into existing ones rather than developing parallel initiatives according to external priorities.

The activities of the Institute for Medical Research (Chapter 6) include early examples of Malaysia's international collaboration on research into tropical disease control and professional training for countries in the region (Ministry of Health Malaysia, 1980). A more recent example is the establishment of the ASEAN Risk Assessment Centre for Food Safety (ARAC) to foster collaboration among Association of Southeast Asian Nations (ASEAN) members to improve food safety (Ministry of Health Malaysia, 2018).

The wide range of Malaysia's engagement in international collaboration comprises the continuing contributions of the WHO Collaborating Regional Centre for Research and Training in Tropical Diseases and Nutrition, and the Collaborating Centre for Ecology, Taxonomy and Control of Vectors of Malaria, Filariasis and Dengue, as well as collaboration in health systems research, among others (World Health Organization, 2002; Barraclough & Phua, 2007; Ministry of Health Malaysia, 2018). Other areas of international collaboration involve co-operation with and support of ASEAN countries on a range of health concerns (Barraclough & Phua, 2007). In addition to food safety, these activities include the control of infectious diseases and oral health, as well as other ASEAN clusters of co-operation on issues such as healthcare coverage and access, human resources and health technology assessment (Ministry of Health Malaysia, 2018).

12.4 Leadership in the Public Health Sector

In addition to exercising intersectoral leadership, the MoH has also needed to provide leadership and governance in the public health system. This includes establishing visions and programmes, evaluating performance, ensuring accountability, addressing systemic issues and developing leadership.

12.4.1 Vision and Programme Setting

The national priorities set by the PMD and the Cabinet and articulated in various Malaysia Plans guide health priorities. For example, a major national aim was to achieve balanced development with greater equity, particularly between urban and rural areas, and poverty alleviation (Chapter 3). Top leadership in the MoH contributed to the ability of the health sector to translate national goals into a health sector vision and inculcate basic values that characterised the delivery of health services in both the public and private sectors. An example of the contribution of personal leadership is, for example, the leadership of the Health DG in the 1970s, who translated the Alma Ata vision for primary healthcare into the Malaysian context, as described in Chapter 4. In later eras, successive DGs translated the national emphasis on improving quality of service into a systematic nationwide programme and culture in the public sector health services, as illustrated in Chapter 5. Leaders demonstrated their commitment to collaborating with peers across organisational boundaries and recognising leadership qualities in their subordinate staff and supporting them. Box 12.1 illustrates how persons occupying top positions in the MoH at various times viewed their own contributions to leadership.

Box 12.1 Reflection on leadership in Malaysia's health sector

'Many factors that influence health are outside the purview of the MoH. Leaders in the Ministry of Health must be able to interact with leaders in other sectors to advocate on health issues.'

'They have to be informative, persuasive and proactive. Leaders should monitor performance of the organisation and insist on evaluating interventions.'

'We have excellent leaders at various levels. For example, I remember a director in Hospital Kota Tinggi who was a quiet, humble person but inspired great teamwork. I respect him.'

'Resisting political pressure is an essential characteristic of leaders. For example, one MB overruled construction of a septic tank by refusing to approve land. Another diverted funds to his own interest group for building a private hospital.'

Tan Sri Abu Bakar Suleiman Director General Health, Malaysia, 1991–2001

'The Minister of Health should advocate rather than be an administrator. I am very proud of my success in advocating and convincing the PM against approving "kiddie packs" of cigarettes.'

'Politicians know that providing healthcare is an easy credit point with their electorate. Hence they will always push for items for which they can claim credit.'

Dato Seri Dr S. Subramaniam Minister of Health, Malaysia, 2013–2018

'A leader needs to be knowledgeable. I am a lawyer who had to make myself knowledgeable about health issues.'

'I was fortunate to have a highly competent DG in Tan Sri Abu Bakar. We had an excellent partnership.'

'My proudest achievement is that I managed to influence the culture in the MoH. During my tenure, we began the tradition of inviting stakeholder views and having regular consultations. This increased the prestige of the MoH. My ministry was recognised as the leader on health topics.'

Dato Chua Jui Meng *Minister of Health, Malaysia*, 1995–2004

'Leadership should be both a top-down and a bottom-up process: leaders need to listen, anticipate and innovate.'

'Leaders in the MoH need to manage the perceptions of the public.'

'We need to embrace technology and use it innovatively to improve healthcare.'

'Communication strategy is important. For example, we now focus on the non-smoker rather than the smoker!'

Datuk Dr Noor Hisham Abdullah *Director General Health, Malaysia*, 2013–present[2]

Leadership also emerged at various levels of the MoH organisation in response to specific challenges, as illustrated in the example of the introduction of the human papillomavirus (HPV) vaccination programme (Table 12.2). Leadership has also emerged from the private sector health service. For example, it was a general practitioner (GP) from the private sector who spearheaded the development of family medicine as a speciality (Rajakumar, 1984).

Most health system programming has been concerned with the organisation of services in the public sector in accordance with national priorities, as detailed in the previous chapters. The health requirements programming in Malaysia follows a top-down and bottom-up approach with a reiterative consultative process that involves a wide variety of officers at national, state, district and hospital levels. MoH programme directors in the various divisions and institutions raise and discuss issues, while similar processes occur at state level. This process involves reviewing and assessing health conditions and trends in Malaysia and identifying the driving factors in order to formulate responses. Current programmes are evaluated, with changes planned to meet evolving circumstances (e.g. Ministry of Health Malaysia, 2012; 2018). Proposed programmes and projects are also evaluated, and those involving large expenditures undergo further assessment for compatibility with development budget estimates. They are submitted for review and approval to the Economic Planning Unit in the PMD for financing and implementation during the period of the proposed Malaysia Plan (Suleiman & Jegathesan, 2000; Ministry of Health Malaysia, 2018).

Issues and priorities identified at the national level are cascaded down to state and district level, which in turn identify local issues and merge them into the national framework and cascade them up to national level for review by a committee of senior managers, with the Division of Planning as the secretariat. This has the advantage of considering perceived major national issues in conjunction with the benefit of emerging local conditions and constraints. In addition, it is a mechanism for developing leadership and governance skills at various levels of the MoH system. However, this process may lead to delays between the identification of health risks and the implementation of responses, such as in the case of dengue and diabetes control (Institute for Public Health, 2015).

Table 12.2 ***Illustrative features of leadership during Malaysia's experience in introducing HPV immunisation***

Context	Organisational leadership by MoH	Personal leadership examples
Rapid increase in HPV vaccination in adolescent girls, 2011–2016	1. Established and sustained mechanisms for collaboration with related agencies and departments. An example is the Joint School Health Committees at national and state level. This: a. facilitated institutional memory, b. enabled continuity of dialogue despite changes in personnel, and c. provided a safe and respected space for dialogue between stakeholders. 2. Partner agencies and the public perceived the MoH as a trusted source for technical leadership. Recognition by professional and international agencies contributed to this trust. 3. Within the MoH system, there was strong leadership at national, state and district level.	1. There was mutual respect for the roles and responsibilities of partner agencies. 2. Staff in various managerial positions had the ability to assume differing leadership roles that were appropriate and relevant to their position. For example, at national level, leaders provided a vision and established a culture of collaboration, while at the operational levels, leaders were supportive and responsible to their staff and clients. 3. Leaders displayed the ability to listen to and be heard by stakeholders, for example, the 360-degree process of 'listen–act–provide feedback'.

Source: Buang et al., 2018.

12.4.2 Data and Evaluation

Governance is first and foremost about achieving results. Monitoring is crucial for identifying constraints encountered in the short term and the attainment of outcomes in the longer term. Reliable and relevant health information is essential in the performance of this governance function (Chapter 10), and relevant follow-up action is a critical partner to monitoring and evaluation. Monitoring and evaluation could be considered necessary but are not sufficient conditions of progress. For example, there has been a lag between monitoring and action in the incidence of dengue. Infectious diseases monitoring has shown a substantial rise in the incidence of dengue since 2000. Although case fatality rates declined due to medical treatment, preventive action lagged and incidence rates were 10 times higher in 2016 than in 2000 (Ministry of Health Malaysia, 2018). Malaysia's systematic planning and evaluation of health development uses information from regular population censuses and comprehensive registration of vital statistics that identifies the population groups most at risk and what degree of progress, or otherwise, has been made over time. Another strength has been the wider people-centred development approach that focused on poverty and human capital, including health, with the collection of data on living conditions (e.g. Department of Statistics, 1959) that identified the population groups most at risk. These were complemented by the registration of health professionals, inventories of health facilities and health service activity information, especially in the public sector, which provided most services. However, it was their analysis in relation to the population that provided the basis for evaluating the results and relative progress. The National Institutes of Health provide research and programme evaluation studies that contribute to the information database. Requests for many of the National Institutes of Health studies come from the MoH, and therefore have a direct link to decision-making.

The evaluation of data and the use of the findings for management purposes demonstrated the importance of health information and research, creating a feedback loop that has led to further investments and improvements in data quality and relevance. In early times, data collection and processing was often carried out by manual methods, before the wider use of computers and what became known as IT (information technology). The substantial investment in the use of IT in managing health services has improved the storage of, access to and analysis of a wide range of health information for monitoring and evaluating progress (Ministry of Health Malaysia, 2005; 2018; Chapter 10). However, it is important to note that improved data collection alone does not guarantee health improvements. The substantial IT thrust has coincided with an increase in the incidence of some non-communicable diseases (e.g. diabetes) during the 2000s and 2010s, stagnation of infant and maternal mortality rates and slower improvements in life expectancy (Chapter 3). Effective ways of understanding and using data to meet these new health challenges need to be developed.

The governance of the health system entails assessment of the current and emerging technologies and practices to evaluate effectiveness, relevance to local conditions and efficient provision. In earlier years, Malaysia depended largely on expertise from international agencies such as the WHO to inform the selection and use of technologies. Examples are the very early adoption of a list of essential drugs and the selection of vaccines to be included in universal childhood immunisation programmes. However, as the complexity of health technology increased and new hospitals were built based on external expertise, technology assessment and use in the Malaysian context became more imperative (Sivalal, 2009; Roza et al., 2019). The MoH established a section for assessing new technologies and reviewing current ones (Malaysian Health Technology Assessment Section, or MaHTAS), and its process relies on systematic reviews of intelligence gathered from other reliable sources and its own evaluation (Ministry of Health Malaysia, 2018). The outputs inform the development of clinical practice guidelines and the purchase of costly technology or medical products by the MoH (Chapter 5). Other examples of the evaluation and use of findings include the assessment of the cost-effectiveness of some of its services, such as neonatal intensive care and diagnostic imaging services, and the effectiveness and improvement of clinical services such as renal dialysis and cataract surgery (Ministry of Health Malaysia, 2002; 2005; Chapter 5). Another example is the evaluation of services that have been outsourced, such as hospital laundry and cleaning services, where the performance of contractual services is a regular feature and has shown increased levels of contractual compliance (Chapter 7).

12.4.3 Accountability

Accountability is an essential feature of governance, although the concept is difficult to define. Accountability involves reporting the actions taken to another who is in a position to assess their appropriateness (Mulgan, 2000). Accountability processes are learning opportunities for corrective action or appropriate shifts. In the Malaysian health system, accountability takes place at different levels and several forms. For example, compliance with rules and regulations, or spending within set budgets, is a form of accountability. Another example is the accountability of professional and other standards of healthcare practice exercised by professionals to their respective statutory registration boards, as described previously. On a different level, accountability is concerned with enhancing the performance and responsiveness of a health service to health conditions and the expectations of the public. This happens on a personal level, through complaints either via official pipelines or the mass media. Alternatively, accountability to the public can occur through political channels.

Several institutional mechanisms support accountability in the health sector. Performance reviews of the various programmes and services take place within the MoH system in a quasi-hierarchical manner, from single service units to state and national level. Accountability of performance and responsiveness to health needs also takes place during the preparation for each five-year Malaysia Plan and their mid-term reviews (Ministry of Health Malaysia, 2012; 2018), reviewed by the PMD and Cabinet. In turn, the Cabinet is accountable to parliament and it to the electorate. At micro and intermediate level, accountability to the public occurs through the mass media, whereby the MoH monitors and reviews every complaint appearing in news media. MoH procedures require a response to the complaint or appropriate remedial action.

Non-regulatory mechanisms can also promote accountability, as seen in the surveillance of practice and follow-up remedial action, particularly in the public sector (Chapters 4, 5 and 7). Examples include the Quality Assurance Programme (QAP) established in the MoH in 1985 that provided leadership to foster service quality (Ministry of Health Malaysia, 1998; 2018); the adoption of the International Organisation of Standardisation (ISO) (9001 version) Quality Management System (QMP) in accordance with government policy (Hashim & Ibrahim, 2016; Ministry of Health Malaysia, 2018); and the establishment of the Malaysian Society for Quality in Health

(MSQH), which provides voluntary accreditation for public and private hospitals using national standards to assess the level of performance through external review and encourages continuous improvement of practice (Malaysian Society for Quality in Health, 2019). Most MoH hospitals have been accredited (Ministry of Health Malaysia, 2018), as have many in the private sector (Aziz & Azizan, 2013). The evolution from regulatory to non-regulatory mechanisms reflects the tacit acknowledgement that regulation is suited only to weed out extreme cases of poor quality (the 'bad apples'). Continuing improvement of the systems-wide quality of healthcare requires systems-wide incentives, including monitoring and feedback, professional and managerial human resources competencies and the development of an organisational culture that values quality.

A systemic challenge to accountability in the public health system is that the MoH is simultaneously the regulator and the provider of public health services in Malaysia. One illustrative example of potential conflict is that all the regulatory boards that govern health professionals have the DG of the MoH as chairperson and the respective programme director as secretary. However, the DG and the respective directors are also the heads of the respective services provided by the MoH, thereby posing a challenge to preserving the principles of accountability.

12.4.4 Structural Challenges and Governance Responses

The divisions of expertise and responsibility necessary for a functional health system also tend to foster the development of silos. The MoH employs task forces and committees that cut across divisions to mitigate this problem. The task forces deal with issues that require time-limited activities, while the joint or national committees deal with issues that require continuing collaboration. Changing demands on the health system have dictated different responses. For example, when maternal and child health were the focus, obstetricians and paediatricians from hospitals joined public health professionals in committees for the investigation of maternal deaths. As the focus moved to non-communicable diseases and emerging infectious diseases, a plethora of other committees and task forces combined the talents of clinicians, epidemiologists, laboratory specialties and healthcare managers to develop national strategies or action plans, as illustrated in Chapters 5 and 6.

Box 12.2 System observations: attempts to bridge silos

The observations of short-term task forces and long-term committees formed to foster cross-division co-operation within the MoH demonstrate the difficulty of sustaining lateral engagement. In the absence of tangible and high-priority goals, the regular system structure and work priorities dominate. It also shows the importance of informal systems (e.g. institutional memory and personal relationships) that are not reflected in an organisational chart. Health systems need both formal and informal linkages to facilitate communication and counteract the tendency toward silos.

Anecdotal evidence suggests that task forces that had to produce tangible products within short timeframes were very successful, as evidenced in the examples in the chapter on disease control (Chapter 6). Committees that had continuing responsibilities over time, such as the MoH/MoE joint committee for school health, tended to become lethargic or dormant until energised periodically by having to respond to new leadership or focus on a new challenge, as seen in the example of introducing the HPV vaccine for schoolgirls. Nonetheless, these committees appear to foster institutional memory that can facilitate rapid and effective collaboration across divisions (Buang et al., 2018).

Another challenge is that human resources in the MoH are part of the larger civil service of Malaysia and are governed by the large and rather unwieldy bureaucracy. As such, the MoH has limited flexibility in adjusting employment conditions to the needs of healthcare services. For example, posts and promotion criteria adhere to general civil service rules (Institute of Health Management, 2006). Another example is the prolonged negotiations required to provide special incentives for selected categories to address brain drain to the private sector. This was partly due to concerns that other categories of professionals in the same grade would demand similar incentives, although there was no reason to provide them.

12.4.5 Leadership Development

Although there is no empirical evidence, it is possible to postulate that several factors have contributed to the development of leadership at various levels in the health system. First, the civil service system of career progression requires, as a precondition to promotion, participation in management training programmes that raise awareness of leadership and its functions and the opportunity to bond with fellow officers from other ministries, thereby facilitating future networking. Second, career progression provides officers with the opportunity to occupy leadership positions at successively higher levels in the system (namely district, state and then national levels), thereby providing invaluable experience in communicating and collaborating with other agencies at progressively more complex levels. Third, within the MoH itself, the system requires clinical specialists, who previously focused only on their own patients, to take leadership for their clinical speciality across the state or the whole country. Participating in cross-disciplinary task forces, they acquire leadership competencies. However, to some extent, clinicians are disadvantaged compared to their colleagues in public health, as the latter acquire managerial experience throughout their career, starting from managing district-level entities and progressing to larger entities. In contrast, clinicians acquire exposure to managerial functions relatively later in their career. Fourth, the devolution of decision-making functions in programme formulation, as described above, provides the opportunity for nurturing leadership within the system.

Box 12.3 System observations: systems perspectives on leadership development

It is often easier to describe the role that leadership plays in a health system than it is to identify how a health system produces good leadership. Indeed, the process of grooming and selecting leaders in a health system, especially top leadership, is often not open to documentation and outside scrutiny.

While leadership is indeed critical to the development of a health system, it too is shaped and constrained by health system structures and policies. Health system culture, needs and rules will strongly influence where in the health system leadership can be exercised and what form that leadership takes (e.g. technical, transformational, etc.). In particular, the appropriate devolution of decision-making is important for enabling leadership at all levels and the continuous development of new leaders.

12.5 Conclusions

Health development in Malaysia offers helpful examples of successes and challenges in governance and leadership.

Some of the lessons from successful practice are:

- The formulation and pursuit of national development policies that prioritised social and human advancement and set health development in that wider synergistic context.
- Sage leadership that stimulated the involvement of local leaders, and associated community participation, in socio-economic development, including health improvements.
- The identification of the people most at risk in the population and the organisation of health services to reach out to them in a manner compatible with the limited human and financial resources available.
- Health development policies and priorities that took guidance from macroeconomic policies and that in turn provided feedback that moulded government policies in relation to wellbeing and human development.
- The MoH provided leadership and technical support in areas of significant importance in health improvement that were the more immediate responsibility of other government agencies.
- Periodic review and evaluation of health outcomes and resource gaps led to related resource enhancement and corrections and shifts in direction in response to feedback from information collected and from stakeholders, including the community.
- The use of a comprehensive but incremental approach to health development in response to community demands and political goals. At no stage was there a radical overhaul of the system.

However, there are also some lessons from the persisting challenges, such as:

- How to garner community participation and involvement in health enhancement practices in a changed urban, industrialised and more affluent society.
- The burden of non-communicable diseases prevalent before old age.
- Responses to the ever-rising expectations of the public for more accessible and improved health services in the face of public funding constraints and the high cost of private health services.

- Reconciliation of the political aim of increasing reliance on the private sector with its higher price with the related higher social cost and rising total health expenditure.

A number of questions could be raised in this context:

- Are there applicable lessons from the past, such as how to address health threats arising from activities in other areas?
- Is there a need for a paradigm shift in the provision of health services? What are the critical elements of such a shift and how can stakeholder support for them be garnered?

In line with Malaysia's incremental and consensual approach, these challenges take time to resolve and achieve further enhancements of health. Significant change in the last decade has remained an unrealised goal.

12.6 Key Messages from Malaysia's Experience

12.6.1 What Went Well?

- Despite the highly centralised structure of the healthcare system, it
  - contains both top-down and bottom-up systems for planning, evaluation and implementation,
  - has good internal feedback loops, and
  - has adaptive capacity at implementation level.
- The system promoted and supported leadership development.
- The centralised nature of the system addressed concerns of equity across administrative state boundaries.

12.6.2 What Did Not Go So Well?

- Limited capacity to deal with determinants of health that are under the purview of other sectors.
- Governance structure and inadequate information limited the ability to respond to some social and environmental issues arising from rapid urbanisation, such as:

  - health in pockets of urban poverty,
  - the health of marginalised groups, and
  - loss of trust in authority and establishments, giving rise to anti-vaccination movements, etc.
- The combination of the roles of provision and governance of healthcare in the public sector creates the appearance of conflicts of interest, such as:
  - regulation of professional bodies, and
  - governance of private sector healthcare.

12.6.3 Trends and Challenges

- The rapid rate of change of the societal ecosystem and technology presents challenges to governance and leadership.

References

Aziz, A. and Azizan, N. A. (2013). The effectiveness of accreditation assessment for quality improvement in health care: Malaysian private hospital experience. *International Journal of Social Sciences & Education*, 3(4), 990–9.

Barraclough, S. and Phua, K.-L. (2007). Health imperatives in foreign policy: the case of Malaysia. *Bulletin of the World Health Organization*, 85(3), 225–9.

Buang, S. N., Ja'afar, S., Pathmanathan, I. and Saint, V. (2018). Human papillomavirus immunisation of adolescent girls: improving coverage through multisectoral collaboration in Malaysia. *British Medical Journal*, 363, k4602.

Chandran, S. D., Mohamed, A. S. P., Zainuddin, A., Puteh, F. and Azmi, N. A. (2017). Medical tourism: why Malaysia is a preferred destination? *Advanced Science Letters*, 3(8), 7861–4.

Chong, M. C., Sellick, K., Francis, K. and Abdullah, K. L. (2011). What influences Malaysian nurses to participate in continuing professional education activities? *Asian Nursing Research*, 5(1), 38–47.

Commissioner of Law Revision. (2014). *Federal Constitution*. Selangor: International Book Services.

Department of Statistics. (1959). *Household Budget Survey of the Federation of Malaya 1957–58*. Kuala Lumpur: Department of Statistics.

Economic Planning Unit. (1991). *Sixth Malaysia Plan 1991–1995*. Kuala Lumpur: Prime Minister's Department.

Economic Planning Unit. (2015). *Eleventh Malaysia Plan 2016–2020: Anchoring Growth on People*. Putrajaya: Prime Minister's Department.

Hartley, J. M. (2008). *Leadership in Healthcare: A Review of the Literature for Healthcare Professional, Managers and Researchers*. Coventry: Warwick Business School, Institute of Governance & Public Management.

Hashim, F. A. H. and Ibrahim, M. (2016). MS ISO 9001 certification: does it effective and beneficial to MARDI. *International Journal of Business and Management Invention*, 5(10), 142–51.

Institute of Health Management. (2006). *Health Workforce Development Strategies*. Putrajaya: Ministry of Health Malaysia.

Institute for Public Health. (2015). *National Health and Morbidity Survey 2015. Volume II: Non-communicable Diseases, Risk Factors and Other Health Problems*. Kuala Lumpur: Ministry of Health Malaysia.

Lim, K. G. (2016). *The History of Medicine and Health in Malaysia*. Kuala Lumpur: Lim Kean Ghee.

Malaysia External Trade Development Corporation. (2018). *Top 10 Major Export Products, 2017*. Online article. www.matrade.gov.my/en/28-malaysia-exporters/trade-statistics/3789-top-10-major-export-products-2017

Malaysia Healthcare Travel Council. (2017). *A Million Medical Tourists for Malaysia in 2017*. Online article. www.mhtc.org.my/mhtc/2017/04/24/a-million-medical-tourists-for-malaisia-in2017

Malaysia Healthcare Travel Council. (2020). *About Us*. Online webpage. www.mhtc.org.my/about-us

Malaysian Medical Council. (2018). *Registration Procedures and Guidelines*. Kuala Lumpur: Malaysian Medical Council.

Malaysian Society for Quality in Health (MSQH). 2019. *Overview Hospital Accreditation Programme*. Online webpage. www.msqh.com.my/home/hospital-accreditation-program

Malaysia Productivity Corporation. (2014a). *Reducing Unnecessary Regulatory Burdens on Business: Private Hospitals*. Petaling Jaya: Malaysia Productivity Corporation.

Malaysia Productivity Corporation. (2014b). *MPC 21st Productivity Report 2013/2014*. Petaling Jaya: Malaysia Productivity Corporation.

Martins, J. M. (2004). *Health Financing: An International Perspective*. In M. Courtney and D. Briggs, eds., *Health Care Financial Management*. Marrickville: Elsevier, pp. 23–61.

Ministry of Health Malaysia. (1975). *Annual Report Ministry of Health Malaysia 1973–74*. Kuala Lumpur: Ministry of Health Malaysia.

Ministry of Health Malaysia. (1980). *Annual Report Ministry of Health Malaysia 1980*. Kuala Lumpur: Ministry of Health Malaysia.

Ministry of Health Malaysia. (1998). *Malaysia's Health 1998*. Kuala Lumpur: Ministry of Health Malaysia.

Ministry of Health Malaysia. (2002). *Malaysia's Health 2002*. Putrajaya: Ministry of Health Malaysia.

Ministry of Health Malaysia. (2005). *Malaysia's Health 2005*. Putrajaya: Ministry of Health Malaysia.

Ministry of Health Malaysia. (2012). *Country Health Plan: 10th Malaysia Plan 2011–2015*. Putrajaya: Ministry of Health Malaysia.

Ministry of Health Malaysia. (2017). *Malaysia National Health Accounts: Health Expenditure Report 1997–2015*. Putrajaya: Ministry of Health Malaysia.

Ministry of Health Malaysia. (2018). *Annual Report Ministry of Health Malaysia 2016*. Putrajaya: Ministry of Health Malaysia.

Mulgan, R. (2000). Accountability: an ever-expanding concept? *Public Administration*, 78(3), 555–73.

Ormond, M., Wong, K. M. and Chan, C. K. (2014). Medical tourism in Malaysia: how can we identify and manage its advantages and disadvantages? *Global Health Action*, 7(1). DOI: https://doi.org/10.3402/gha.v7.25201

Pidgeon, M. (2012). Soggy politics making water 'public' in Malaysia. In M. Pidgeon, D. A. McDonald, O. Hoedeman and S. Kishimoto, eds., *Remunicipalisation: Putting Water Back into Public Hands*. Amsterdam: Transnational Institute, pp. 90–104.

Pourbohloul, B. and Kieny, M.-P. (2011). Complex systems analysis: towards holistic approaches to health systems planning and policy. *Bulletin of the World Health Organization*, 89, 241–316. DOI: http://102471/BLT.11.087544

Prime Minister's Department. (2017). *National Transformation Programme Annual Report 2017*. Putrajaya: Prime Minister's Department.

Rajakumar, M. (1984). A proposal for the training of physicians in primary care for the rural areas of Malaysia. *Family Practitioner*, 7(1), 58–61.

Roza, S., Junainah, S., Izzuna, M. M. G. and Nurhami, K. A. R. K. (2019). Health technology assessment in Malaysia: past, present and future. *International Journal of Technology Assessment in Health Care*, 35(6), 446–51.

Sivalal, S. (2009). Health technology assessment in Malaysia. *International Journal of Technology Assessment in Health Care*, 25(Supplement 1), 224–30.

Suleiman, A. B. and Jegathesan, M., eds. (2000). *Health in Malaysia: Achievements and Challenges*. Kuala Lumpur: Ministry of Health Malaysia.

Wahab, N. A. (2011). *Overview of the Water Services Industry in Malaysia.* Putrajaya: Ministry of Energy, Green Technology and Water. Online document. www.mlit.go.jp/common/000135515.pdf

Ward, S. (2019). *What Is Leadership? And Can You Learn to Be a Good Leader?* Online article. www.thebalancesmb.com/leadership-definition-2948275

Washington, M., Boal, K. and Davis, J. (2008). Institutional leadership: past, present, and future. In R. Greenwood, C. Oliver, R. Suddaby and K. Sahlin, eds., *The SAGE Handbook of Organizational Institutionalism.* Thousand Oaks, CA: SAGE, pp. 721–35.

West, M. A., Armit, K., Loewenthal, L., Eckert, R., West, T. and Lee, A. (2015). *Leadership and Leadership Development in Health Care: The Evidence Base.* London: King's Fund, Faculty of Medical Leadership and Management.

World Health Organization. (2002). *Malaysia: Country Cooperation Strategy.* Online document. www.who.int>countries>cooperation_strategy_mys_en

World Health Organization. (2019). *Health Systems Topics: Governance.* Online document. www.who.int/healthsystems/topics/stewardship/en

System Analysis Case Study 12.1: Leadership Enabled Affordable Treatment of Hepatitis C in Malaysia

Chee Han Lim, Faizul Nizam bin Abu Salim and David T. Tan

This case study illustrates the role of leadership in the complex negotiations that resulted in Malaysia obtaining an affordable price for medication for hepatitis C.

Background

Hepatitis C is a liver disease caused by a bloodborne virus (hepatitis C virus, or HCV) and is a major cause of liver cancer. The most common modes of infection are through exposure to small quantities of blood. This may happen through injection drug use, unsafe injection practices, unsafe healthcare, transfusion of unscreened blood and blood products, and sexual practices that lead to exposure to blood. There is currently no effective vaccine against hepatitis C; nevertheless, research in this area is ongoing. Antiviral medicines can cure more than 95% of persons with hepatitis C infection, thereby reducing the risk of death from cirrhosis and liver cancer, but access to diagnosis and treatment is low (World Health Organization, 2019). As the pool of infected persons is large, the risk of spreading the infection is high. The World Health Assembly resolution 63.18 'recognised viral hepatitis as a global public health problem and the need for governments and populations to take action to prevent, diagnose and treat viral hepatitis'.

The HCV disease burden is a major concern in Malaysia. In 2009, the MoH estimated that 453,700 people were living with HCV infection in Malaysia (McDonald et al., 2014) and that there would be a cumulative total of 63,900 HCV-related deaths by 2039 (McDonald et al., 2015). The incidence rate of HCV infection increased from 2.56 per 100,000 population in 2010 to 9.54 per 100,000 population in 2017 (Ministry of Health Malaysia, 2019), with about 2,000–3,000 newly diagnosed patients added to the patient burden every year (Hiebert et al., 2019).

After more than a decade of multiple research initiatives, an effective medicine, sofosbuvir (the generic name), was developed and patented. This drug has cure rates ranging from 30% to 97% (depending on the genotype treated) and has relatively few adverse effects. However, the price of medication in Malaysia for the requisite 12-week treatment was RM 300,000 (US$70,000) (Drugs for Neglected Diseases Initiative, 2017). The high price was a serious barrier to patient access to effective treatment and prevented its inclusion in the MoH drug formulary, thereby making it unavailable to the highly subsidised public sector.

A Conflict of Interest

Malaysia was seriously concerned about the need to manage the pool of infected patients effectively to prevent spread. A conflict situation was emerging between the price dictated by the foreign pharmaceutical company and the Malaysian desire for affordable medication to contain the public health risk of the large pool of patients capable of spreading hepatitis C.

Essential Features of the Conflict Situation

International pharmaceutical companies are for-profit agencies. They justify the high cost of patented drugs by citing the need to recover the costly process of developing new drugs. The World Trade Organization (WTO) and the Agreement on Trade-Related Aspects of Intellectual Property Rights (TRIPS) granted authority for patenting innovative products to protect the rights of the patent holder. Patents last for a specific number of years (see Box 12-A). Enforcement against violations of intellectual property rights (IPR) are usually through trade sanctions by the patent holder's host country against the violating country.

Gilead Science[3] is the patent holder for sofosbuvir (trade name Sovaldi), and the patent will be valid at least until 2024. Compulsory licensing allowed 11 Indian companies to produce and export a generic version of the medicine at a much lower price to 100 low-income countries, but this arrangement excluded Malaysia because it is an upper-middle-income country.

Price Control Tools: Paradigms and Risks

There is an intuitive and widely held paradigm that affordable medical treatment should be available to all. Such beliefs are reinforced when treatment prices become a barrier to access

Box 12-A Essential vocabulary regarding rules governing international trade of medicines

The **WTO** is an international body that deals with the global rules of trade between nations.

TRIPS is an international legal agreement between all the member nations of the WTO. It sets down minimum standards for the regulation by national governments of many forms of intellectual property as applied to nationals of other WTO member nations (World Trade Organization, n.d.).

A **patent** is an exclusive right granted for an invention, which is a product or a process. The patent owner has the exclusive right to prevent others from commercially exploiting the patented invention. Usually the patent lasts for about 20 years. Thus other manufactures cannot produce and market a patented medicine at a lower cost.

Compulsory licensing (an exception granted by the WTO) authorises third parties to produce medicines for government use without authorisation by the patent holder. The intention is to enable low-income countries to access patented drugs by giving them the right to produce generic versions of the drugs. *However*, the national legal process must deem it not anti-competitive and it must be for public health (World Trade Organization, 2018).

Voluntary licensing is an arrangement whereby a patent holder may allow others to manufacture, import and/or distribute its patented drug (Amin, 2017).

The **Medicines Patent Pool (MPP)** is a UN-backed public health organisation working to increase access to, and facilitate the development of, life-saving medicines for low- and middle-income countries. The MPP negotiates with patent holders for licences on life-saving medicines for low- and middle-income countries (Medicines Patent Pool, 2019).

(Figure 12-A). This paradigm has been instrumental in creating protections and price control tools, especially for developing countries, such as TRIPS and the Medicines Patent Pool. These tools are

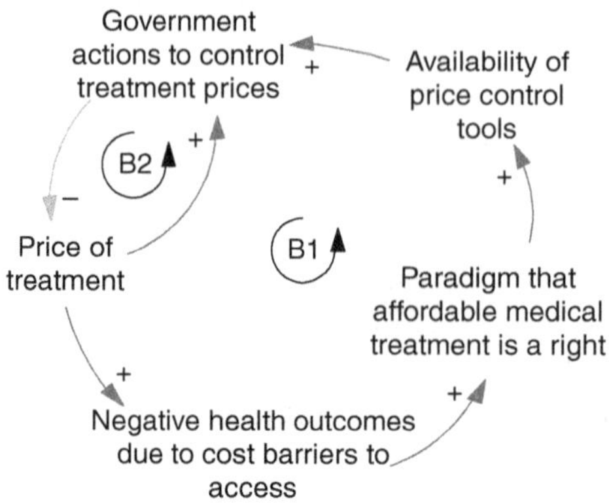

Figure 12-A The paradigm that affordable medical treatment should be a right has led to the creation of tools meant to limit the price of treatment (B1 loop). These tools have provided governments with important leverage to negotiate treatment prices with suppliers (B2 loop).

meant to provide governments with the ability to negotiate and control treatment prices.

There is a competing paradigm, however, that medical treatment is best developed through market mechanisms (Figure 12-B). The private sector has indeed been an important engine for developing new medical products. For those who benefit from these products and the existing system, either medically or monetarily, price control tools may threaten to disincentivise private investment, slowing or even halting the development of new medical products. These actors thus challenge the paradigm of affordable medical treatment as a right. They also advocate trade agreements and IPR that restrict countries' abilities to make use of price control tools.

As a result, government actions to control treatment prices incur risks in the form of political pressure, sanctions, etc., limiting government willingness to take action to reduce treatment prices (Figure 12-C, B4 loop). Using these tools requires political and technical leadership at local and international scale to manage these risks.

The Negotiation Process

Facilitated by the United Nations (UN)-backed Medicine Patents Pool, Malaysia embarked on a nine-month negotiation with the patent

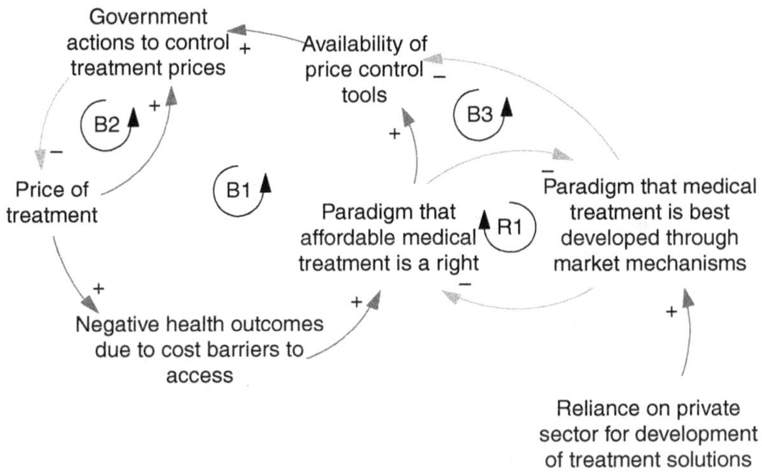

Figure 12-B Reliance on the private sector for developing treatment solutions creates a competing paradigm that distrusts interference with market mechanisms (R1 loop). This paradigm undermines the availability of price control tools (B3 loop).

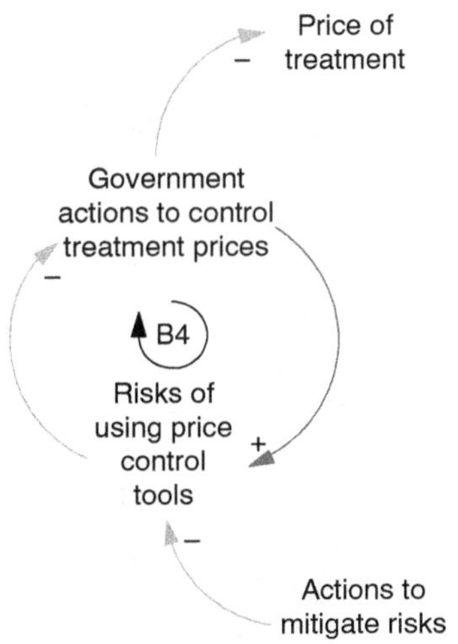

Figure 12-C Advocates for market-driven development of medical products have pushed for trade agreements, IPR protection and the use of political pressure and sanctions that increase the risk of using price control tools to limit government actions to control treatment prices (B4 loop). For governments to successfully utilise these tools, they must take a variety of actions to mitigate against these risks.

holder to award voluntary licensing to Malaysia. At the end of this period, the patent holder reduced the quoted price per 12-week treatment per person from US$70,000 to US$12,000. However, Malaysia regarded this as unaffordable.

Therefore, Malaysia decided to explore the route of obtaining compulsory licensing. The country had previous experience in using this route to obtain generic medicines for HIV/AIDS by using a specific clause in TRIPS that specifies flexibility (World Health Organization Regional Office for South-East Asia, 2014). 'The key TRIPS flexibility, as highlighted in the Doha Declaration on TRIPS and Public Health (the Doha Declaration) (World Trade Organization, 2001), is the right of WTO Member States to include in their patent legislation a provision for use without authorization of the patent holder, as provided in Article 31' (Nicol & Owoeye, 2013).

Malaysia already had the Patents Act 1983 (Intellectual Property Corporation of Malaysia, n.d.). The Act authorises the issue of a compulsory licence without agreement of the patent holder in a national emergency, stipulating no sale to others and no commercial exploitation.[4] The major risk in this approach would be retaliation through negative trade sanctions.

Meanwhile, in a parallel development, an Egyptian producer (Pharco Pharmaceuticals) applied through the auspices of the DNDi[5] to Malaysia (and Thailand) to conduct clinical trials of a new combination medication (ravidasvir/sofosbuvir) that promised to be highly effective against several strains of HCV. Being a founder member of the DNDi, the MoH had strong connections with the organisation, and Malaysia had a strong ecosystem for conducting clinical trials.

Learning of this initiative, the patent holder initiated the next phase of consultations and negotiations between various stakeholders. Table 12-A provides a summary of the stakeholders' positions. The patent holder adopted a 'carrot and stick' approach by offering voluntary licensing that also dictated the price of the medicine while simultaneously mobilising trade associations and representatives of the US government to pressure Malaysia against adopting the compulsory licensing route. In response, Malaysia focused on rallying the various domestic players who either feared or supported the compulsory licensing route and on consolidating political, commercial and professional support for whichever route

Table 12-A *Stakeholder concerns and contributions*

Malaysian stakeholders and their key concerns and contributions in the negotiation process	
MoH: Disease Control Division	• Concerned about public health and the need to increase access to care. Provided epidemiological and cost-effectiveness data.
MoH: Pharmacy Division	• Knowledge of drug registration, procurement and international drug pricing. Concerned about ensuring competitive price.
Director General Health	• Established Malaysia's position as solely to address a serious public health concern, namely preventing the spread of infections. Provided repeated assurance that Malaysia would not use it as a precedent for other medicines, such as oncology and rare diseases that could not be regarded as of public health concern.
Ministry of International Trade (MyIPO)	• Responsible for IPR and preserving favourable international trade conditions for the country – concerns about negative trade impact.
Attorney General's Chambers	• Knowledge of provisions and precedents in the national and international legislation. Concern is to ensure that any measure taken has a firm legal basis.
Ministry of Domestic Trade and Consumer Affairs	• Concerned for trade deals, fair price for consumers, protection of competitive practices – ensuring fair trade practice.
Minister of Health, Malaysia	• Concerned that pressing for compulsory licensing would generate negative public image during the upcoming general election, but provided strong support when he realised the price difference and potential savings and health benefit. Worked collaboratively with the Health DG to gain the understanding and support of the prime minister and key colleagues in the Cabinet.
Top political leaders in the Malaysian government (prime minister, deputy prime minister, ministers of domestic trade and consumer affairs, and international trade and industry) and the Deputy Minister of Economic Affairs provided sustained political support for the position advocated by the MoH.	

Table 12-A (*cont.*)

International stakeholders and their concerns and contributions in the negotiation process	
Médecins Sans Frontières (MSF, an independent, private medical aid organisation)	• Concerned about 'finding long-term, sustainable solutions to the lack of essential medicines', they participated in a workshop in Malaysia early in the negotiation process to raise awareness and share ideas on potential solutions.
Third World Network	• Concerned about pricing of and access to affordable DAA (direct-acting antivirals) for treating hepatitis C and finding options available to promote access to these new HCV medicines at an affordable price in Malaysia. Co-organised a national workshop to bring together national stakeholders as well as international experts to exchange information on the national and global situation. The workshop inspired the MoH to take the lead later in pushing for the issuance of compulsory licensing. Provided legal expertise and advice on using TRIPS flexibility for the access to medicine.
DNDi	• Regarding hepatitis C: 'a key challenge: the existing system of biomedical innovation has failed to deliver safe, effective, quality products that are affordable to poor populations'. Business model is 'supportive' and 'engagement is tailored and appropriate to need'.
Gilead Science	• As the patent holder, was anxious to retain its monopolistic position in relation to hepatitis C medication.
The USA – represented by the White House Coordinator for Intellectual Property and the Office of the US Intellectual Property Enforcement Coordinator, and supported by the American–Malaysia Chamber of Commerce (AMCHAM), the US Chamber of Commerce and the Global Innovation Policy Centre	• Concerned about safeguarding the rights of intellectual property owners to ensure future private investment in research and development. • Concern that the use of compulsory licensing for hepatitis C would be a prelude to extending its use to a wide variety of other drugs.

Trade Associations such as the Pharmaceutical Research and Manufacturers of America (PhRMA) and the Biotechnology Innovation Organisation	• Called for Malaysia to be placed on the US Trade Representative's Priority Foreign Countries watch list in its 2018 Special 301 Report.
Eleven Indian companies that operated under compulsory licensing for sofosbuvir	• Collaboration with the patent holder to maintain profit margins.
Pharco Pharmaceuticals (an Egyptian producer)	• Keen to break into a new market (Malaysia and Thailand) with a new product (a pan-genotype combination product of ravidasvir/sofosbuvir).

Box 12-B Relevant quotes

1. Letter to the Honourable Minister of Health dated 10 December 2018 by 74 NGOs: 'we strongly support the Government Use Licence (GU) that offers the Government the best option for urgently procuring HCV treatment at a price that enables MoH to sustainably scale up and make treatment available . . .'
2. MSF support letter to Malaysia dated 11 February 2019: 'we are writing to express our support for the "government use" licence to accelerate the MoH's effort to scale HCV treatment . . .'
3. 26 February 2018, DG of the World Health Organization at the WHO-WIPO-WTO Technical Symposium on Sustainable Development Goals: Innovative technologies to promote healthy lives and wellbeing: 'We must not tolerate systems that put the protection of intellectual property ahead of the protection of health. Patients must always come before patents.'

would enable Malaysia to obtain the medicine at the best competitive price.

Having launched the clinical trials, Malaysia learnt informally that the price of the medication could be much lower than that offered by the patent holder through voluntary licensing. This enabled Malaysia to sustain a strong stand in resisting pressure while bargaining for the best price using the market forces rationale.

After 12 months of intense negotiations, Malaysia adopted compulsory licensing, using its Patents Act, and obtained the medicine at about US$300 for a 12-week treatment, an almost 100% drop from the original treatment prices.

Leadership

This case study analyses leadership using the concepts of leadership as demonstrated by 'the personal qualities of leaders, leadership positions in the organization and social interactions and relationship of the

Table 12-B *Leadership characteristics and outcomes*

The leader(s)	Characteristics and source of influence	What they did and evidence of success
Director General of Health, Malaysia	• A dedicated and visionary health professional who believes in teamwork. • Had excellent international and regional contacts in the health sector by virtue of his position.	• Established the purpose and rationale of the exercise. • Mobilised professional resources within the MoH and the Attorney General's Chambers. • Interacted with and obtained active support from international networks (Table 12-A). • Built political support through well-researched messages that recognised the concerns of various stakeholders (Table 12-A). • Recognised the window of opportunity provided by the competing interest of a rival initiative (Table 12-A, Pharco Pharmaceuticals). • Sustained a long negotiation process with a cordial relationship while building and sustaining a strong bargaining position.
Leadership from Malaysian professional resources		
Director, Disease Control Division, MoH	• Health professional who applied knowledge of epidemiology and management to analyse the situation and advise the DG on management options.	• Researched and shared up-to-date knowledge on hepatitis C, its public health implications and options for management. • Supported the DG in creating appropriate messages for various audiences.

Table 12-B (*cont.*)

The leader(s)	Characteristics and source of influence	What they did and evidence of success
Director, Pharmaceutical Division, MoH	• Health professional who applied knowledge of drug registration, procurement and pricing.	• To advise the DG on international pricing and regulations. • Mobilised international networks in the pharmaceutical field.
Legal department of the MoH and Attorney General's Chamber, Malaysia	• Legal professionals who researched domestic laws and international agreements to advise the DG on legally acceptable measures.	Identified: • The flexibility provided in TRIPS (Doha Declaration). • The empowerment provided by the Malaysian Patents Act 1983. Supported the MoH in applying the relevant legal provisions.
MoH Malaysia	• The MoH has credibility and a reputation for technical competence both domestically and internationally.	In particular, Malaysia gained kudos for being the first country to use the flexibilities in the TRIPS (Doha Declaration) to obtain anti-retroviral drugs in 2003.
Malaysian political leadership		
Minister of Health	• Politician with a health background and interest in affordability of healthcare.	• Grasped the complexity of the negotiations. • Used his technical expertise and the credibility of the MoH to obtain sustained support from top political leaders to withstand pressure from international sources mobilised by the patent holder.

leaders ... The person, position and process approach to leadership' (Hartley, 2008). Malaysia is a small upper-middle-income country with little political or economic advantage. Therefore, individuals within the Malaysian system served as leaders, using their personal qualities and organisational positions to leverage networks and knowledge bases. Working in collaborative team modes or as individuals, these various leaders steered the MoH and the country through the complex environment of international trade, IPR and conflicts between commercial interests and social goals to reduce the financial barriers to accessing a medical product. Their success is evident, not only in having overcome price barriers but also in setting an example from which other countries sought to benefit.

Systems Lessons

Systems analysis demonstrates how two competing paradigms on healthcare generate conflicting views on acceptable mechanisms for making critical patented medicines affordable. Such conflicts create risks for national governments seeking to ensure access to medicines. This case study shows how innovative leadership can mitigate these risks while intervening for public health purposes.

References

Amin, T. (2017). *Voluntary Licensing Practices in the Pharmaceutical Sector: An Acceptable Solution to Improving Access to Affordable Medicines?* Online document. https://apps.who.int/medicinedocs/documents/s19793en/s19793en.pdf

Drugs for Neglected Diseases Initiative. (2017). *DNDi Welcomes Malaysia's Move to Secure Access to More Affordable Treatments for Hepatitis C.* Online article. www.dndi.org/2017/media-centre/press-releases/dndi-welcomes-malaysia-move-access-affordable-treatments-hepc

Hartley, J. M. (2008). *Leadership in Healthcare: A Review of the Literature for Healthcare Professional, Managers and Researchers.* Coventry: Warwick Business School, Institute of Governance & Public Management.

Hiebert, L., Hecht, R., Soe-Lin, S., Mohamed, R., Shabaruddin, F. H., Syed Mansor, S. M. et al. (2019).A stepwise approach to a national hepatitis C screening strategy in Malaysia to meet the WHO 2030 targets: proposed strategy, coverage, and costs. *Value in Health Regional Issues*, 18, 112–20. DOI: http://10.1016/j.vhri.2018.12.005

Intellectual Property Corporation of Malaysia (MyIPO). (n.d.). *Laws of Malaysia. Act 291. Patents Act 1983*. Kuala Lumpur: Intellectual Property Corporation of Malaysia.

McDonald, S. A., Mohamed, R., Dahlui, M., Naning, H. and Kamarulzaman, A. (2014). Bridging the data gaps in the epidemiology of hepatitis C virus infection in Malaysia using multi-parameter evidence synthesis. *BMC Infectious Diseases*, 14, 564.

McDonald, S. A., Dahlui, M., Mohamed, R., Naning, H., Shabaruddin, F. H. and Kamarulzaman, A. (2015). Projections of the current and future disease burden of hepatitis C virus infection in Malaysia. *PloS One*, 10 (6), e0128091.

Medicines Patent Pool. (2019). *Who We Are: MPP*. Online webpage. https://medicinespatentpool.org/who-we-are

Ministry of Health Malaysia. (2019). *National Strategic Plan for Hepatitis B and C 2019–2023*. Putrajaya: Disease Control Division, Ministry of Health Malaysia.

Nicol, D. and Owoeye, O. (2013). Using TRIPS flexibilities to facilitate access to medicines. *Bulletin of the World Health Organization*, 91, 533–9.

World Health Organization. (2019). *Fact Sheets: Hepatitis C*. Geneva: World Health Organization.

World Health Organization Regional Office for South-East Asia. (2014). *Access to Affordable Medicines for HIV/AIDS and Hepatitis: The Intellectual Property Rights Context*. Geneva: World Health Organization.

World Trade Organization. (n.d.). *What Is the WTO?* Geneva: World Trade Organization.

World Trade Organization. (2001). *WTO | Ministerial Conferences: Doha 4th Ministerial – TRIPS Declaration*. Geneva: World Trade Organization.

World Trade Organization. (2018). *WTO | Intellectual Property (TRIPS) – TRIPS and Public Health: Compulsory Licensing of Pharmaceuticals and TRIPS*. Geneva: World Trade Organization.

Notes

1. Public goods are those from which consumption by an individual cannot restrict others from benefiting.
2. Interviews conducted by authors during January 2019.
3. Gilead Science is a pharmaceutical company based in the USA.
4. Section 84 of the same Act deals with the rights of the government to exploit a patented invention even without the patent holder's permission, provided there is a national emergency or where the public interest – in particular, national security, nutrition, health or the development of

other vital sectors of the national economy as determined by the government – so requires or a judicial or relevant authority has determined that the manner of exploitation by the patent owner or their licensee is anti-competitive.

5. The DNDi is a collaborative, patients'-needs-driven, non-profit drug research and development organisation that is developing new treatments for neglected diseases.

SECTION III

13 Lessons from a Health System in Evolution

DAVID MCCOY, INDRA PATHMANATHAN, DAVID T. TAN, JO. M. MARTINS AND SHIANG CHENG LIM

13.1 Introduction

Section II of this book analysed the evolution of the Malaysian health system over 60 years. Using the World Health Organization (WHO) health systems framework (World Health Organization, 2007) as a starting point, we analysed the interactions and feedback loops between the so-called building blocks of the health system and traced the evolution in terms of access, equity, quality and safety, and outcomes in terms of health status, financial protection and client satisfaction (Figure 13.1).

Recognising the limitations of the WHO framework, this chapter sets out to identify the key messages and lessons that cut across the individual chapters of this book. In doing so, it seeks to illuminate the multi-directional interactions between the various building blocks of the WHO health system framework and the interaction between the health system and its context in understanding the story of Malaysia's health system and its future challenges.

The chapter begins with a discussion of the context of Malaysia's health system and its importance to health systems development and evolution. Next, it focuses on the health system, including its different building blocks, and seeks to identify lessons from the historical evolution of Malaysia's health system. It then goes on to look at more recent developments and the current challenges facing both the healthcare system and the state of population health. Finally, the chapter provides a critique of the WHO health systems framework and proposes a set of generic issues that may be relevant to other countries who wish to analyse their own health systems.

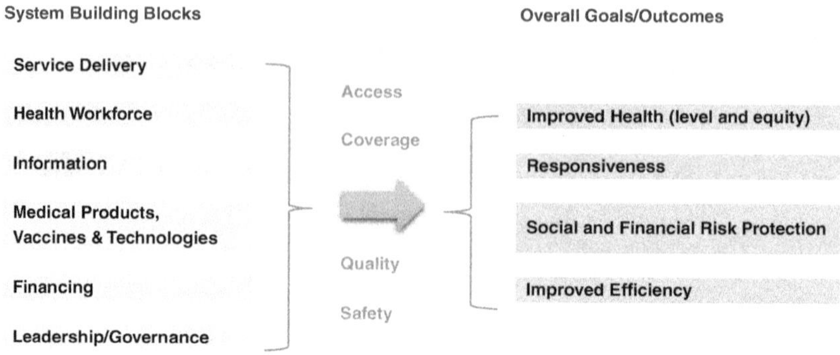

Figure 13.1 The WHO health system framework.
Source: World Health Organization, 2007.

13.2 The Importance of Context

As noted in Chapter 1, health systems are situated within a wider social, political, economic and geographic context. Furthermore, as open systems, they interact with this context and its changes and transitions over time. The health needs and expectations of the population are part of this context, and they too evolve over time to place changing demands on the health system. The importance of the inter-relationships between the health system, its context and the population is evident from Malaysia's experience as well as from a consideration of the future challenges to the health system.

For example, Malaysia's relative political stability and rapid social and economic development after independence were important in providing the basis for rapid improvements in health and the emergence of an effective health system. Sustained long-term economic growth, steady progress in poverty reduction and improvements in education were important contextual factors that not only improved health but also helped generate public revenue (from a mix of taxes, the sale of natural resources, and state-owned industries) with which to build a health system *and* allow many services to be provided free at the point of use. With a growing economy, total health expenditure (THE) has been able to consistently grow in both relative and absolute terms (Chapters 3 and 9 provide details).

Another important contextual factor, especially in the first few decades after independence, was the interventionist role played by the government in social and economic development. This included the government playing a central and proactive role in the building of a national health system as part of a wider nation-building exercise. The Ministry of Health (MoH), in particular, led a successful supply-led approach to health systems development that involved the production and deployment of health personnel across the country; the building and improvement of clinics and hospitals; and the establishment of disease control, family planning and nutrition supplementation programmes (Suleiman & Jegathesan, n.d.). Chapters 4–8 and 10–12 provide details.

The government also played a critical role in shaping an approach to health improvement that was appropriate and effective (this approach was similar to but preceded the Primary Health Care Approach codified by the WHO at the 1978 Alma Ata Conference). This included ensuring effective multi-sectoral collaboration and community engagement, developing human resources that were affordable yet effective in delivering prioritised, simple but effective interventions such as growth monitoring, effective oral rehydration techniques, breastfeeding support, basic immunisation coverage, female literacy, school health, family planning, food and nutrition, and water and sanitation programmes (Chapters 4, 6, 7 and 8 provide details). As a modern and predominantly urbanised upper-middle-income country with a high human development index (United Nations Development Programme, 2018), Malaysia has now met *most* basic needs.

However, the role of the state in driving socio-economic development has become less central in more recent decades. Malaysia is now part of a more liberalised and integrated world economy that has shifted many governments towards encouraging greater marketisation, consumer choice and privatisation across society. As a consequence, although the government still produces five-year plans with explicit social and human development objectives, its role relative to that of markets and the private sector has diminished.

This shift in approach with respect to the health sector was first expressed explicitly in the Fifth Malaysia Plan, which noted the limited financial capacity of the public sector and the need for wealthier households to make direct contributions towards the cost of their own healthcare (Prime Minister's Office, Malaysia, 1986). Private health finance has subsequently risen from being about 25% of THE in 1983 (Westinghouse Health Systems, 1985) to now being about

50% of THE (Ministry of Health Malaysia, 2017), and the role of private providers has similarly grown in the health system.

Another important contextual variable is the population served by health systems and for whom they provide services. In some instances, the population directly influences the health system. For example, urbanisation and a growing upper and middle class with increasing levels of disposable household income helped create a greater demand for private healthcare and more sophisticated secondary and tertiary services (Chapters 5 and 9 provide details). In other instances, demographic, epidemiological and nutrition transitions have required the health system to evolve and respond to new challenges such as the growing prevalence of chronic diseases and a rising prevalence of conditions of old age (Chapter 6). Similarly, the growing number of migrants in Malaysia (documented and undocumented) is posing several new challenges to the health system (Chapter 3).

13.3 Achieving Universal Health Coverage: Lessons Learnt

Malaysia has to a great extent attained the goal of achieving universal health coverage (UHC), especially in relation to meeting basic needs and ensuring that all Malaysian citizens and permanent residents have access to essential and affordable healthcare (Ng et al., 2016; World Health Organization Western Pacific Region, 2018). Although all countries face the challenge of continually expanding the depth and breadth of UHC coverage while also extending financial protection, a number of lessons can be learnt about Malaysia's past success.

To begin, during the first four decades after independence, improvements in health were largely the consequence of broader socio-economic development and a commitment to reducing disparities within the country. Improvements in water and sanitation, nutrition status and literacy not only improved living standards but also contributed to reductions in mortality and morbidity. Developments of the health system also made important contributions to health improvement by rapidly increasing vaccination coverage, reducing maternal mortality from obstetric causes of death, improving completed tuberculosis (TB) treatment rates and providing access to essential drugs and vaccines.

Importantly, the health system improved health in ways that were *efficient* and *equitable*. Efficiency can be seen from the relatively low levels of THE. For example, in 1973, during the phase of rapid health system development and declining mortality and morbidity, THE was still only about 2% of the gross domestic product (GDP), two-thirds of which was spent in the public sector (Roemer, 1985). A notable aspect of the early history of health systems development in Malaysia was the active targeting of investments and services towards the poorer and rural communities of the country, which produced notable reductions in geographic and socio-economic disparities in health (Chapter 3 provides details).

But what can be learnt from the experience of Malaysia about how the building blocks of the health system combined to improve health? We have drawn five key lessons from it.

The first lesson is that governance and leadership played a central role, especially during the early decades when public sector financing enabled the government to build the human and physical infrastructure of the health system. The health system was predominantly public in nature. The MoH played a particularly important role in implementing a set of supply-side interventions to increase population coverage of key programmes and services. Crucially, the supply-side ingredients of the health system were combined with community engagement and an appropriate mix of vertical and horizontal programmes. For example, effective community mobilisation by allied environmental health officers and technical expertise from engineers trained in public health are credited as two key factors in the success of the rural water supply and sanitation programme (Chapter 7 provides details). Similarly, the provision of credible and easily accessible basic obstetric care, with prompt and effective referral mechanisms for obstetric complications, combined with partnership with traditional birth attendants are credited for the rapid reduction in maternal mortality (Chapter 4). All of these services were provided free to the clients.

A corollary to governance and leadership was that the system was sufficiently flexible to enable leadership to modify the course of development in response to feedback. For example, after 15 years of investment in expanding the rural health infrastructure, the MoH commissioned a community survey that showed that a high proportion of rural villages remained under-served (Noordin, 1978). This resulted in a change in policy to focus on the rapid production and deployment of community nurse-midwives and nurses, rather than awaiting the slower pace of construction of new rural health facilities (Chapter 4).

The second lesson is that while governance and leadership were important, effective management was critical, especially in relation to the operational building blocks. For example, of particular importance to the successful and rapid expansion of health services was the development and implementation of strategic health workforce development plans. Chapter 8 describes how the key ingredients were the production and use of an appropriate mix of health workers, including allied health workers, and the provision of non-financial incentives to help ensure good retention rates (especially in remote and rural areas) and high levels of morale and motivation. For example, because the rapidly expanding rural health programmes needed large numbers of new health workers close to rural communities and because the interventions needed were not technically complex, the MoH concentrated on producing allied health personnel.

Indeed, task shifting has been successfully practised in all phases of development, in accordance with service needs and accompanied by on-the-job training (e.g. surgical and anaesthetic procedures by medical assistants, emergency obstetric care by nurse-midwives, renal dialysis by nurses). Career and service development pathways were also integrated into workforce plans so that the workforce expanded and became increasingly skilled and specialised as the scope and quality of services improved (Chapter 8).

Similarly, there were well-designed plans for expanding healthcare infrastructure and promoting equitable access to speciality services. Chapter 5 describes the case of hospitals, where the MoH adopted a systematic approach based on regionalisation, with all hospitals categorised into one of three levels: Level 1 consisted of five basic specialities; Level 2 had six additional specialities; Level 3 consisted of sub-specialities (e.g. cardiologists and neurologists within the broader specialism of internal medicine).

Since independence, concerns regarding social and living conditions resulted in regular population surveys, complemented by reliable population and vital statistics, to monitor progress, at least in Peninsular Malaysia where most people lived. The early establishment of a health and management information system and the recognition of the importance of data also allowed the MoH to monitor and evaluate indicators of access, utilisation and health outcomes across rural and urban areas and between the different ethnic communities of the country. Chapter 10 illustrates how the MoH used a variety of sources such as routine data, supplementary surveys, research and evaluation, complaints and surveys of satisfaction, and media feedback. It also used different types of information, such as digitalisation, national health accounts and technology assessment, to support decision-making. The willingness and ability of policymakers and managers to use data and information, including community feedback, to refine or shift their strategies and plans was key to the success of many programmes.

Part of this success came from paying attention to developing managerial competency. Management training programmes were established from the very beginning for national, state, and district and facility managers. This was also accompanied by the appropriate devolution of decision-making to enable leadership development at all levels. Chapter 12 describes how attention was also paid to senior leadership training and competence. Appointment to senior posts within the MoH followed structured career development pathways that required prior management experience at different levels of the health system so that senior personnel could draw from a wide range of experience and a network of former colleagues and contacts. The early emphasis on managerial competencies later evolved into the development of formal institutes of training with good international reputation, including the National Institute of Public Administration (known as INTAN) and the Institute of Health Management.

The third lesson is that many of the successes in the development of the health system arose from incremental and steady improvements and the avoidance of sudden and radical reforms. Improvements were both incremental and phased through a set of sensible and logical steps. This slow but steady and incremental approach made it easier for the different building blocks of the health system to establish positive synergies with each other. Chapters 4 and 5 describe how this approach enabled the development of mutually beneficial relationships between the primary, secondary and tertiary levels of the system, and Chapters 6 and 7 describe how it enabled the integration of vertical disease control programmes and environmental health services into the rest of the health system.

Low dependence on foreign funding sheltered domestic policies and considerations from the influence of the vagaries of donor-driven agendas. However, a desire for international recognition meant a willingness by the MoH to use external expertise strategically to build local expertise in a way that avoided overdependence on foreign expertise.

It is possible to discern a common stepwise pattern in the development of the different components of the health system: progression from first improving access to healthcare, then improving quality and efficiency, to optimising the features of health systems responsiveness. For example, Chapter 11 describes the case of medicines, vaccines and technologies. The initial emphasis was on establishing secure and efficient storage, supply and distribution systems. This was followed by developing the infrastructure to test and monitor the quality and safety of medicines, for example, through adverse event monitoring. Subsequently, attention focused on issues such as price and cost control, for example, through the local production of generics and the use of international price referencing, bulk procurement and TRIPS (the Agreement on Trade-Related Aspects of Intellectual Property Rights) exemptions.

A similar pattern can be seen in the case of Malaysia's rapid reduction of maternal mortality rates, which has been hailed as an international success story. Having established a national commitment to reducing maternal mortality rates, plans and strategies were established to first increase the supply and availability of skilled birth attendants and safe birth facilities. This was accompanied by a systematic stepwise service improvement plan that incorporated engagement with communities, including partnerships with traditional birth attendants and respect for non-harmful traditional practices, and the use of health service– and population-based information systems to monitor the quality and impact of maternal healthcare (Pathmanathan et al., 2003) (Chapter 4).

The fourth lesson is that organising the health system around a set of clearly demarcated and contiguous geographic units was an important basis for effective health management, monitoring and evaluation. For example, the rural health service (RHS) was built around a number of basic units (health centres and satellite community clinics), each intended to serve 50,000 population. Each health district had a number of such configurations and a district hospital that embodied primary healthcare (PHC) principles in that the hospital provided support for national disease control programmes such as those for malaria, TB and leprosy and for the rural health services. Ambulances ferried patients, staff and laboratory samples and linked primary and secondary levels of care. The progress in infrastructure development as well as the performance of health programmes was monitored on a district-by-district basis in a way that commanded the attention of politicians and civil service administrators at all levels of national and state government.

The fifth lesson is that adequate public financing, enabled by a progressive tax-funded system, was important (Chapter 9). It not only paid for the development of the health system's infrastructure but also allowed services to be provided free at the point of use for the large segments of the population living in poverty or on low incomes. Furthermore, because the health system was predominantly financed by public revenue, developments were able to take advantage of economies of scale and the government was able to play an unencumbered governance and leadership role. By contrast, the growth of private finance and private provision in more recent decades has compromised the government's ability to manage the performance of the health system as a whole.

13.4 Achieving UHC: Current and Future Health Systems Challenges

Achieving UHC is not necessarily synonymous with sustaining it over time or in the face of new challenges. In fact, all health systems are faced with new challenges even while improvements in health status are being made. While earlier sections have told the story of Malaysia's rapid improvements in health and access to healthcare, some data suggest that population health improvements have stalled and plateaued. There are also data indicating that levels of avoidable mortality are higher than in comparator countries (Ministry of Health Malaysia & Harvard T. H. Chan School of Public Health, 2016). Furthermore, a set of new and emerging health challenges threaten to bring the 'success story' of Malaysia's health system into question.

In this section, we summarise our analysis of two broad health systems issues as they relate to the health challenges facing the country. These issues are evident in all the chapters that describe the Malaysian experience. The first is the relationship between the public and private sectors. Although the WHO building blocks framework ignores the public–private mix as a dimension of a health system, it is critical to understand how public–private interactions impact on each other and on the health system as a whole. The second is the set of challenges facing the public sector specifically.

13.4.1 The Public–Private Mix

Malaysia's health system has evolved from one that had been predominantly driven by the public sector to one in which the private sector and market are more prominent. The evolution began passively, mainly with the growth of private general practitioner (GP) clinics in urban areas and growing demand from an increasingly affluent segment of the population that sought to bypass waiting times and overcrowded facilities in the public sector. This was followed later on by specialist doctors leaving the public sector and helping to grow a private secondary and tertiary care (STC) sector.

However, in recent decades, the government has also actively encouraged private sector growth, especially in STC (Chee & Barraclough, 2007; Chee, 2008). For example, the government has enabled private sector workers to use some of their social security contributions to purchase private healthcare (Ng, 2005) and has allowed for private medical expenses and the purchase of voluntary health insurance to be tax-deductible (Chee & Barraclough, 2007). Private finance makes up approximately half of THE, mainly from out-of-pocket payments (OOPPs) made to the private sector (Ministry of Health Malaysia, 2017).[1]

Finance capital investment in the health sector has been another driver of the growth of the private STC sector and the fact that profit-maximising corporations mainly own private hospitals. A significant amount of finance capital in Malaysia comes from sovereign wealth funds. Many private hospitals are thus wholly or partially owned by government-linked companies (GLCs).[2] The proportion of all acute hospital beds in private hospitals grew from 5.8% in 1980 to 27.3% in 2017, and about 30% of all acute hospital admissions now occur in private hospitals (Ministry of Health Malaysia, 2018b). However, GLCs own more than 50% of private hospital beds, supporting the government's interest in seeing private hospitals maximise profits. More recently, this has included the growing market in health tourism (Ng, 2019).

Within this context, the rapid growth of private medical and nursing schools is noteworthy (Chapter 8). Similarly, the outsourcing of public services (e.g. clinical waste management, renal dialysis, sewage and sanitation, air quality monitoring (Chapter 7), and pharmaceuticals procurement, supply and distribution (Chapter 11)) to private enterprises are indications of this trend.

Passive and active privatisation has thus been an important aspect of health system development in the past 30 years or so; inevitably, this raises questions about the impact it has had on the health system. As previously noted, some aspects of privatisation are viewed as success stories, mainly in relation to unlocking capital investment through the outsourcing of certain services and functions. It is also argued that private finance has increased overall health expenditure, that private providers have reduced the burden of care in the public sector, and that consumer choice and market competition have improved patient satisfaction and quality and helped contain costs.

Equally, there are some concerns about the public–private mix. The high level of OOPPs suggests that health finance may not be progressive and that user fees could limit access to healthcare. In reality, free or low-cost public sector hospital and outpatient services appear to have avoided significant financial barriers to healthcare and helped keep levels of catastrophic health expenditure (CHE) low in Malaysia (Chapter 9).[3]

However, a tiered system of healthcare has emerged, with the lower-income population groups being disproportionately reliant on the public sector for ambulatory and inpatient care. In comparison, wealthier sections utilise the private sector (Health Policy Research Associates et al., 2013). This runs the risk of widening the social inequalities in health by institutionalising a lower-quality public service for the poor and a better-resourced private sector for the wealthy. For example, we already see a proliferation of high-cost technology and a higher concentration of STC in the more affluent regions of the country (Suleiman & Jegathesan, n.d.). This is one of the reasons the health system as a whole has become unbalanced, with a disproportionately high level of expenditure at STC level (Suleiman & Jegathesan, n.d.).

Some aspects of the public–private mix are also likely to produce health sector inefficiencies. For example, the high level of OOPPs in the STC should raise concerns about the potential for market failures and high levels of supplier-induced demand for unnecessary or overpriced healthcare. Commercial pressures may also result in cost-cutting and compromises on the quality of care, or the private sector cherry-picking profitable elements of healthcare while leaving the public sector to look after patients and conditions that are unprofitable. Additionally, the private sector can drain the public sector of human resources that are in short supply, most notably medical specialists.

Elsewhere in the health system, the multiplicity of primary care providers, including private GPs, pharmacies, specialist practitioners and traditional medicine providers competing with each and with public sector clinics, results in healthcare provision being fragmented, inefficient and characterised by poor continuity of care as patients hop between different providers. The lack of communication and effective referral systems between private primary care providers and STC facilities are not only another example of fragmentation but also an indicator of substandard and inefficient care. The lack of co-ordination between the public and private sectors is also evident in the mismatch between the production of new medical and nursing graduates by private institutions and the lack of post-graduate training and employment opportunities in the public sector. Another example is the financial barrier to patients coming from the private sector to the public sector.

For any health system to function optimally, the public and private sectors need to work in a co-ordinated and positively synergistic manner. But for this to happen, regulation is required to correct any market failures that may emerge within the system and to ensure that private actors have the right mix of incentives and sanctions to prevent unwanted behaviour. It is also necessary to be able to monitor and evaluate the nature and impacts of the public–private mix. Thus, for both the primary and the STC sector, the general direction of travel should be towards improving data and knowledge on the public–private dynamics within the health system and subsequently implementing regulations to optimise health systems performance.

The first concerns the fragmentation and inefficiency of the primary care system and the fact that private primary care providers could be deployed to deliver more cost-effective care. Some improvements could be made by adjusting the fee schedule for private GPs so that they would be incentivised to spend time and effort on health promotion while also ending their over-reliance on the dispensing of medicines for their income. Requiring private primary care providers to adhere to a national health and management information system (HMIS) would also make it possible for primary care to be adequately monitored and evaluated. A more ambitious aim would be to incorporate private GPs into public service contracts by which they would form part of a single and integrated primary care system that would include public sector services.

Regarding the STC sector, better data and information are required to help us understand the quality, safety and outcomes of care in private hospitals. In addition, the tension between the government's economic objectives – increasing foreign income from medical tourism and ensuring healthy returns to the state's investment in private hospitals – and its social goals of providing practical, equitable and efficient healthcare for all may need to be assessed and addressed more explicitly.

The third issue relates to the need for better alignment between the production of new health workers, driven by a growing number of private institutions, and the design and implementation of a medium- to long-term health workforce plan based on projected population health and health systems needs. Ideally, both public and private institutions producing new health workers will be responsive to the workforce needs of the health system, rather than the health system being expected to accommodate the training and career development needs of students and graduates. A related concern is the government encouragement of the development of education in the private sector, including education of health professionals, partly as an export industry. Limited capacity to cope with related internships has led to problems in providing quality supervision (Wong & Abdul Kadir, 2017).

The final issue concerns medical inflation or the propensity for healthcare costs to keep growing due to costly medical and technological advancements and because of the growing number of people living with chronic medical conditions. Rising healthcare costs not only result in pressures on government and household budgets but may also increase disparities in access to healthcare due to wealthy households being able to afford the higher costs of medical care. While medical inflation is a global challenge for the health sector as a whole, it is particularly important to regulate private sector actors that have an interest in encouraging medical inflation. Of particular importance is the need to engage with trade-related policies and laws that govern the price of medicines and other technologies and that set limits on the abilities of governments to regulate markets and market actors.

13.4.2 Public Sector Strengthening

The MoH has a long and impressive track record of ensuring that the public sector works effectively and efficiently. Furthermore, although the private sector consumes nearly half of THE, the public sector is the largest provider of inpatient and ambulatory care, employing 65% of all doctors and 76% of all nurses in 2015 (Planning Division, MoH, 2016). Together with the fact that it has the primary responsibility of managing public health threats, these are clear reasons why a well-performing public sector is essential.

One aspect that needs attention concerns public financing. Presently, public revenue as a proportion of the GDP is declining in Malaysia and is low compared to other upper-middle-income countries (Organisation for Economic Co-operation and Development, 2019). This places constraints on government health budgets and the MoH's ability to strengthen the public sector healthcare system. The reason for the reduction in public sector revenue (as a proportion of GDP) is not apparent.

Another issue requiring attention relates to the health challenges associated with rapid (and thereby informal and less well-planned) urbanisation. The challenges include a higher proportion of undocumented residents who may be living in poor and crowded conditions, a lack of healthcare organisation with services being more fragmented, higher levels of population mobility, and increased susceptibility to disease outbreaks. While there are good data on disparities between states, monitoring systems have been slow to adapt to the challenges posed by rapid urbanisation. Currently, with 70% of the population living in urban configurations, information systems are not sufficiently sophisticated for monitoring social inequities in health and being able to identify high-need households and communities. Thus, for example, the routine nationwide monitoring of childhood nutrition status was unable to pick up the high prevalence of childhood stunting in dwellers in urban low-cost housing in one city (United Nations Children's Fund, 2018).

In terms of the challenges of improving the overall performance of the public sector, the MoH is already implementing several initiatives such as developing multi-disciplinary health centres to provide cost-effective and seamless preventive and curative care in ambulatory settings (within family and community perspectives). However, to really enable the critical role of PHC within the health system, levels of PHC spending will need to increase. It is estimated that only 17% of THE is spent on primary care (Ministry of Health Malaysia & Harvard T. H. Chan School of Public Health, 2016) and that public expenditure on primary care is even lower (only 11% compared to 65% on STC).

The need to strengthen PHC is highlighted by a study that found that the prevalence of hypertension and diabetes among adults was 30.3% and 17.5%, respectively (Institute for Public Health, 2015), with about half of these adults being unaware of their condition.

Another issue is the significant underutilisation of small district hospitals with bed occupancy rates below 50%. The reasons for this are both the overprovision of hospital beds in some cases and the scale of operation of small hospitals that limits their capacity to provide more critical services and updated surgical practices. Recent experience with clustering some smaller hospitals with larger ones for the provision of elective surgery in the smaller hospitals increased the occupancy rates of the smaller hospitals slightly from an average of 48% to only 54% (Institute of Health Management, 2017). While the use of telemedicine and the pooling of budgets and management through the formation of hospital clusters have helped plug skills and service gaps in these hospitals, there remains a need to keep reviewing the role and performance of district hospitals within the health system.

13.5 Contextual and External Threats

Three external and contextual factors act as potential threats to both human health and the functioning of the health system. While these issues lie outside the health sector, the MoH has previously demonstrated its ability to catalyse actions by other agencies to address health issues (e.g. efforts to improve urban sanitation and reduce environmental health hazards, as described in Chapter 7). The challenge is to adapt and apply this former experience to address each of these current and future threats.

The first threat is a set of environmental health hazards that includes particulate matter, chemical pollutants and microplastics, which pose direct threats to health. In addition, global warming, which involves rising sea levels, flooding, extreme weather events and disruptive weather patterns, will produce direct and indirect threats to health that may include declining food security, forced migration and conflict. While these threats cannot be addressed by the health sector alone, health systems will need to mitigate the effects of global warming and ecological degradation and play a role in moving society away from its dependence on fossil fuel and unsustainable patterns of consumption. There are now a growing number of initiatives and programmes aimed at greening the health sector in various countries across the world, including the WHO green hospitals initiative (Global Green and Healthy Hospitals, n.d.).

The second threat concerns the growing prevalence of diseases caused by the unhealthy consumption of alcohol, tobacco and so-called 'junk' food. The growing prevalence of these diseases have been termed industrial epidemics because of their association with various commercial industries. In 2016, non-communicable diseases (NCD) accounted for 74% of all deaths globally (World Health Organization, 2018), while NCD-related morbidities increased by 80% between 1990 and 2013 (Ministry of Health Malaysia & Harvard T. H. Chan School of Public Health, 2016). Evidence points to the need to change the environments in which people live to tackle these diseases, rather than to rely on individual behaviour change. This will require taking public health approaches to regulating the food and retail sector, as well as other social and economic drivers of unhealthy behaviours.

Furthermore, as medical technology advances inexorably and as populations grow older and more morbid, healthcare needs and demands will place ever greater pressure on health systems. While new forms of affordable care and technology may help meet this challenge of growing need and demand, health systems need to prevent disease in order to 'compress' the period during which people are living with chronic diseases.

The third threat concerns the continued existence of pockets of intractable poverty and a growing number of people who live unsettled, migratory and marginalised lives. This includes high levels of stunting and maternal anaemia in the urban poor, existing side by side with child obesity (United Nations Children's Fund, 2018), as well as a large number of undocumented migrants who lack safe access to essential healthcare. Not only does this harm the moral wellbeing of society, it creates vulnerabilities in the population and the health system as a whole in terms of emerging diseases (e.g. HIV, dengue, Nipah virus, SARS (severe acute respiratory syndrome)) and re-emerging diseases (e.g. TB, polio, measles, malaria).

13.6 The Applicability of the WHO Building Blocks Framework

Notwithstanding their loosely bound nature and the influence of contextual factors, health systems are also discrete and organised entities in their own right. The WHO framework provides a useful *starting point* for the analysis of a health system by identifying the key components of the system and suggesting desirable outcomes. However, the experience of applying the WHO framework to a historical analysis of the Malaysian health system has led to several observations about its utility.

First, as others have suggested, the framework can be better organised to describe some of the key relationships between the different building blocks. We propose a framework (Figure 13.2) that identifies 'governance and leadership' and 'financing' as foundational building blocks. In fact, governance and leadership not only determine the overall structural design and institutional framework (laws, regulations and policies) of a health system but also influences the second foundational building block (health financing), which in turn sets the priorities and determines how the health system is resourced and how the costs and benefits of the health system are distributed across society. 'Governance and leadership' and 'financing' are also fundamental to determining the social, cultural and political characteristics of a health system, as highlighted in Chapter 1.

The next three building blocks can be depicted as operational building blocks: people (the health workforce), intelligence (the health information system) and products (medicines, vaccines and technologies). These three blocks can also be seen as providing the inputs for the final building block (service delivery), which is therefore also best understood as a cross-cutting building block. This representation of the WHO framework is shown in Figure 13.2.

Second, while this description of the WHO framework suggests a linear set of relationships between different building blocks that are logically arranged to deliver services in an organised and planned manner, in reality, health systems are complex and unpredictable, and the different building blocks often interact with each other in a non-linear and unpredictable manner. For example, two operational building blocks (health workforce and health information) play critical roles in enabling good governance and leadership. This is illustrated, for example, by how leadership capacity was developed in the Malaysian system (Chapter 12) and how leadership played crucial roles in influencing the development of environmental health services (Chapter 7) or the delivery of primary care services (Chapter 4). Similarly, the ethos, values and nature of 'service delivery' can influence

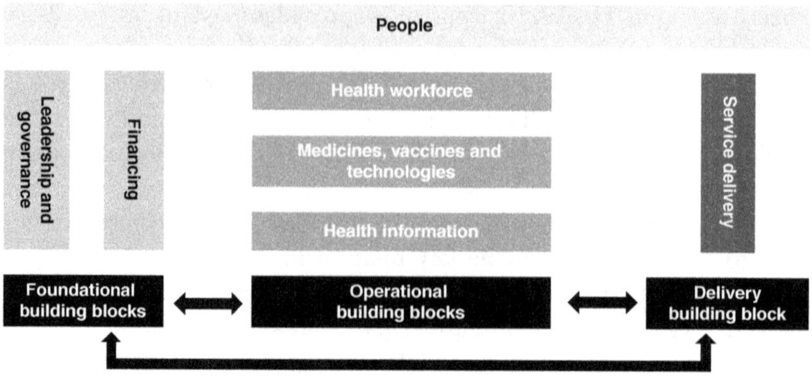

Figure 13.2 Proposed revised layout of the WHO building blocks depicted in Figure 13.1.

the way in which the other building blocks operate or function (Chapter 5 provides an illustrative example of these interactions).

Third, the interaction between the health system and its wider context includes separate interactions between the wider context and the individual building blocks of the health system. For example, Chapter 11 provides illustrative examples of how the 'medicines, vaccines and technology' building block is strongly influenced by national and global intellectual property rights regimes. Chapter 8 illustrates how the 'health workforce' building block is influenced by labour migration patterns between public and private sectors, as well as the way in which the education sector is financed and structured. In other countries, supranational migration patterns would be an additional factor. Chapter 12 describes how health sector 'governance and leadership' is influenced by national governance and the state of the wider political economy, including the forces of globalisation.

Fourth, any study of the evolution of a health system, including the interactions between its building blocks, requires a historical and longitudinal approach that employs both qualitative and quantitative data. While cross-sectional analyses of health systems may provide a useful snapshot of how they are organised and how well they perform, it is important to be able to tell the story of how health systems have evolved and developed over time to be able to fully understand them.

Finally, while the WHO framework notes the need to assess health systems performance in terms of a set of intermediate goals (access, coverage, quality, safety) and outcome goals (health status, responsiveness, financial risk protection, improved efficiency), it does not consider some of the other purposes of a health system. These include its contribution to the wider economy, its importance in shaping and reflecting socio-cultural norms and values, and its role in mitigating social inequality. It is important therefore to ensure that the WHO health systems framework is used as an evaluative framework in combination with other frameworks (Chapter 1).

13.7 Looking Beyond the Health System and the Building Blocks Framework

As noted in Chapter 1, the WHO building blocks framework does not cover all aspects of the performance of a health system. These include the economic, social and cultural functions and effects of the health system.

It is surprising that the economic function and effects of the health system are not highlighted in the WHO framework, given that this aspect of a health system is well recognised as important. For example, we can assume that healthy growth and nutrition in early childhood will contribute to broader socio-economic development, and there is evidence that health services provided free to the poor contribute substantially to poverty reduction (Hammer et al., 1995).

Analysis of the Malaysian health system opens windows to several other issues that are not usually covered in the discussion of health systems. For example, the health system may be expected to contribute to the country's economy by earning foreign income. For example, in Malaysia, as in many other developing economies, the fledgling medical tourism industry and the domestic pharmaceutical industry are viewed as opportunities to grow the country's exports. Health systems are also important generators of employment in society. In addition, they create jobs in areas that may otherwise be economically marginalised. This function is rarely considered by health systems planners, who may be more concerned with issues of health systems productivity and the desire to minimise human resource costs.

As countries progress along the developmental scale, the boundaries blur between health issues and issues typically assigned to the realm of social protection. This realm includes activities that make large contributions to health, such as care of the elderly, the provision of social and physical activities, and the integration of people with special needs into mainstream society. However, in Malaysia, as in many middle-income countries, social services are less developed than health services. Unless adequate attention and funding is focused on such services, there is a risk that the health system will end up having to fill the gaps.

The social and cultural aspects of a health system are also often neglected in health systems research and analysis even though they are important purveyors of social, cultural and moral norms and values. For example, the early decades of health systems development in Malaysia reflected a social commitment towards equitable development and uplifting the rural poor. It also stressed the importance of social equity and solidarity by explicitly seeking to reduce disparities in health. The more recent growth of corporatisation and market forces in healthcare delivery could pose implicit challenges to the earlier norms and values, but they are seldom the topic of discussion and debate.

By and large, the health system has also been developed as a secular institution that has worked across racial and religious differences, and it may therefore be seen as contributing to social tolerance and harmony. It also acts as a platform upon which gender norms are reflected and shaped. Further, the manner in which it interacts with traditional medicines and health practices will influence the way traditional cultures are viewed and respected. Equally, the modernisation and commercialisation of the health system will produce new cultural norms.

13.8 Key Messages: Summary of Generic Issues

13.8.1 Generic Lessons Derived from the Historic Evolution of Malaysia's Health System

- The provision of health services to the poor free of charge is an important element in alleviating poverty and enhancing productivity.
- People in rural areas can be reached with targeted, effective and low-cost basic health services with improved health outcomes.
- Effective and efficient environmental health services are an important corollary to PHC.
- The co-ordinated development of the various components of the health system depicted by the WHO building blocks creates strong synergy.

- Specific attention to management training and leadership development is key to the ability of the health system to implement initiatives effectively, using information from a variety of sources and responding to new challenges.

13.8.2 Generic Issues Arising from Current Challenges

- Rising affluence and urbanisation, associated with the public–private divide in healthcare, could lead to higher THE not associated with improved health outcomes.
- Health system managers need competence in using a wide range of governance mechanisms to address such issues.
- The major current health challenges have their roots outside the health system. The health system needs to develop innovative approaches to provide acceptable leadership in a multi-sectoral context.

References

Chan, C. K. (2014). The Malaysian health system in transition: the ambiguity of public and private, Occasional Paper No. 26. In D. A. Mcdonald and G. Ruiters, eds., Municipal Services Project. Ontario: Municipal Services Project. Online paper. www.municipalservicesproject.org/sites/municipalservicesproject.org/files/publications/OccasionalPaper26_Chan_Malaysian_health_system_in_transition_Aug2014.pdf

Chee, H. L. (2008). Ownership, control, and contention: challenges for the future of healthcare in Malaysia. *Social Science & Medicine*, 66, 2145–56.

Chee, H. L. and Barraclough, S. (2007). The growth of corporate health care in Malaysia. In Chee, H. L. and Barraclough, S. (eds.), *Health Care in Malaysia: The Dynamics of Provision, Financing and Access*. New York: Routledge, pp. 19–39.

Global Green and Healthy Hospitals. (n.d.). *Global Green and Healthy Hospitals: Acting Together for Environmental Health*. Online paper. www.greenhospitals.net

Hammer, J. S., Nabi, I. and Cercone, J. (1995). Distributional effects of social sector expenditures in Malaysia, 1974 to 1989. In D. van de Walle and K. Nead (eds.), *Public Spending and the Poor: Theory and Evidence*. Washington, DC: World Bank, pp. 521–54.

Health Policy Research Associates (HPRA), Institute for Health Systems Research (IHSR) and Institute for Health Policy (IHP). (2013). *Malaysia*

Health Care Demand Analysis: Inequalities in Healthcare Demand and Simulation of Trends and Impact of Potential Changes in Healthcare Spending. Putrajaya: Ministry of Health Malaysia.

Institute for Public Health (IPH). (2015). *National Health and Morbidity Survey 2015 – Volume II: Non-communicable Diseases, Risk Factors and Other Health Problems*. Putrajaya: Ministry of Health Malaysia.

Institute of Health Management. (2017). *Compilation of Reports of the Hospital Cluster Implementation*, 2nd ed. Putrajaya: Ministry of Health Malaysia.

Ministry of Health Malaysia. (2017). *Malaysia National Health Accounts: Health Expenditure Report 1997–2015*. Putrajaya: Ministry of Health Malaysia.

Ministry of Health Malaysia. (2018a). *Annual Report, 2016*. Putrajaya: Ministry of Health Malaysia.

Ministry of Health Malaysia. (2018b). *Health Facts 2018*. Putrajaya: Ministry of Health Malaysia.

Ministry of Health Malaysia and Harvard T. H. Chan School of Public Health. (2016). *Malaysian Health Systems Research Volume 1: Contextual Analysis of the Malaysian Health System March 2016*. Putrajaya: Ministry of Health Malaysia.

Ng, C. W. (2005). *Contributions of the Employees Provident Fund and the Social Security Organisation towards Affordable Health Care*. Kuala Lumpur: University of Malaya.

Ng, C. W. (2019). Price setting and price regulation in health care: case study of Malaysia. In S. L. Barber, L. Lorenzoni and P. Ong, eds., *Price Setting and Price Regulation in Health Care: Lessons in Advancing Universal Health Coverage*. Geneva: World Health Organization, Organisation for Economic Co-operation and Development, pp. 165–96.

Ng, C. W., Mohd Hairi, N. N., Ng, C. J. and Kamarulzaman, A. (2016). Universal health coverage in Malaysia: issues and challenges. In Tey, N. P., Cheong, K. C. and Rasiah, R. (eds.), *Revisiting Malaysia's Population-Development Nexus*. Kuala Lumpur: University of Malaya Press, pp. 175–90.

Noordin, R. A. (1978). Primary health care approaches in the underserved areas with special reference to Malaysia, Proceedings of Intercountry Workshop on Primary Health Care in Malaysia and Republic of Korea. Kuala Lumpur: Ministry of Health Malaysia and World Health Organization, 13–18 November.

Organisation for Economic Co-operation and Development (OECD). (2019). *Revenue Statistics in Asian and Pacific Economies 2019: Key Findings for Malaysia*. Paris: Organisation for Economic Co-operation and Development (OECD).

Pathmanathan, I., Liljestrand, J., Martins, J. M., Rajapaksa, L. C., Lissner, C., de Silva, A. et al. (2003). *Investing in Maternal Health: Learning from Malaysia and Sri Lanka*. Washington, DC: World Bank.

Planning Division, MoH. (2016). *Human Resources for Health Country Profiles 2015, Malaysia*. Putrajaya: Ministry of Health Malaysia.

Prime Minister's Office, Malaysia. (1986). *Fifth Malaysia Plan, 1986–1990*. Kuala Lumpur: Government of Malaysia.

Roemer, M. I. (1985). *National Strategies for Health Care Organization: A World Overview*. Ann Arbor, MI: Health Administration Press.

Suleiman, A. B. and Jegathesan, M. (eds.). (n.d.). *Health in Malaysia: Achievements and Challenges*. Putrajaya: Ministry of Health Malaysia.

United Nations Children's Fund. (2018). *Children Without: A Study of Urban Child Poverty and Deprivation in Low-Cost Flats in Kuala Lumpur*. Putrajaya: UNICEF Malaysia.

United Nations Development Programme (UNDP). (2018). *Human Development Indices and Indicators: 2018 Statistical Update*. New York: UNDP.

Westinghouse Health Systems. (1985). *Malaysia Health Services and Financing Study*. Kuala Lumpur: Asian Development Bank/Westinghouse Overseas Service Corp.

Wong, R. S. Y. and Abdul Kadir, S. Y. (2017). Medical education in Malaysia: quality versus quantity. *Perspectives on Medical Education*, 6, 10–1.

World Health Organization. (2007). *Everybody's Business: Strengthening Health Systems to Improve Health Outcomes: WHO's Framework for Action*. Geneva: World Health Organization.

World Health Organization. (2018). *Noncommunicable Diseases (NCD) Country Profiles: Malaysia*. Geneva: World Health Organization.

World Health Organization Western Pacific Region. (2018). *UHC and SDG Country Profile 2018: Malaysia*. Manila: World Health Organization Western Pacific Region.

Notes

1 In 2014, private voluntary health insurance (PVHI) as a share of THE increased to 8.8%. In 2017, an estimated 45% of the population had some health insurance cover. Direct financing by private corporations dropped from 7.2% of THE in 1997 to 2.3% in 2017. Managed care organisations increased their participation in managing private sector funds from 0.5% to 4% of private funds during a five-year period (2012–2017).

2 GLCs are companies that have a primary commercial objective in which the government has a direct controlling stake (Chan, 2014). Such

companies include IHH Healthcare Berhad, a subsidiary of Khazanah Nasional Berhad, the federal government sovereign wealth fund; and KPJ Healthcare Berhad, a public-listed company belonging to the investment arm of the Johor state government. The Terengganu and Melaka state governments are also involved in providing private healthcare. Sime Darby is another GLC that owns hospitals through a joint venture with Ramsay Health Limited, an Australian company.

3 Data suggest that levels of CHE are higher in wealthier households compared to poorer ones: it was estimated in 2009 that while 0.2% of households in the poorest quintile made CHE, the proportion was 0.55% in the richest quintile (Health Policy Research Associates et al., 2013).

14 Toward a Systems Thinking Theory for Health Systems*

DAVID T. TAN

14.1 Lessons from the Case Study Approach

Thus far, we have utilised a problem-based approach in applying systems thinking to health systems. We have surveyed the historical development of the Malaysian health system for adaptive behaviours, unintended consequences, tipping points for change and other systems lessons and presented in-depth systems understandings of problems or interventions in 11 case studies co-developed with health experts (HEs). In addition to providing insights for health systems, described in Chapter 13, this exercise draws out lessons for the application of systems thinking to health system strengthening.

Challenges to developing and applying system insights in health system improvement and elsewhere have been discussed extensively (Trochim et al., 2006; Plsek & Greenhalgh, 2001; Basile & Caputo, 2017). In the process of researching and co-developing the materials for this volume, several obstacles stood out. First, in both interviews and surveys of written documents, we often encountered a plethora of facts with no organising hypothesis. That is, the development of the health system was often described simply as a series of events without critical reflection on how these events were connected and what the key enablers or alternative development possibilities were. While such event descriptions are an important source of data for mapping out the system of interest, this level of synthesis is insufficient for drawing out meaningful lessons.

Where an organising hypothesis was present, there was still a tendency toward simple narratives and universal solutions that frequently obscured complex interactions. For example, health system interventions were often presented as self-contained activities implemented by visionary leaders; much probing was necessary to uncover the contextual factors that allowed a change to occur, that shaped the form of the intervention and that mediated the intervention pathway. Finally, restricted views of the problem space, and of the health system itself, limited the ability to recognise causal pathways — a common reason for the health system shortcomings described in the case studies.

Overcoming these obstacles to understanding complexity is challenging and time-consuming; acting on these insights adds further challenges because co-operation from multiple actors is typically necessary. Thus without tools and incentives to support efforts to pursue systemic understandings, health system actors are likely to base their understanding and decision-making on simplistic mental models.

This is not to say, however, that health system actors are unaware of the complexity of health issues and health systems. Indeed, in the co-production of the case studies, the HEs readily recognised the system effects suggested to them, observed these effects themselves, or had already utilised system principles in making operational decisions. Nonetheless, systemic insights rarely emerged at the outset of the case study collaborations. Instead, the linear cause-and-effect analysis was typically prevalent in initial explorations of health system problems and interventions. While the HEs had, or could readily reach, systemic insights when asked about the broader context of the case studies, they often found it difficult to articulate these insights in understandable ways. Indeed, several proponents had experienced difficulty getting other health system actors to see the issues in the ways they did. This difficulty in communicating systems understandings hinders learning by making it difficult to blend the mental models of the broad range of stakeholders.

Narratives are powerful communication tools, with stories and case studies often being more persuasive than more 'robust' forms of evidence in persuading policymakers (Sallis et al., 2016). However, narratives are used for more than communication; the construction of narratives is a sense-making process in which we build understanding. Indeed, we need narratives to make sense of evidence even as we use evidence to construct more accurate narratives (Schlaufer, 2018; Rickinson et al., 2019). And, because narratives can be rich and multi-layered and hold competing ideas in tension, they are a useful tool for addressing complexity. However, because they are easier to develop and propagate, many narratives are relatively simple. This is good to the extent that the understandings they communicate are useful. However, for many complex problems in health systems, simple narratives are unable to capture important features of the problem, leading to poor understanding and decision-making. The case studies in this volume are experiments in creating experience-based systemic narratives that better capture the key features of health system complexity and make the related insights more accessible to a broad audience.

It is not possible to prove that a given systemic narrative is accurate; any such 'proof' rests on *a priori* assumptions about what is and is not useful for understanding and decision-making. Nonetheless, we observe that the process of co-producing the systems diagrams developed in the case studies was useful for organising a wide array of data into narratives that captured important interlinkages and placed key feedback at the centre of the story. The diagrams captured intervention-context systems more holistically, typically extending beyond the initial scope proposed by the HEs. When these narratives were presented to stakeholders for feedback, the diagrams provided frameworks that kept the focus on the core hypotheses. Critically, they worked to hold the multi-faceted stories together. In several contentious case studies, the cause-effect pathways portrayed in the systems diagrams helped the team identify points of disagreement and facilitated discussion of the nature of interlinkages and causal mechanisms. These observations are evidence of the utility of the systemic narratives for generating and communicating understanding.

Co-production was critical to the process of narrative-building in the case studies. It required HEs with knowledge about the historical details of the subject, time and commitment to work with systems thinkers (STs) on the systems thinking approach and develop an understanding of the dynamic interactions, and it also required access to the necessary evidence to support the study. Also important was a willingness on the part of the HEs to follow key causal pathways in working out the proper scope of the system, which in some cases resulted in substantial shifts in focus or topic. A few promising case studies were excluded due to the absence of one or more of these key criteria. As with all methodologies that rely on participatory and co-production approaches, effective utilisation of systems thinking for health systems strengthening will require the capacity for engagement and adequate incentives for the necessary actors to participate.

One goal the case study approach did not achieve on its own was creating a clear picture of health systems structures. The case studies presented selected problems or issues in each of the World Health Organization (WHO) health system building blocks. Each case study illustrated multiple relationships between these building blocks, with linkages central to the narratives shown in Table 14.1 to illustrate the nature of the linkages. However, a systems model for representing a generic health system and the key relationships between its component building blocks was not readily apparent from the compilation of examples. In retrospect, this is unsurprising. Just as each case study required an organising hypothesis to make sense of events and data, so a model of a health system would require an organising hypothesis to synthesise the insights from the case studies. This pointed to a need for an *a priori* theoretical framework and narrative that would help us organise the practical insights from the case studies. Based on this, we began developing a macro-level health system model to serve as a working hypothesis as the basis for further evaluation, critique and development.

14.2 Building a Macro-Level Model

In constructing a macro-level model of a health system, we re-visited what it should accomplish. We thought that a useful macro-level systems model of a health system should: (1) improve on existing ways of thinking about the health system and its component building blocks by (2) focusing on the influence pathways that form high-level feedback loops to (3) identify the proper boundaries of the health system. We assumed that the health system building blocks were a reasonable approximation of the scope of the health system and asked what key feedback loops shape each building block. To identify high-level feedback loops, we considered whether the various health system building blocks were subject to different influences and could be categorised accordingly. In this process, we noted that health systems are often described as open systems subject to exogenous forces (Gray, 2017) and that many of the feedback pathways 'travel' outside the health system. A larger view that includes populations and societies opens up new avenues for advancing health (Frenk, 2010). Thus we drew on the Cultural Adaptation Template (CAT) developed by Dyball and Newell (2015) as the framework for developing a health systems in society model that would encompass these feedbacks and 'exogenous forces'.

Table 14.1 *Key linkages between building blocks in the case studies*

Linkage	Case study	Description
Service delivery → financing[1]	Dialysis services	The model for the provision of dialysis services provides short-term benefit through mobilising private sector resources. In the longer term, however, the strategy threatens to create a major financing challenge in the face of rising rates of diabetes.
Service delivery → health information	Telehealth	Local implementation of telehealth systems was driven by perceived needs and constrained by infrastructure and capacity of the service delivery staff.
Human resources → service delivery	REAP-WISE	The team approach for service delivery was constrained by the career development paths of individual team members.
	Rural drinking water	Large community-engaged workforce enabled the Ministry of Health (MoH) to engage in small-scale drinking water and sanitation solutions that the Public Works Department was not positioned to carry out.
Human resources → leadership and governance	Managed care	General practitioners are insufficiently organised and motivated to successfully advocate for governance action to ensure holistic regulation of managed care organisations (MCOs).
Financing → service delivery[2]	Dialysis services	Capital financing as a constraint to the expansion of dialysis services in the public sector.
	Clinical waste management	Capital financing as a constraint to upgrading clinical waste management services to meet environmental standards.
	Managed care	Strict caps on reimbursement by certain MCOs leads to general practitioners adopting sub-optimal service delivery practices.
Financing → health information	Clinical waste management	Private sector clinical waste management contractors are paid by the weight of clinical waste, generating cost information to incentivise good practices by hospital administrators.

Table 14.1 (*cont.*)

Linkage	Case study	Description
	Adoption of case-mix	Adoption of case-mix approach would allow the generation of valuable information on medical cases and hospital performance through financing data.
Health information → leadership and governance	Harm reduction approach	Importance of monitoring and reporting stipulated in international agreements for drawing attention to marginalised groups and precipitating change.
Health information → human resources	House officer crisis	Lack of monitoring of local and foreign medical student intakes slowed responsiveness of the health system to the influx of medical graduates seeking house officer positions.
Health information → financing	Adoption of case-mix	Adoption of case-mix approach would allow better finance planning by hospital administrators and health ministry staff.
Medical products → financing	Hepatitis C drug	The system of intellectual property rights to incentivise the development of medical products also shapes the cost of treatment and the burden on public financing systems.
Medical products → leadership and governance	Hepatitis C drug	International trade agreements and intellectual property rights on medical products provide governments with the tools and constraints to negotiate prices and seek alternatives.
Leadership and governance → service delivery	REAP-WISE	Leadership is necessary to make changes to and invest in the healthcare ecosystem to adopt an integrated care approach in primary clinics.
	Harm reduction approach	Role of health system actors in engaging different government ministries and non-government stakeholders to generate support and co-ordination for harm reduction approach.
	Rural drinking water and sanitation	The MoH took on the responsibility of addressing rural drinking water and sanitation, areas traditionally outside its purview. Leadership was necessary to

		overcome internal and external resistance to the shift in the scope of service delivery responsibilities.
Leadership and governance → financing	Managed care	Gaps in the jurisdiction have left MCOs largely unregulated by the government.
Leadership and governance → health information	House officer crisis	Despite the experience of the house officer crisis, there remains no mechanism for tracking local and foreign medical student intakes. The cross-ministry nature of this problem may complicate solutions.
	Clinical waste management	Government actors recognised the importance of a hospital waste information system to ensure accountability of private sector service providers and hospital management.
	Telehealth	High-level health system leadership was necessary for the extensive implementation of telehealth. The lack of technical expertise at that level created conditions that gave rise to interoperability problems.
Leadership and governance → medical products	Regulation of traditional medicines	The development of a regulatory framework for traditional medicines has shaped their manufacture and sale.

[1] In many case studies, shortcomings in service delivery were the impetus for leadership actions and financing solutions.

[2] Linkage from financing to service delivery typically involved the human resource and/or medical product building blocks as an intermediate step for supporting service delivery.

Table 14.2 ***Examples of health-related components of sub-systems in the cultural adaptation template***

Sub-system	Examples
Societal institutions	The health system, political lobbyists, legislation on workplace practices, international trade, patent systems, civil society groups
Cultural paradigms	Belief in universal healthcare, preference for private over public service providers, openness to immigration, level of trust in government
Human health and wellbeing	Prevalence of obesity, suicide rates, incidence of malaria, sense of security, job satisfaction, level of anxiety
Environment	Intensity of the urban heat island, air quality, access to healthy diets, amount of green space, level of societal acceptance or hostility

The CAT contains four major sub-systems (Table 14.2): societal institutions, cultural paradigms, human health and wellbeing, and the environment. In our macro-level model, the health system is the key societal institution of interest. Cultural paradigms are the worldviews, paradigms and beliefs held by society. Cultural paradigms, which reflect our understandings of the way the world is and how it ought to be, inform the ways we organise and operate our societal institutions. Human health and wellbeing encompass physiological and psychological health and the holistic meeting of needs critical to human flourishing. The health system contributes to this through the provision of healthcare, while shortcomings in the state of human health and wellbeing place demands on the health system. We have expanded the 'ecosystem' contained in the original cultural adaptation template to 'environment'. The former was limited to the natural and built biophysical environments; here, we include social environments to more fully represent how the state of the environment shapes the state of human health and wellbeing via the social determinants of health. In doing so, we distinguish between societal institutions and the social environments they create, while recognising that the two are not always neatly parsed.

Model construction began with identifying the relationships between the six health system building blocks and the feedback process that shapes them. An influence diagram format was chosen for its ability to represent broad, high-level concepts. We observed a natural division of the health system based on key drivers. The patient-facing portion of the health system, which we term the 'provider sub-system', is directly subject to and shaped by public health needs and demands. The second portion of the health system, which we call the 'enabler sub-system', plays a supporting and administrative role and is typically less visible to the public.

In considering the operation of the health system, the six building blocks are not co-equal. Service delivery is the means by which the health system achieves the goal of improving the state of human health and wellbeing; meanwhile, leadership and governance determines how the remaining health system building blocks operate to achieve good service delivery. We thus equate service delivery with the provider sub-system and leadership and governance with the enabler sub-system. The human resources and medical products and technology building blocks belong to the patient-facing portion of the provider sub-system whereas the financing and health information building blocks are less visible and thus placed in the enabler sub-system. 'Programmes and strategies' and 'infrastructure' have been added to the provider sub-system as key components of service delivery not covered by human resources or medical products and technology based on building block indicators proposed by the WHO and observations from the corresponding chapters in this publication; similarly, 'policies' and 'capacity for decision-making' have been added to the enabler sub-system (World Health Organization, 2010).

In mapping out important feedback loops shaping the health system building blocks, we propose five types of feedback loops that shape the health system and health outcomes (Figure 14.1). Each of these feedback loop types can be adaptive (i.e. leading to better practices and outcomes) or maladaptive (often due to incorrect understandings of causal relationships or actions that make sense locally but have negative consequences at a higher system level). Adaptive feedback is more likely when actors are aware of the full scope of the system, have good data, work across boundaries and seek global rather than local optimisation.

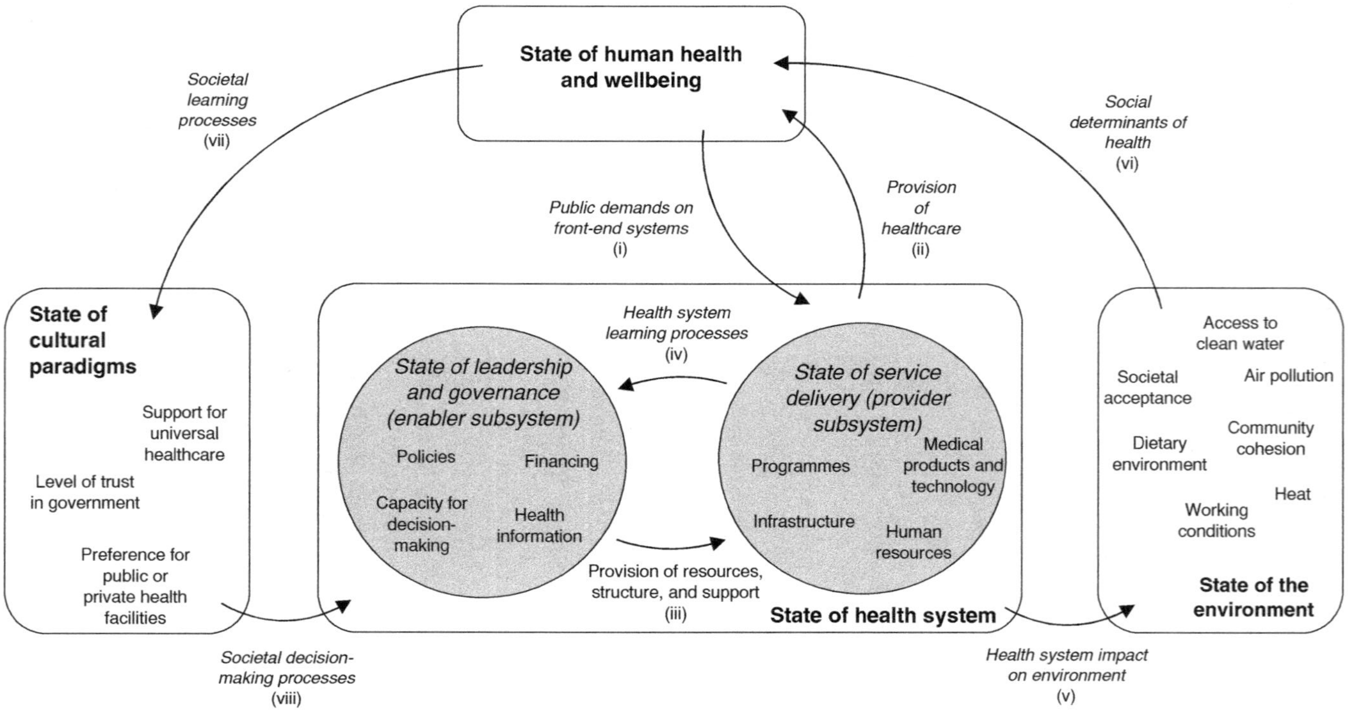

Figure 14.1 The health systems in society model contains eight linkages that form the macro-level feedback loops that shape the health system and its component building blocks.

Type I feedback loops occur due to 'natural' interlinkages within a health system building block or between multiple health system building blocks. For example, the purchase of expensive diagnostic medical equipment (medical products and technology) tends to lead to high use of the equipment to justify its purchase (service delivery); apparent demand for that diagnostic service encourages further investment in similar equipment. Some Type I feedback loops are well recognised while others are hidden in the fabric of the health system.

Type II feedback loops stem from direct public demands on health systems resulting from human health and wellbeing (i) and the response of health systems to meet these demands (ii). Public demands are typically directed at the visible provider sub-system. Due to political (for the public health system) and profit (for the private health system) pressures, shortcomings in the provider sub-system are often quickly identified and readily addressed where feasible, making Type II feedback loops relatively responsive.

Type III feedback loops are learning loops within the health system and are often linked to demands generated by Type II feedback loops. Improvements to service delivery frequently require support from the enabler sub-system (iii), while long-term demands and experiences from the provider sub-system shape leadership and governance of the health system (iv). The efficacy of Type III feedback loops often depends on the quality and flow of health information (Scott et al., 2018) and whether rules, structures and incentives align to support or obstruct adaptive learning (Committee on Quality of Health Care in America and Institute of Medicine, 2001; Carroll & Edmondson, 2002; Edmondson, 2004).

Type IV feedback loops are intertwined with social determinants of health. Health systems have been primarily organised as healthcare systems delivering services to individuals. Therefore, with a few notable exceptions, the structures, capacity and resource allocation in health systems are not designed to address social and physical environments (v), which in turn play a large part in human health and wellbeing (vi) (Friedman & Banegas, 2018; Solomon & Kanter, 2018). Despite the rapid rise of non-communicable diseases (NCDs), effective, large-scale solutions for health promotion and preventative care remain elusive (Baugh Littlejohns et al., 2018). To engage in Type IV feedback loops effectively, health systems will need to recruit and develop new types of expertise and learn to engage issues and stakeholders that have historically been outside its purview.

Type V feedback loops include cultural paradigms, being related to societal learning (vii) and decision-making (viii) processes. These often involve drivers that have been regarded as exogenous to health systems, such as education levels and national budgets. Societal learning shapes crucial beliefs, such as who should pay for healthcare, whether it should be delivered by public or private practice, the level of education required of the health workforce, etc. This learning comes not only from societal perceptions of the state of human health and wellbeing and experiences of the health system; rather, lessons are interpreted and filtered through value systems and *a priori* beliefs and are in dialogue with other societal narratives. Health systems will never have full control over Type V feedback loops (indeed, health system actors often have less control even over feedback loops within the health system than we would like to think). Nonetheless, health system actors have not only the right but the responsibility to engage with Type V feedback loops — a task that is severely underexplored in the literature and in practice.

This macro-level model highlights the importance of thinking about the larger societal context in which health systems exist. Much of the focus in health systems strengthening has been in improving processes within the health system (i.e. Types I, II and III feedback loops), with a lack of priority placed on intersectoral co-operation (Munir & Worm, 2016). Expanding the view of health systems strengthening, however, raises the question of *what else* health systems should be doing, *who else* they need to engage and how they need to be structured and strengthened to do so.

There are limitations in the health systems in society model. The first is related to categorisation and depiction of the variables and their relationships. For example, the health information building block is critical to health system learning processes, and we have postulated that the leadership and governance building block should influence societal learning processes; however, these relationships are not easily represented within an influence diagram. Also, certain variable boundaries are blurry, as noted previously regarding the division between societal institutions and social environments. However, we believe that these limitations do not substantially detract from the insights that can be derived from the analysis of the feedback loops.

Another set of limitations relates to the ways in which this macro-level model can be used. As a conceptual model, it is useful for visualising relationships to formulate broad hypotheses about leverage points for strengthening the health system. It can also be a reference point when constructing more detailed systems diagrams around a particular problem, as a check on whether all the appropriate variables have been considered. It does not, however, provide predictive power. More detailed relationships that can support causal loop diagrams and stock-and-flow models are needed to develop trends and scenarios that have utility for prospective analysis.

Finally, the model remains a hypothesis in need of testing and improvement. We begin such testing in the following section; the health system community needs to do more work to determine if and to what extent the health systems in society model improves the way we think about the health system and how the model can be further developed to better inform various aspects of health system interactions.

14.3 The Case Studies and the Macro-Level Model

Construction of the model began with developing a high-level narrative to interpret the evidence from the case studies. The insights from interpretation were used in turn to evaluate the utility and limitations of the model. There is, of course, a danger that the macro-level model limits the dataset used to evaluate itself, potentially screening out data inconsistent with the assumptions used to build it. This problem is inherent in any theoretical approach, however. We also recognise that the case studies are not representative of the entirety of the Malaysian health system, and that the selection and analysis of the case studies was influenced by the availability of the participating authors and the understandings that they brought. With these caveats, we will draw some observations here.

To investigate whether the findings in the case studies support the health systems in society systems model, we classified each feedback loop from the case studies according to the five feedback loop types present in the model (Table 14.3). All of the feedback loops were readily categorised into at least one of the five types, although some crossed multiple categories. One such example was the efforts to adjust the health system to compensate for the unexpected influx of house officers, which was driven by both experiences within the health system (Type III) and political and societal pressures (Type V) and which created knock-on effects that affected the training process (Type I).

Table 14.3 *Feedback loop types in the case studies*

Case study	Feedback loop number	Feedback loop type	Description
REAP-WISE approach	R1 and R2	I and III	Re-alignment of health clinic structures, practices and career incentives to achieve an integrated care approach.
Managed care	B1, B1b and B3	V	Employer–employee interactions that shape employee health benefits and how MCOs change this dynamic.
	B2 and R1	I and III	Adaptive practices by general practitioners in response to financial pressures by MCOs, which threaten quality of care.
	B4 and B5	V	Inadequacy of societal learning mechanisms to effect regulation of MCOs.
Dialysis services	B1 and B2	II	Health system attempts to keep up with demand for dialysis services.
	R1a and R1b	V	Health needs for dialysis are unable to align with market forces to meet dialysis demand without government intervention in the market.
	B3 and B4	I	Linkage between proliferation of dialysis services and health workforce.
Harm reduction approach	B1	II	Health system efforts to curb spread of HIV among drug users through education and rehabilitative efforts.
	R1	III	Success of harm reduction programme creating acceptance and ownership within the health system.
	B2	V	Willingness to take risks in search for effective solutions to HIV spread among drug users due to persistence of problem and the risk of missing Millennium Development Goals (MDG) targets.
Rural drinking water and sanitation	B1	IV and V	Lack of response by the Public Works Department to rural health issues due to water and sanitation infrastructure strategy; MoH expansion of functions to address issue.

	B2	II	Health system effort to provide educational services in response to prevalence of rural waterborne disease.
Clinical waste management	B1	III	Focus on direct patient services to the exclusion of waste management hinders learning processes that would improve clinical waste management.
	B2 and B3	V	Interaction between environmental regulations, perceptions of these regulations and hospital practice of clinical waste management.
House officer crisis	B1 and B2	V	Increasing access to medical education as a response to societal demand for career path for deserving students.
	R1 and B3	I, III and V	Efforts to adjust the health system to compensate for unexpected influx of house officers and resulting political pressure and the knock-on effects experienced.
	R2a and R2b	I	Training of medical doctors by specialists creates a potential bottleneck to creating new specialists.
	B4a, and B4b	V	Reactive responses to the education system to reduce intake of new medical students; continued lack of proactive data collection to enable response to future trends.
Adoption of case-mix	B1 and B2	I and III	Efforts to strengthen learning capacity of health system to improve hospital performance.
	R1 and R2	V	Government accounting norms as a barrier to the adoption of case-mix accounting methodology.
Regulation of traditional medicines	B1	II	Regulation of traditional medicines in response to negative health outcomes from improper manufacture and use.
	B2 and R1	V	Race between regulators and businesses to close or exploit regulatory loopholes.
Hepatitis C drug	B1, B2, B3 and R1	V	Competing paradigms around drug development and affordability and their impact on price control tools available to governments to regulate the price of treatment.

After categorising these feedback loops, we examined the frequency of each type (Table 14.4) to determine if particular portions of the systems model were over- or under-represented and what the implications might be for the model and for how we think about health systems.

A key hypothesis in developing the health systems in society systems model was that societal learning processes are important to understanding a health system. This hypothesis is supported by the case studies, in which 9 of the 11 case studies have a systems diagram containing at least one Type V feedback loop, a higher representation than any of the other types (Table 14.4). In each case, a Type V feedback loop was initially an obstacle to achieving a desired change or the precipitator of a disruption to the health system. The two exceptions (REAP-WISE and telehealth) focused on the role of Type I feedback loops in the implementation of a systemic change. The prominence of the Type V feedback loop in key developments in the Malaysian health system point toward this feedback pathway as a critical component with which health systems need to engage. However, health systems often lack leadership and governance capable of initiating and maintaining effective intersectoral collaboration to disrupt maladaptive Type V feedback loops (Baugh Littlejohns et al., 2018).

Among the case studies in this volume, only one, that is, rural drinking water and sanitation, contains a Type IV feedback loop (Table 14.4). This is despite the widely recognised importance of the social determinants of health, especially in the face of rising NCDs. Several linkages between the health system and the environment are apparent in reviewing the historical development of the Malaysian

Table 14.4 *Feedback loop type frequencies in the case studies*

Feedback loop type	Number of case studies containing at least one example
I	5
II	4
III	6
IV	1
V	9

health. There are a few positive examples, with (1) the Malaysian health system being an international leader in addressing rural water and sanitation issues, (2) current engagement in cross-sector efforts in formulating and implementing a National Environmental Health Action Plan, and (3) innovating in community intervention through KOSPEN (*Komuniti Sihat Pembina Negara*, or Healthy Community Builds the Nation), though rigorous evaluation of its efficacy and impact is still pending. Other examples that we were unable to cover in the book include tobacco control and promotion of good infant feeding practices. Nonetheless, the development of the Malaysian health system — mirroring health systems worldwide — has been almost entirely geared toward the delivery of clinical services. While the clinical services paradigm of health systems has delivered important advances for health in Malaysia and globally, this alone seems unable to support a health system structure that can deliver effective promotive and preventative care today.

In summary: (1) a survey of the case studies shows examples of all five types of feedback loops hypothesised in the model; (2) examples of the health system addressing the environment and social determinants of health were under-represented in our sample, which seems consistent with the composition of the health workforce and expenditure in the health system; (3) societal learning processes were over-represented and played pivotal roles in our sample. These observations, which need to be confirmed by other health system researchers, suggest that effective use of systems tools for health systems strengthening will need to account for wider societal issues and learning processes in feedback analysis.

14.4 Toward the Use of Systems Thinking in Health Systems

We see a variety of opportunities for the use of systems thinking in health systems strengthening, ranging from hypothesis generation and scenario-building to systems action. The creation of systems diagrams for mapping a system of interest is hypothesis generation. This is exemplified in the macro-level model of the health system proposed in this book, which raises questions around what drives health systems and whether the current concept of the role of a health system is adequate. Systems maps also posit causal chains that may be checked against experience and historical data, as with the case studies in this publication. This can be done prospectively as well, through qualitative analysis of feedback loops to identify potential trends or through the construction of quantitative models. From here, scenarios of possible futures can be generated for long-term planning. All these functions can be done top down, beginning with high-level questions and theory about the health system, or bottom up, beginning with very concrete problems.

Problem definition is a crucial part of systems analysis of a health system. Without some means of creating a problem boundary, the vast number of interconnections and causal chains quickly makes any attempt to make sense of a system untenable. A clear problem statement allows a system of interest to emerge; major and minor relationships can be distinguished. A problem-based approach does not limit the scale of issues that can be addressed through systems thinking. Problems exist on multiple scales, although larger problems tend to be more difficult to define well. Indeed, the macro-level model of the health system emerged when we were able to frame a problem statement, which was identifying the types of feedback loops that shape each health system building block.

A corollary to adopting a problem-based approach for systems analysis is the importance of the process of problem-framing. Improper frames overly limit the scope of analysis and cause relevant feedback loops that shape system behaviour to be missed out. For this reason, problem scopes should not be predetermined and problem identification should not be rushed. Instead, problem definition should be iterative and open to re-examination as the system of interest is mapped.

It is also important that problem definition and systems mapping be a co-produced process involving stakeholders from a range of disciplines and perspectives. It may be tempting to outsource systems analysis to an expert ST. However, the process of co-production creates a shared language, understanding and narratives necessary for collective action as knowledge is produced. Furthermore, bypassing the co-production process reduces the benefits to model-users, as they miss out on the learning that takes place in model construction and are usually unaware of the strengths and limitations of the model.

The use of systems thinking in health systems does not require everyone in a health system to be an ST thinker, nor does it require all health system experts to be expert system dynamic modelers. However, health systems experts will have to be capable of understanding the interlinkages across organisational silos. Managing these interlinkages effectively will require at least the basic concepts of feedback dynamics in health systems. Tools and methodologies for systems thinking in health systems are well-developed and widely available. Investment in such expertise is critical to overcoming fragmentation and working toward coherence in a health system.

Apart from systems expertise, skills and resources to convene and engage the relevant actors across and beyond the health system are necessary to utilise systems thinking in health systems. The fact that systems problems invariably cut across organisational boundaries can make systems analysis and action a very political process. This is itself a systems problem! Ownership of the process at high leadership levels and facilitation by external parties may help address some of these barriers. In the long term, building horizontal linkages within the health system and increasing the capacity of the health system for external engagement will be necessary to sustain the use of systems tools.

Finally, there remains a need for useful models of a generic health system and examples of how such models can be contextualised and applied in a particular setting. We have proposed and begun testing of such a model, but much more input is needed from the systems thinking community. Areas for such work include a more detailed mapping of common feedback dynamics among health system building blocks, evaluation of whether the WHO health system building blocks are sufficient for describing a health system — especially in light of the changing needs in health — and consideration of how health system actors can manage feedback dynamics that extend beyond the traditional boundaries of a health system. We look forward to seeing how such work will contribute to the development and practice of health systems.

References

Basile, G. and Caputo, F. (2017). Theories and challenges for systems thinking in practice. *Journal of Organisational Transformation & Social Change*, 14 (1), 1–3. DOI: https://doi.org/10.1080/14779633.2017.1291148

Baugh Littlejohns, L., Baum, F., Lawless, A. and Freeman, T. (2018). The value of a causal loop diagram in exploring the complex interplay of factors that influence health promotion in a multisectoral health system in Australia. *Health Research Policy and Systems*, 16(1), 126. DOI: https://doi.org/10.1186/s12961-018-0394-x

Carroll, J. S. and Edmondson, A. C. (2002). Leading organisational learning in health care. *BMJ Quality & Safety*, 11(1), 51–6. DOI: https://doi.org/10.1136/qhc.11.1.51

Committee on Quality of Health Care in America and Institute of Medicine. (2001). Formulating new rules to redesign and improve Care. In *Crossing the Quality Chasm: A New Health System for the 21st Century*. Online publication. www.ncbi.nlm.nih.gov/books/NBK222277

Dyball, R. and Newell, B., eds. (2015). *Understanding Human Ecology: A Systems Approach to Sustainability*. New York: Routledge.

Edmondson, A. C. (2004). Learning from failure in health care: frequent opportunities, pervasive barriers. *BMJ Quality & Safety*, 13(Supplement 2), ii3–9. DOI: https://doi.org/10.1136/qshc.2003.009597

Frenk, J. (2010). The global health system: strengthening national health systems as the next step for global progress. *PLOS Medicine*, 7(1), e1000089. DOI: https://doi.org/10.1371/journal.pmed.1000089

Friedman, N. L. and Banegas, M. P. (2018). Toward addressing social determinants of health: a health care system strategy. *The Permanente Journal*, 22. DOI: https://doi.org/10.7812/TPP/18-095

Gray, M. (2017). Population healthcare: designing population-based systems. *Journal of the Royal Society of Medicine*, 110(5), 183–7. DOI: https://doi.org/10.1177/0141076817703028

Munir, K. and Worm, I. (2016). Health systems strengthening in German development cooperation: making the case for a comprehensive strategy. *Globalization and Health*, 12(1), 81. DOI: https://doi.org/10.1186/s12992-016-0215-3

Newell, B. (2015). Towards a shared theoretical framework. In R. Dyball and B. Newell, eds., *Understanding Human Ecology: A Systems Approach to Sustainability*. New York: Routledge, pp. 214–39.

Plsek, P. E. and Greenhalgh, T. (2001). The challenge of complexity in health care. *British Medical Journal*, 323(7313), 625–8.

Rickinson, M., Walsh, L., de Bruin, K. and Hall, M. (2019, May). Understanding evidence use within education policy: a policy narrative perspective. *Evidence & Policy*, 15(2), 235–52. DOI: https://doi.org/info:doi/10.1332/174426418X15172393826277

Sallis, J. F., Bull, F., Burdett, R., Frank, L. D., Griffiths, P., Giles-Corti, B. et al. (2016). Use of science to guide city planning policy and practice: how to achieve healthy and sustainable future cities. *The Lancet*, 388(10062), 2936–47. DOI: https://doi.org/10.1016/S0140-6736(16)30068-X

Schlaufer, C. (2018). The narrative uses of evidence. *Policy Studies Journal*, 46(1), 90–118. DOI: https://doi.org/10.1111/psj.12174

Scott, P. J., Dunscombe, R., Evans, D., Mukherjee, M. and Wyatt, J. C. (2018). Learning health systems need to bridge the 'two cultures' of clinical informatics and data science. *BMJ Health & Care Informatics*, 25(2), 126–31. DOI: https://doi.org/10.14236/jhi.v25i2.1062

Solomon, L. S. and Kanter, M. H. (2018). Health care steps up to social determinants of health: current context. *The Permanente Journal*, 22. DOI: https://doi.org/10.7812/TPP/18-139

Trochim, W. M., Cabrera, D. A., Milstein, B., Gallagher, R. S. and Leischow, S. J. (2006). Practical challenges of systems thinking and modeling in public health. *American Journal of Public Health*, 96(3), 538–46. https://doi.org/10.2105/AJPH.2005.066001

World Health Organization. (2010). *Monitoring the Building Blocks of Health Systems: A Handbook of Indicators and their Measurement Strategies*. Online publication. www.who.int/healthinfo/systems/WHO_MBHSS_2010_full_web.pdf

Note

[*]We acknowledge and thank Barry Newell for his input to and feedback on this chapter.

Appendix IV

Detailed Acknowledgements

Name	Designation and organisation
Ministry of Health (MOH)	
MOH Divisions and Departments	
Datuk Dr Noor Hisham Abdullah	Director General of Health
Dr Faizul Nizam Abu Salim	Special Officer, Director General Office
Datuk Dr Hj Rohaizat bin Hj Yon	Deputy Director-General of Health (Medical)
Dato' Dr Chong Chee Keong	Deputy Director General of Health (Public Health)
Dr Hj Nordin bin Salleh	Director, Planning Division
Dr Hajah Faridah binti Abu Bakar	Director, Family Health Development Division (FHDD)
Dr Norhayati binti Rusli	Director, Disease Control Division
Ir. Tauran Zaidi bin Ahmad Zaidi	Director, Engineering Services Division
Dato' Dr Haji Bahari bin Dato' Tok Muda Haji Awang Ngah	Director, Medical Development Division
Dr Goh Cheng Soon	Director, Traditional and Complementary Medicine Division
Dr Rokiah binti Mohd	Deputy Director, FHDD (Family Health)
Dr Nazrila Hairizan binti Nasir	Deputy Director, FHDD (Primary Healthcare)
Dr Feisul Idzwan Mustapha	Deputy Director, Non-communicable Disease Section, Disease Control Division
Dr Azuana binti Ramli	Deputy Director, Pharmacy Policy and Strategic Planning, Pharmaceutical Services Division

Name	Designation and organisation
Mr Dzulkifli bin Mohamad	Deputy Director, Engineering Services Division (Regulatory)
Dr Md Khadzir bin Sheikh Ahmad	Deputy Director, Health Informatics Centre, Planning Division
Dr Mastura binti Mohamed Tahir	Public Health Physician, Planning Division
Dr Malar Velli Segarmurthy	Senior Principal Assistant Director, Planning Division
Dr Rusilawati binti Jaudin	Senior Principal Assistant Director, Planning Division
Dr Mohd Safiee bin Ismail	Senior Principal Assistant Director, FHDD (Primary Healthcare)
Dr Lily Rafidah binti Mohamed Zaki	Principal Assistant Director, FHDD (Primary Healthcare)
Dr Norli binti Abdul Jabbar	Principal Assistant Director, Disease Control Division
Dr Fazidah Yuswan	Principal Assistant Director, Disease Control Division
En. Fahmi bin Hassan	Principal Assistant Director, Division of Pharmacy Practice and Development, Pharmaceutical Services Division
Ms Wong Shui Ling	Principal Assistant Director, Medicines Pricing Division, Pharmaceutical Services Division
Mr Voon Kok How	Senior Principal Assistant Director, Engineering Services Division
Ms Ashila binti Razmi	Principal Assistant Director, Engineering Services Division (Regulatory)
Ms Bariah binti Bakri	Principal Assistant Director, Engineering Services Division (Regulatory)
Ms Idda Elfazana binti Albar	Assistant Director, Engineering Services Division (Regulatory)
Mr Khairul Anwar bin Shahimi	Assistant Director, Engineering Services Division (Regulatory)
Dr Chai Koh Meow	Senior Principal Assistant Director, Traditional and Complementary Medicine (T&CM) Division
Dr Muhammad Naufal bin Nordin	Medical Officer, Health Informatics Centre, Planning Division

Name	Designation and organisation
Dr Ridhwan bin Hassan	Medical Officer, Health Informatics Centre, Planning Division
Mohd Salim bin Hj Dulatti	Senior Director, Food Safety and Quality Division
MoH National Institutes of Health	
Dato' Dr Goh Pik Pin	Director, National Institutes of Health (NIH)
Dr Nor Hayati binti Ibrahim	Director, Institute for Health Management (IHM)
Dr Nor Izzah binti Hj Ahmad Shauki	Director, Institutes for Health Systems Research (IHSR)
Dr Nor Haniza Bt Zakaria	Deputy Director, IHM
Datin Dr Sheamini Sivasampu	Head, Healthcare Statistic Unit, Institute for Clinical Research (ICR)
Dr Sondi Sararaks	Head, Health Outcomes Research Division, IHSR
Dr Zulkarnain Abdul Karim	Head, Centre for Health Services Research, IHSR
Dr Zalilah binti Abdullah	Head, Centre for Health Policy Research, IHSR
Political leaders	
Datuk Dr Seri S. Subramaniam	Former Minister of Health
Dato' Chua Jui Meng	Former Minister of Health
Professional leaders	
Tan Sri Dato' Mohd. Sheriff Mohd. Kassim	Former Secretary General, Ministry of Finance
Tan Sri Dato' Dr Abu Bakar Suleiman	Former Director General of Health
Tan Sri Dato' Seri Dr Haji Mohd Ismail Merican	Former Director General of Health
Previous key officers in the MoH	
Tan Sri Dr M. Jegathesan	Former Deputy Director-General of Health (Research and Technical Support)
Prof. Datuk Dr Haji Megat Burhainuddin	Former Deputy Director-General of Health (Medical)
Datuk Seri Dr Jeyaindran Tan Sri Sinnadurai	Former Deputy Director-General of Health (Medical)

Name	Designation and organisation
Dato' Dr Maimunah bt A Hamid	Former Deputy Director-General of Health (Research and Technical Support)/Professor, currently International Medical University (IMU)
Datuk Dr Lokman Hakim bin Sulaiman	Former Deputy Director-General of Health (Public Health)/Professor, currently International Medical University (IMU)
Dato' Jagjit Singh a/l Nashatar Singh	Former Finance Division Secretary
Dato' Dr Narimah Awin	Former Director, FHDD
Dr Ramli bin Zainal	Former Director, Pharmaceutical Services Division
Dr Amiruddin Hisan	Former Director, Telehealth Division
Wee Bee Wah	Former Director, Food Safety and Quality Division
Safiah Yusof	Former Director, Nutrition Division, MoH
Datin Dr Hjh. Noriah binti Bidin	Former Director, IHM
Dato' Dr Fadzilah Kamaludin	Former Director, Institute for Medical Research
World Health Organization (WHO) – Representatives of the Office for Malaysia, Brunei Darussalam and Singapore	
Dr Ying-Ru Jacqueline Lo	WHO Representative for Malaysia, Brunei Darussalam and Singapore
Dr Taketo Tanaka	Technical Officer
Dr Karina Razali	Consultant
Academia (universities)	
Prof. Dr Sharifa Ezat Wan Puteh	Deputy Dean of Network and Resources, Faculty of Medicine, National University Malaysia
Dato' Prof. Dr Adeeba binti Kamarulzaman	Dean, Faculty of Medicine, University Malaya
Dr Khor Swee Kheng	Senior Fellow, Health Systems and Policy, University of Malaya (UM)
Assoc. Prof. Dr Farizah binti Mohd Hairi	Department of Social Preventive Medicine, UM

Name	Designation and organisation
Dr Ahmad Syamil Mohamad	Department of Social Preventive Medicine, UM
Prof. Daniel D. Reidpath	Professor, Jeffrey Cheah School of Medicine and Health Sciences, Monash University Malaysia/ Senior Director, Health Systems and Population Studies Division, International Centre for Diarrhoeal Disease Research, Bangladesh
Dr Barry Newell	Australia National University
Dr Katrina Proust	Australia National University
Professional Medical Associations	
Dr Thirunavukarasu Rajoo	Honorary General Secretary, Malaysian Medical Association (MMA)
Dr Sivanaesan Letchumanan	Chairman, Private Practitioner Section (PPS), MMA
Dr Steven Chow Kim Weng	President Federation of Private Medical Practitioners' Associations, Malaysia
Pharmaceutical private sector agencies	
Mr Ewe Kheng Huat	Executive Director, PhAMA
Mr Lim Shi Hao	Policy Manager, PhAMA
Mr Keh Song Hock	Executive Director, Malaysian Organisation of Pharmaceutical Industries (MOPI)
Managed Care Organization	
Mr Adzahar Abdul Wahid	CEO, PMCare Sdn Bhd

United Nations University International Institute for Global Health (UNU-IIGH): Officers who provided support for the editorial team and the stakeholder consultations:

Dr Michael J. Penkunas	Research Fellow
Ms Agnes Siew Fern Wong	Intern
Dr Hena Lee	Intern
Ms Jane Fui Ching Lam	Intern
Dr Ellie Hyeon Gyeong Park	Intern
Ms Yap Yee Chern	Intern
Ms Yap Jia Xuan	Intern

Index

bold locators are tables and italics are figures.

CPSIA information can be obtained
at www.ICGtesting.com
Printed in the USA
LVHW081534150921
697863LV00002B/60

9 781108 845205